Cardiopulmonary Physiotherapy in Trauma

An Evidence-based Approach

Cardiopulmonary Physiotherapy in Trauma

An Evidence-based Approach

Editors

Heleen van Aswegen

Department of Physiotherapy,
University of the Witwatersrand, Johannesburg, South Africa

Brenda Morrow

Department of Paediatrics and Child Health,
University of Cape Town, South Africa

ICP

Imperial College Press

Published by

Imperial College Press
57 Shelton Street
Covent Garden
London WC2H 9HE

Distributed by

World Scientific Publishing Co. Pte. Ltd.

5 Toh Tuck Link, Singapore 596224

USA office: 27 Warren Street, Suite 401-402, Hackensack, NJ 07601

UK office: 57 Shelton Street, Covent Garden, London WC2H 9HE

Library of Congress Cataloging-in-Publication Data
Cardiopulmonary physiotherapy in trauma : an evidence-based approach / edited by
Heleen van Aswegen, Brenda Morrow.
p. ; cm.
Includes bibliographical references and index.
ISBN 978-1-78326-651-7 (hardcover : alk. paper)
I. Van Aswegen, Heleen, editor. II. Morrow, Brenda, 1973– , editor.
[DNLM: 1. Wounds and Injuries--therapy. 2. Heart Diseases--therapy. 3. Physical Therapy
Modalities. 4. Respiratory Tract Diseases--therapy. 5. Wounds and Injuries--complications. WO 700]
RE831
617.7'13--dc23

2015005248

British Library Cataloguing-in-Publication Data
A catalogue record for this book is available from the British Library.

Typeset by Stallion Press
Email: enquiries@stallionpress.com

Printed in Singapore by B & Jo Enterprise Pte Ltd

Contents

Preface

Trauma in its various forms remains a serious public health problem worldwide and is the leading cause of death among adults and children, particularly those between the ages of one and nine years. The Global Status Report on Road Safety (2009) states that 20–50 million people worldwide sustain injuries related to motor vehicle accidents annually. The Global Burden of Armed Violence (2011) reported that 526,000 people worldwide lose their lives due to violence each year and that many more people suffer from a range of physical and mental health problems due to violence. According to the World Health Organisation (2014), the majority of trauma occurs in low-income and middle-income countries. Burns, sustained as a result of interpersonal violence or suicidal attempt, remain a serious public health problem in some countries, and fire-related deaths rank among the 15 leading causes of death worldwide. Motor vehicle accidents and war injuries are among the top ten projected leading causes of disability-adjusted life years in 2020. In light of these facts, trauma-related injuries are likely to remain one of the leading causes of high hospital admission rates and health care costs associated with care provided to patients in acute care settings worldwide.

For the purpose of this book, trauma is defined as damage to any body part as a result of physical impact or accident. Such injuries can range from mild (not requiring hospitalisation) to life threatening. The interdisciplinary health care team usually involved in the management of patients who have sustained life-threatening trauma-related injuries includes physiotherapists who work in the acute care and rehabilitation settings. In the acute care setting (intensive care unit, high care unit, hospital ward), the main roles of the physiotherapist are the prevention or management of respiratory complications or existing respiratory conditions and the prevention of musculoskeletal complications that may develop secondary to injury and immobility. This book has been written by physiotherapists for physiotherapists and physiotherapy students to encourage evidence-based cardiopulmonary physiotherapy management of adult and paediatric survivors of trauma in the acute care setting. The elements of evidence-based clinical practice are often described as a combination of: (a) best available research evidence; (b) professional expertise and judgement; and (c) the needs and preferences of the patient. In this book, information obtained from published research is shared with the reader as well as the clinical expertise of the writers in cases where evidence to support the use of certain treatment interventions in the management of patients with trauma is still lacking.

This book provides information on physiological responses to trauma to provide the physiotherapist with a better understanding of the mechanisms behind muscle protein breakdown and weakness and delayed recovery, so often observed in patients who suffer critical illness due to trauma-related injuries. A chapter that describes the anatomical differences between children and adults is included to demonstrate that children are not just small adults and illustrates how their management differs. Immunosuppressive diseases such as human immunodeficiency virus (HIV) and acquired immunodeficiency syndrome (AIDS) are prevalent worldwide; the chapter on trauma and immunosuppressive diseases describes the pulmonary and extrapulmonary complications associated with HIV and AIDS and antiretroviral therapy, and highlights important points to be considered in the management of patients with HIV or AIDS who are involved in trauma. This is followed by a chapter that provides an overview of various cardiopulmonary physiotherapy treatment interventions, subjective and objective markers and outcome measures that may be used in the care of patients with traumatic injury. The clinical chapters are dedicated to specific types of life-threatening trauma commonly encountered in patients in the acute care setting. These chapters are structured in a similar format and include: an overview of causes and mechanisms of injury; medical and surgical management; physiotherapy treatment aims; suggested treatment interventions; contraindications and precautions to physiotherapy intervention; and clinical case scenarios and suggested further reading. Differences in management between adults and children involved in trauma are highlighted. Towards the end of the book, quality of life of patients who survived trauma is discussed, as well as the role of exercise therapy to aid such survivors' recovery. Key messages boxes, which contain important clinical information for the reader to be aware of, appear throughout many of the chapters.

The focus of this book is mainly on the physiotherapy treatment of adults, children and infants with trauma-related injuries in the acute care setting. The reader is referred to other published medical, physiological and physiotherapy texts for detailed information on the assessment of patients in the acute care setting. The reader is also referred to other published physiotherapy texts for detailed information on rehabilitation of trauma survivors in the chronic health care setting.

H. van Aswegen

B.M. Morrow

Bibliography

Global Burden of Armed Violence (2011). Chapter 2: Trends and patterns of lethal violence. [Online]. Available at: http://www.genevadeclaration.org/fileadmin/docs/GBAV2/GBAV2011-Ch2-Summary.pdf [Accessed 13 November 2014].

World Health Organisation (2009). Global Status Report on Road Safety: Time for Action. [Online]. Available at: http://www.who.int/violence_injury_prevention/road_safety_status/2009/en/ [Accessed 01 August 2014].

World Health Organisation (2014). *Violence and injury prevention: injury-related disability and rehabilitation.* [Online]. Available at: http://www.who.int/violence_injury_prevention/disability/en/ [Accessed 13 November 2014].

List of Contributors

Heleen van Aswegen (PhD)
Associate Professor
Department of Physiotherapy,
Faculty of Health Sciences,
University of the Witwatersrand,
Johannesburg, South Africa.

Brenda Morrow (PhD)
Associate Professor
Department of Paediatrics,
Faculty of Health Sciences,
University of Cape Town,
Cape Town, South Africa.

Susan Hanekom (PhD)
Associate Professor
Division of Physiotherapy,
Department of Interdisciplinary Health Sciences,
Faculty of Medicine and Health Sciences,
Stellenbosch University,
Stellenbosch, South Africa.

Witness Mudzi (PhD)
Associate Professor
Department of Physiotherapy,
Faculty of Health Sciences,
University of the Witwatersrand,
Johannesburg, South Africa.

Natascha Plani (MSc Physiotherapy)
Senior Physiotherapy Clinician
Sklaar, Laidler and Associates Physiotherapists,
Netcare Union Hospital,
Alberton, South Africa.

Ronel Roos (PhD)
Lecturer
Department of Physiotherapy,
Faculty of Health Sciences,
University of the Witwatersrand,
Johannesburg, South Africa.

Elizna van Aswegen (MBBCh; DipPEC (SA))
Medical Doctor
Head Emergency Centre,
Mediclinic Bloemfontein,
Bloemfontein, South Africa.

Moira Wilson (Diploma in Physiotherapy)
Senior Physiotherapy Clinician
Netcare Milpark Hospital,
Johannesburg, South Africa.

Chapter 1

Physiological Response to Trauma

Written by H. van Aswegen

Trauma is sometimes referred to as the hidden epidemic, as it tends to get much less media attention than the human immunodeficiency virus/ acquired immunodeficiency syndrome (HIV/AIDS) pandemic but has an equally high mortality rate (Thomson, 2003). Trauma kills young people in the prime of their economically productive lives, and those that survive severe trauma often suffer from long-term health disabilities that impact their quality of life.

This chapter provides the physiotherapist with information about:

- The human immune system and its response to injury and inflammation.
- The impact of inflammation and sepsis on muscle function and structure.
- The response of the body to shock, different types of shock and the management of shock.
- The effect of shock and critical illness on blood oxygen content.
- The effect of trauma on blood glucose levels.
- The classification of patients with traumatic injuries to determine severity of illness, risk for mortality and morbidity estimation.

1.1. Human Immunity and its Response to Injury and Inflammation

Bodily injury sustained through traumatic events invariably leads to bleeding. Injury to blood vessel walls leads to haemostasis and coagulation to reduce the amount of blood lost from the circulation, followed by fibrinolysis in order to restore blood flow. Both of these processes are discussed in Sections 1.1.1. and 1.1.2. The coagulation system and immune system overlap, as bacteria that invade the body can be trapped inside blood clots that form during haemostasis. Immunity is the ability of the human body to protect itself against infiltration from infectious matter and foreign cells. The immune system is a complex system made up of many different immune system cells that continuously patrol the body to detect invasion of its barriers. An in-depth discussion of human immunity is beyond the scope of this book and the reader is referred to other texts for such detailed information. The immune system consists of non-specific as well as specific defences, which are discussed in Sections 1.1.3. and 1.1.4.

1.1.1. *Haemostasis*

The normal physiological response to blood loss as a result of injury to the vascular wall is a process called haemostasis. Blood changes from a liquid to a solid state during haemostasis. Haemostasis is made up of a sequence of events that are initiated within 20 seconds of vascular wall injury. The first step in this sequence is blood vessel constriction to reduce blood flow. This is followed by adherence of circulating platelets to the vessel wall at the site of injury. Platelets are activated by the endothelial cell injury and form a cluster to initiate the formation of a clot. A series of enzyme reactions occur, which involve coagulation proteins produced through intrinsic and extrinsic coagulation pathways to produce the enzyme thrombin. Thrombin is the key enzyme for coagulation. Fibrin is subsequently produced to form a stable haemostatic clot. The main function of haemostasis is therefore to maintain the integrity of the circulatory system. The haemostatic process can, however, be disrupted by inflammation and infection, resulting in uncontrolled bleeding and may lead to significant morbidity and even mortality (see septic shock in Section 1.2.3.3.3.) (Chan and Paredes, 2013).

1.1.2. *Fibrinolysis*

Fibrinolysis is the process of the restoration of blood flow by changing blood from a solid to a liquid state. As the integrity of the blood vessel wall is restored, endothelial cells secrete tissue plasminogen activators to start dissolving the clot. Plasminogen breaks up the fibrin in the clot and dissolves the clot, and during this process blood flow is restored. The fibrinolytic system can also be disrupted by inflammation and infection, resulting in uncontrolled thrombus formation and may lead to significant morbidity and mortality (see septic shock in section 1.2.3.3.3.) (Chan and Paredes, 2013).

1.1.3. *Non-specific defence systems*

Non-specific defences of the body include barriers such as the skin and mucous membranes, inflammatory reactions characterised by the stimulation of phagocytes, mast cells, eosinophils and natural killer cells. Protective proteins (such as interferon) also form part of the non-specific defences of the body and are activated when microbes enter the body. Protective proteins attract phagocytes to the scene of the infection in order to devour these microbes (Kapasi, 2006; Van Dyk, 2008) (Fig. 1.1).

1.1.4. *Specific defence systems*

The specific defences of the body consist primarily of white cells, of which the T-lymphocyte and B-lymphocyte activities are most important. The T-lymphocytes represent the cellular immune system and B-lymphocytes represent the humoral immune system. T-lymphocytes are responsbile for the destruction of foreign cells and coordinate the overall immune response of the body. Stimulation of the T-lymphocytes leads to the release of CD4 cells, which migrate via the blood stream to the site of infection and destroy the foreign invaders. CD4 cells also stimulate other immune system cells to mount the attack against the foreign cells. B-lymphocytes are responsible for the production of antibodies. These anitbodies, immunoglobulins, are deposited onto antigens (foreign substances that invade the defence barriers of the body), neutralise their actions and mark them for destruction by other immune system cells (Kapasi, 2006; Van Dyk, 2008) (Fig. 1.1).

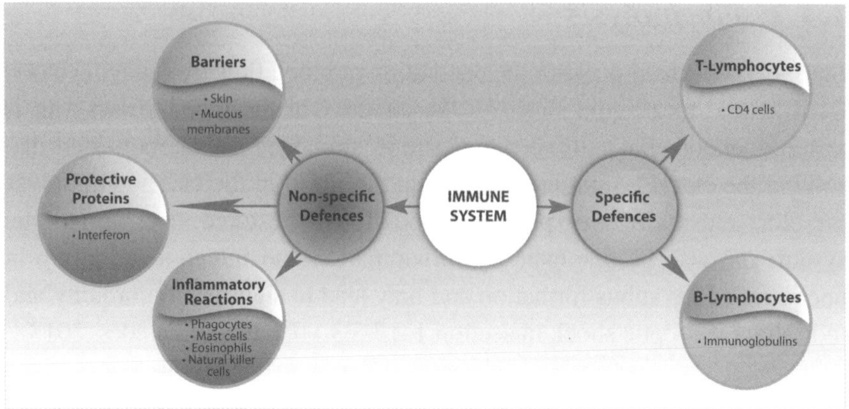

Fig. 1.1: Defence systems of the human body.

1.1.5. *Activation of the body's defence systems*

Local and systemic responses to trauma are activated by various factors, such as injury, surgery, dehydration, sepsis and acute medical illness. Traditionally it was thought that acute injury led to the loss of lean body and skeletal mass and preceded the process of recovery and wound repair. Recently the traditional view of the systemic response to injury has been expanded. Inflammation, as a result of injury, plays an important role in changing muscle structure and function during critical illness and is expanded on below. Inflammation consists of humoral and cellular responses, as mentioned above, and is driven by cytokine activity.

1.1.5.1. *Cytokines*

Cytokines are cell-signalling protein molecules that are secreted by a large number of cells of the immune system. Cytokines are produced by T-lymphocytes, macrophages, endothelial and epithelial cells. These cytokines include interleukin (IL) 1, IL-6 and tumour necrosis factor-alpha (TNF-α). Certain cytokines have a pro-inflammatory effect (IL-1, IL-6 and TNF-α) and others have an anti-inflammatory effect (IL-4, IL-10, IL-13 and IL-1 receptor antagonist). Cytokines have a systemic immunomodulating effect and, during infection or inflammation, pro-inflammatory cytokines signal T-cells and macrophages to travel to the

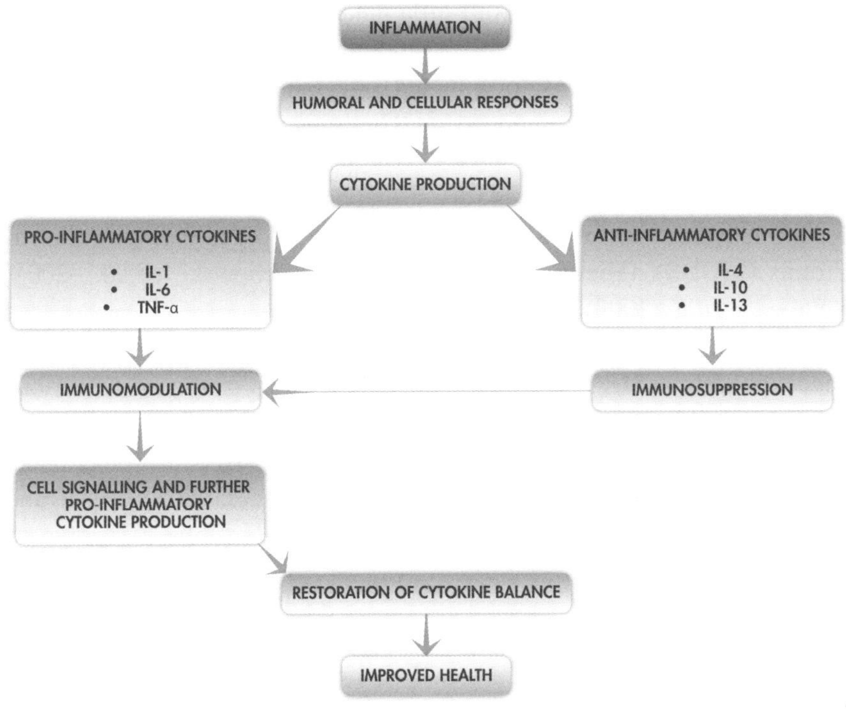

Fig. 1.2: Cytokine interactions during inflammation in healthy individuals.

site of infection and, in turn, as a result of the cell stimulation, the T-cells and macrophages produce more pro-inflammatory cytokines. Under healthy conditions this feedback loop is kept in check by the body through the release of anti-inflammatory cytokines that have an immunosuppression effect (Fig. 1.2); however, this balance between pro-inflammatory and anti-inflammatory activity is lost as a result of severe injury (Mukhopadhyay *et al.*, 2006; Schroeder *et al.*, 2009).

1.1.5.2. *Systemic inflammatory response syndrome and sepsis*

Worsening (exacerbation) of the inflammatory reaction in patients with trauma-related injuries can lead to the development of systemic inflammatory response syndrome (SIRS) due to an imbalance in the production of pro-inflammatory cytokines. Anti-inflammatory cytokines are released to restore this imbalance, but over-activation leads to either a compensatory anti-inflammatory response or a mixed antagonist response, which leads to post-traumatic immunosuppression (Hietbrink *et al.*, 2006; Osuchowski *et al.*, 2006; Schroeder *et al.*, 2009). The patient's immune system is in disarray and the body becomes very susceptible to infection, which might result in septic syndrome and ultimately multiple organ dysfunction syndrome (MODS) (Hietbrink *et al.*, 2006; Osuchowski *et al.*, 2006; Schroeder *et al.*, 2009) (Fig. 1.3).

The American College of Chest Physicians and Society of Critical Care Medicine define SIRS as a systemic inflammatory response to various severe clinical insults such as burns, haemorrhage, ischaemia, inflammation and trauma. It is not always related to infection. Sepsis, on the other hand, is defined as a systemic response to infection (Clarke, 2003). Sepsis and SIRS are diagnosed according to the criteria outlined in Table 1.1; although

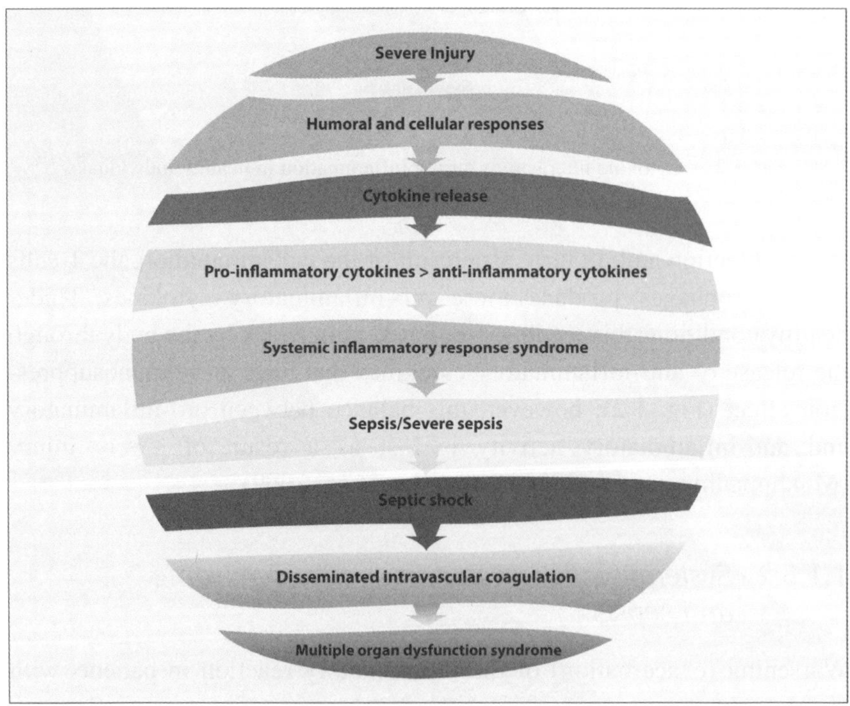

Fig. 1.3: Aetiology of multiple organ dysfunction syndrome.

Table 1.1: Criteria for diagnosis of SIRS and sepsis.

- Temperature >38°C or <36°C
- Heart rate >90 beats/minute
- Respiratory rate >20 breaths/minute or partial pressure of carbon dioxide in arterial blood ($PaCO_2$) <32 mmHg
- White blood cell count >12,000 cells/mm3 or <4,000 cells/mm^3

SIRS is diagnosed in the presence of two or more of the above after severe clinical insults to the body. Sepsis is diagnosed in the presence of two or more of the above in the presence of infection.

the criteria are similar for both, diagnosis is made under different clinical circumstances, as mentioned above.

The presence of sepsis together with dysfunction of one or more organs is defined as severe sepsis. Organ dysfunctions can include: acute lung injury; blood clotting abnormalities; thrombocytopenia; altered mental status; failure of the kidneys, liver or heart; or the presence of lactic acidosis with hypoperfusion. Severe sepsis is caused by bacteraemia in 50% of cases, but in up to 30% of cases no microbial cause may be found for the sepsis. Severe sepsis in the presence of cardiovascular failure is defined as septic shock (Nguyen *et al.*, 2006) (refer to Section 1.2.3.3.3. for a detailed description of septic shock).

1.1.6. *Musculoskeletal changes associated with inflammation*

It is normal for the body to have a surge in circulating cytokine levels during its immune response to injury or infection. These elevated cytokine levels, however, trigger secondary organ reactions that promote tissue damage and dysfunction. Sepsis is directly related to the development of myopathy, which involves the peripheral as well as respiratory muscles.

1.1.6.1. *Muscle protein breakdown and atrophy*

Pro-inflammatory cytokines such as IL-1 and TNF-α contribute to the development of symptoms such as fever, malaise and loss of appetite and lead to 'capillary leak'. These cytokines contribute to muscle protein breakdown, cell death and reduction of muscle mass in the critically ill patient. Interleukin-6 concentrations are higher in patients with greater tissue trauma (high injury severity scores) and higher IL-6 concentrations are associated with adverse patient outcomes. Interleukin-6 levels also tend to be higher in patients with septic shock than in those with other types of shock. Interleukin-6 has been shown to stimulate the production of IL-1 and TNF-α until the patient's condition becomes chronic, and then changes activity by slowing down the production of these cytokines; however, persistently high levels of IL-6 in the blood circulation have been associated with increased mortality in patients who are critically ill due to trauma-related injuries. Low levels of anti-inflammatory cytokines such as IL-10 in critically ill patients has been associated with excessive inflammation and muscle damage (Winkelman, 2004; Winkelman *et al.*, 2007; Callahan and Supinski, 2009; Jawa *et al.*, 2011).

1.1.6.2. *Muscle weakness*

Reactive oxygen species (ROS) are chemically reactive molecules that contain oxygen. They are produced as a natural byproduct to the metabolism of oxygen in the body. Small amounts of ROS form part of the internal defence system of the healthy human body. During illness, elevated levels of ROS that circulate through the body, as a result of cytokine stimulation, have been linked with decreased myofilament function at the muscular level, leading to muscle weakness (Fig. 1.4). Tumour necrosis factor-α has been linked with similar effects on muscle function, due to induced contractile dysfunction at the myofilament level. Reactive oxygen species mediate mitochondrial dysfunction in the skeletal muscle of patients with sepsis, which leads to muscle weakness (Winkelman, 2004; Callahan and Supinski, 2009).

The imbalances between pro-inflammatory and anti-inflammatory cytokine activity and elevated levels of circulating ROS and their effects on the musculoskeletal system offer an explanation for the commonly observed atrophic appearance of critically ill patients in addition to the effects of immobility on muscle function. Winkelman *et al.* (2007) suggested that low levels of physical activity in critically ill patients (rolling in bed, passive range of motion exercises) may assist with restoration of the imbalance between pro-inflammatory and anti-inflammatory cytokines.

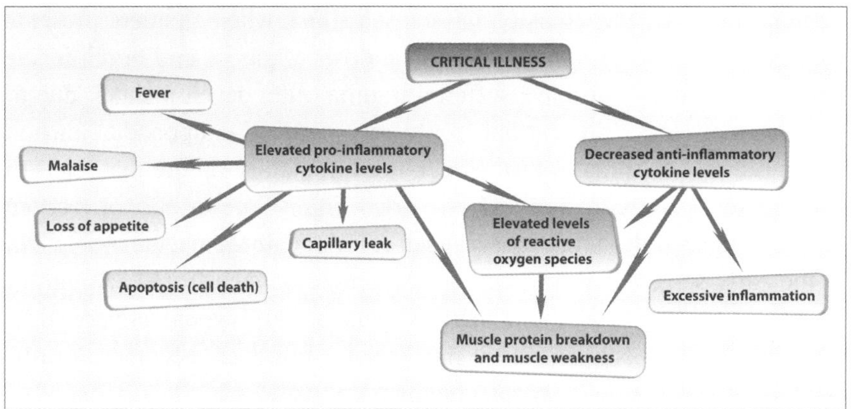

Fig. 1.4: Consequences of cytokine imbalance during critical illness.

This suggestion is, however, based on a small sample size, and confirmation of findings are needed through large clinical trials.

The information shared in this section underscores the importance of the implementation of an appropriate early rehabilitation plan for a patient who suffers traumatic injury and critical illness. Such a plan should aim to address issues related to muscle weakness and joint range of motion as soon as the patient wakes up from sedation and is able to cooperate and participate in rehabilitation.

1.2. Shock and its Effects on the Human Body

1.2.1. *What is shock?*

The cardiovascular system is made up of the heart, the vascular network consisting of arteries, capillaries and veins, and blood. The heart propels the blood (with blood pressure as the driving force) and the vascular network distributes and collects it. These various components of the cardiovascular system are dependent on each other, and if one area malfunctions, the others compensate to return blood pressure to normal. One of the first signs of the development of shock is the presence of hypotension. Hypotension is a sign of cardiovascular insufficiency and indicates that either the heart is not working properly, there is not enough blood in the cardiovascular system or there is a malfunction of the distribution of blood through the body. Hypotension has caused shock when a patient presents with confusion, oliguria and/or lactic acidosis (signs of end organ insufficiency). Patients who have suffered trauma often develop shock due to severe blood loss, myocardial contusion, cardiac tamponade, tension pneumothorax or spinal injury. Shock is a circulatory failure that leads to inadequate tissue perfusion and end organ injury due to lack of oxygen supply at the cellular level. Generalised cellular damage occurs as a result. In the early stages of shock, cells extract more oxygen from each unit of blood and are able to maintain their oxygenation as oxygen delivery starts to decrease. This compensatory mechanism, however, becomes insufficient when oxygen delivery falls below a critical level.

1.2.2. *Organ responses to blood loss*

The ability of organs to withstand blood loss varies according to the amount of blood lost and the success of resuscitation and surgical interventions. The prognosis of the patient depends on their severity of injury, age and pre-existing illnesses (Schroeder *et al.*, 2009).

1.2.2.1. *Cardiovascular system*

The heart rate and blood pressure responses to blood loss are directly related to the amount of total blood volume loss that occurs. Small children are more dependent on heart rate than blood pressure maintenance to compensate for blood loss. A loss of up to 15% of total blood volume in an adult has minimal physiological effects on the cardiovascular system. A loss of 15–30% total blood volume results in an elevated heart rate as well as an elevation in diastolic blood pressure (Garrioch, 2004). The rise in diastolic blood pressure occurs as a result of vasoconstriction, induced by the sympathetic nervous system. Blood loss of 30–40% total volume results in tachycardia and a reduction in systolic and diastolic blood pressure. If more than 40% total blood volume is lost, the patient may present with bradycardia and, in extreme situations, unrecordable blood pressure. Such a situation would be life-threatening (Garrioch, 2004).

In relation to the myocardium, myocardial contractibility may be influenced by traumatic injury, tamponade, mitochondrial calcium losses or nitric oxide production, and this might contribute to a reduction in cardiac output as well as stroke volume. Inappropriate vasodilatation as a result of sepsis or spinal shock might give rise to a reduction in peripheral vascular resistance, leading to a hypotensive state (McLuckie, 2003).

Inadequate restoration of circulating blood volume (low-perfusion state) is associated with the development of inflammation and the release of inflammatory cytokines throughout the circulatory system. The increased cytokine activity causes membrane injury to many vessels in the body, leading to leakage of plasma into the interstitium, which results in a loss of circulating volume and development of generalised oedema (Garrioch, 2004).

1.2.2.2. *Central nervous system*

A loss of more than 30% of total blood volume is accompanied by mental confusion and anxiety and, in severe cases, unresponsiveness (Garrioch, 2004).

1.2.2.3. *Pulmonary system*

In relation to the pulmonary system, hyperventilation occurs early during shock and is related to the development of lactic acidosis. Respiratory rate may increase to more than 20 breaths per minute as a result of lack of tissue oxygenation when 15–30% of total blood volume is lost. Persistently high respiratory rates would accompany blood loss of more than 30% total blood volume (Garrioch, 2004).

Persistent low-perfusion states, which may result from inadequate restoration of circulating blood volume, will lead to the development of inflammation, as discussed above. Systemic inflammatory response syndrome results in capillary leak associated with the development of acute respiratory distress syndrome (ARDS) manifested by progressive posterior lung segment atelectasis (Schroeder *et al.*, 2009). Acute respiratory distress syndrome is defined as a syndrome of acute, diffuse lung inflammation and increased alveolar-capillary membrane permeability associated with clinical signs of decreased oxygenation, decreased lung compliance and increased physiological dead space. Characteristic radiological changes are bilateral radiographic opacities. Oxygenation is impaired in the absence of cardiac dysfunction (Costa and Amato, 2013). Respiratory muscle fatigue from muscle hypoperfusion and increased energy expenditure from breathing with heavy fluid-filled lungs may lead to respiratory failure.

1.2.2.4. *Peripheries*

In adults who have lost 15–30% total blood volume, a degree of peripheral shut down may be observed, which is characterised by cool extremities and peripheral cyanosis. Blood volume loss of more than 30% leads to the development of poor peripheral perfusion, and the patient will present with a pale appearance (Garrioch, 2004).

1.2.2.5. *Renal system*

With regard to the renal system, oliguria occurs due to renal ischaemia when autoregulation fails, or due to antidiuretic hormone and aldosterone secretion, which might result in fluid retention. Blood loss of more than 30% total volume results in negligible urine output (Garrioch, 2004).

1.2.2.6. *Skeletal and splanchnic systems*

In the early stages of shock the skeletal muscles and splanchnic organs (visceral organs such as gastrointestinal tract, liver, pancreas and spleen) are adversely affected by oxygen deprivation. The shock state delays mitochondrial activity and blocks the pathways of cellular energy production. This results in the development of lactic acidosis, which is a sign of widespread inadequate tissue perfusion. Splanchnic ischaemia occurs as vital organs such as the brain, heart, lungs and liver are preferentially perfused (Garrioch, 2004).

1.2.3. *Types of shock*

A person who has suffered trauma-related injuries is at risk of the development of shock. Various types of shock can be identified.

1.2.3.1. *Cardiogenic shock*

A person who has suffered trauma may be at risk for the development of cardiogenic shock when left ventricular function is impaired by injury, such as contusion of the ventricle during a motor vehicle accident or as a result of a fall from a height. Impaired left ventricular function leads to decreased stroke volume, decreased cardiac output, low blood pressure and inadequate tissue perfusion. The sympathetic nervous system response to low blood pressure is vasoconstriction, so increased systemic vascular resistance develops. Clinical presentation of the patient includes cool peripheries, decreased urine output and sweating (Parrillo and Dellinger, 2008).

1.2.3.2. *Hypovolaemic shock*

Hypovolaemic shock may develop in a person who has suffered trauma due to blood loss from organ and tissue injury or loss of blood plasma from burns. The decreased intravascular volume leads to decreased venous return, decreased stroke volume, decreased cardiac output, decreased blood pressure and results in inadequate tissue perfusion. Systemic vascular resistance is increased due to the sympathetic nervous system response to low blood pressure. The clinical presentation of the patient is similar to that described in Section 1.2.3.1. for cardiogenic shock (Parrillo and Dellinger, 2008).

1.2.3.3. *Distributive shock*

Distributive shock occurs when peripheral vascular dilatation causes a drop in systemic vascular resistance. The most common causes of distributive shock are neurogenic shock, anaphylactic shock and septic shock. A description of each of these types of shock is provided below. The clinical presentation of a patient with distributive shock includes warm peripheries, bouncing pulses, altered mental status, oliguria and lactic acidosis (Parrillo and Dellinger, 2008).

1.2.3.3.1. Neurogenic shock

A person who has suffered acute spinal cord injury or traumatic brain injury is at risk for the development of neurogenic shock. Neurogenic shock is the loss of sympathetic control of blood vessels, which results in massive dilatation of arterioles and venules throughout the body. Arteriolar dilation leads to reduced peripheral vascular resistance, resulting in arterial blood pooling which contributes to the decreased amount of blood returning to the heart. Venous dilation leads to venous blood pooling, which results in decreased stroke volume, decreased cardiac output and blood pressure and inadequate tissue perfusion.

1.2.3.3.2. Anaphylactic shock

A person who has suffered trauma may be at risk for the development of anaphylactic shock if he/she has an allergic reaction to blood products or drugs given during resuscitation in the emergency department, theatre or intensive care unit (ICU). Anaphylactic shock is caused by severe allergic antigen–antibody reactions. The patient presents with massive interstitial oedema due to increased capillary permeability as well as hypovolaemia due to venous and arteriolar vasodilation.

1.2.3.3.3. Septic shock

Sepsis is a systemic response to gram negative or gram positive bacterial or fungal infection, as discussed previously. Septic shock is defined as severe sepsis in the presence of persistent hypotension unexplained by other causes (cardiovascular failure). The patient's immune system attempts to fight this infection by activating monocytes, macrophages and neutrophils. These cells interact with the vascular endothelial cells. The cellular activation and endothelial disruption leads to the release of multiple chemicals into the blood stream, including cytokines, ROS, nitric oxide, platelet-activating factor and vasodilators. Certain toxins such as endotoxins and exotoxins are produced, which contribute to the damage of organs and tissues. The toxins and chemicals cause microvascular injury, vasodilation of the capillary bed, capillary leak and interstitial oedema, thrombosis, tissue ischaemia and decreased circulating blood volume. Microvascular injury leads to decreased oxygen delivery and consumption at both cellular and tissue levels. Tissue ischaemia leads to various organ dysfunctions, as mentioned in Section 1.2.2. Thrombocytopenia (diminished platelet count) often leads to the development of disseminated intravascular coagulation. This signifies the disarray of the coagulation and fibrinolytic systems, which lead to spontaneous bleeding from organs, tissues, cavities and any venupuncture sites, as well as microvascular occlusion from excessive fibrin formation. Disseminated intravascular coagulation is associated with MODS and poor patient outcome (Nguyen *et al.*, 2006; Nguyen and Smith, 2007) (Fig. 1.3).

1.2.3.4. *Obstructive shock*

This type of shock is caused by obstruction to cardiac filling. One of the most common causes of obstructive shock is cardiac tamponade, such as occurs with wounds to the heart from penetrating injury. The collection of blood in the pericardium prevents the ventricles from expanding fully. Obstructive shock may also develop due to tension pneumothorax or massive pulmonary embolus (Parrillo and Dellinger, 2008).

1.2.3.5. *Refractory shock*

Refractory shock is also referred to as irreversible shock. At this stage organs have failed and shock cannot be reversed, despite the administration of seemingly adequate therapy. Cardiac function is impaired by inadequate myocardial blood supply and by toxins released by inadequately perfused organs and tissues. Brain damage and cell death ensues (Parrillo and Dellinger, 2008).

1.2.4. *Management of shock*

The initial management of a patient with shock consists of the restoration of oxygen delivery to tissues in the form of oxygen therapy and, if required, mechanical ventilation with low tidal volumes. Restoration of blood volume involves the intravenous administration of crystalloid or colloid fluids and transfusion of red blood cells if indicated. The administration of vasoactive medication assists with the restoration of blood pressure and inotropic drugs assist with the restoration of stroke volume. Early goal-directed therapy is recommended in the emergency department management of a patient with septic shock. This is a management algorithm that is usually instituted and completed within the first six hours of the patient's presentation in the department. Early goal-directed therapy is shown to improve patient outcome significantly. Early detection of the site of infection and implementation of source control measures assists with the further improvement of patient outcome. Source control includes: drainage of an abcess or effusion, wound debridement and initiation of antimicrobial therapy. Patients with refractory shock may be given low-dose corticosteroid therapy in addition to the therapy mentioned above in an attempt to reverse the shock state. The addition of recombinant human-activated protein C therapy for patients with septic shock who present with an APACHE II >25 (see Section 1.6.1.1. for a discussion on APACHE score) has improved survival rates significantly. Recombinant human-activated protein C is used to restore balance to the abnormal coagulation and fibrinolytic pathways associated with septic shock (Nguyen *et al.*, 2006; Nguyen and Smith, 2007).

1.3. Factors that Influence Blood Oxygen Content

Shock, as well as critical illness, can affect the oxygen content of blood due to loss of blood and anaemia. The oxygen content of blood is determined by the amount of oxygen dissolved in the blood plasma and the amount of oxygen bound to haemoglobin. In healthy individuals, low levels of haemoglobin are quickly corrected by an increase in the production of erythropoietin, a glycoprotein hormone that regulates the production of red blood cells (erythropoiesis). Dietary iron is bound to a protein called transferrin and circulates through the body. Excess iron is stored intracellularly through binding with another protein called ferritin. Scharte and Fink (2003) studied red blood cell physiology in critical illness in depth and have stated that a decrease in erythropoietin production response has been observed in patients who suffered trauma. They also stated that low levels of serum iron and transferrin and high levels of ferritin are associated with critical illness, which means that less free iron is available for the production of red blood cells. This reduction in serum iron levels has been linked to the activity of pro-inflammatory cytokines such as IL-1, IL-6 and TNF-α. These cytokines directly provoke the production of ferritin and thereby enhance iron storage intracellularly, which further limits the availability of iron for red blood cell production. Oxygenation is also influenced by phlebotomy (line insertion, sampling for arterial blood gas analysis) in the ICU, which accounts for up to 20% of total blood loss (Scharte and Fink, 2003). This illustrates that a person who has suffered trauma and become critically ill as a result might present with hypoxaemia not only related to chest injuries sustained but also due to a reduction in total blood volume resulting from the processes described around critical illness and ICU procedures.

1.4. Effect of Trauma on Blood Glucose Levels

The initial response of the human body to trauma is to access energy from internal (endogenous) fat oxidation. Fat provides most of the body's energy requirements during the period in which no food is ingested. Fat is mobilised from fat stores and converted to free fatty acids and glycerol. These are then circulated to tissues such as the large muscles, which can burn the fatty acids directly. Blood sugar, however, starts to rise slowly and insulin production from the pancreas is inhibited. It has been reported that hyperglycaemia may contribute to a patient's mortality rate (Schroeder *et al.*, 2009). Poor glycaemic control is associated with increased morbidity and mortality in critically ill trauma patients and is more prevelant in non-diabetic patients (Gale *et al.*, 2007). A greater occurrence of urinary tract infections and complications in non-diabetic trauma patients with poor glycaemic control has also been found (Eakins, 2009). Hyperglycaemia plays a role in the activation of blood coagulation pathways and may put the patient at risk of developing acute thrombosis. Tight glucose control through the administration of insulin therapy has been shown to have a beneficial effect on short-term morbidity and mortality in critically ill patients (Pittas *et al.*, 2004) and today should form part of the standard ICU care of adult patients who have suffered trauma.

In light of this information, an important role of the physiotherapist in the ICU is daily screening of the patient for signs and symptoms of the development of deep venous thrombosis and bringing this to the attention of the interprofessional ICU team.

1.5. Clinical Case Scenario

This scenario incorporates information from all the sections discussed above to demonstrate acute care management of a patient with traumatic injury.

A 33-year-old woman made use of public transport as she travelled home from work. On the way home, the minibus taxi that she was travelling in burst a rear tyre and collided with an oncoming bus. The woman sustained a pelvic fracture and blunt injuries to her abdominal region. She was transported by ambulance to the nearest trauma centre.

In the casualty department she presented with hypovolaemic shock due to internal blood loss from the pelvic fracture and blunt abdominal trauma. Oxygen therapy was started using a partial re-breathing mask as she was still awake and alert. Early goal-directed therapy was initiated and she was taken to theatre for surgical intervention. She was intubated in theatre and central venous and arterial lines were inserted. The pelvic fracture was surgically managed with an external fixator and a laparotomy incision was made to gain access to organs in the abdominal cavity and control the internal bleeding. Afterwards she was transferred to the ICU for monitoring and further management.

In the ICU she remained intubated and was mechanically ventilated with low tidal volumes in order to prevent ventilator-associated lung injury. She presented with low blood pressure due to blood loss from her injuries and surgical interventions in theatre. Intravenous fluids were administered together with vasoactive drugs to restore her blood pressure to acceptable levels. Analgesic and sedative medications were administered, as well as insulin therapy to maintain glucose control. During her stay in the ICU, arterial blood samples were taken every four hours for blood gas analysis and on several occasions blood samples were taken for full blood count, urea and electrolyte analysis and microbiological cultures. As a result of her injuries and the resultant surgery she presented with SIRS, which escalated to sepsis due to wound infection six days after admission to the ICU. This was managed with the administration of antimicrobial therapy, to which she had a favourable response.

Physiotherapy intervention in the ICU while this patient was sedated would consist of prevention or management of respiratory complications, optimisation of oxygenation, passive maintenance of muscle length and joint end of range motion (within precautions and contraindications posed by the pelvic fracture; see Chapter 7) and regular screening of the patient for the development of deep venous thrombosis. As she regains consciousness, the focus of physiotherapy management would shift to active patient participation in rehabilitation in order to address issues related to muscle atrophy and weakness as a result of critical illness and prolonged immobilisation. Active weightbearing through the pelvis with mobilisation would be considered after discussion with the orthopaedic team. The patient would be monitored closely for signs of shortness of breath and unexpected changes in vital signs during chest physiotherapy, exercise rehabilitation and mobilisation.

1.6. Classification of Patients with Traumatic Injuries

The classification of patients with severe injuries on admission to hospital is important. The determination of their severity of illness and risk for mortality guides medical and surgical decision-making in their care pathways. The classification of patients is also important for data capturing in ongoing research studies at trauma centres worldwide in order to objectively compare patient populations and treatment outcomes. Physiotherapists may encounter these classification scoring systems during their daily work in an ICU setting or when reading critical care and trauma literature, and therefore an explanation of the commonly-used scores in the trauma care environment is provided below.

1.6.1. *Severity of illness scoring systems*

The risk of mortality after admission to the ICU is influenced by increasing age, severity of acute illness, pre-existing medical conditions such as cancer, renal failure or immunosuppression, and emergency admission to the ICU. The severity of illness scoring systems were developed in the 1980s to help predict the outcome of patients with critical illness.

1.6.1.1. *APACHE II and SAPS III*

The Acute Physiology and Chronic Health Evaluation (APACHE) score was developed in 1981 to describe accurately the severity of illness of various groups of patients. This was done utilising 34 individual variables (Wong and Knaus, 1991). The APACHE II was developed in 1985 and represented a simplified version of the APACHE score. APACHE II is the most widely used and studied scoring system to date. It is composed of three parts, namely: a) the acute physiology score, composed of 12 laboratory and physical variables; b) the patient's age; and c) a chronic health evaluation. The APACHE II is calculated within the first 24 hours of ICU admission and the maximum score is 71. The higher the score, the greater the risk for mortality (a score of 25 is associated with a predicted mortality of 50%). Unfortunately the APACHE II does not have a component for anatomical injury and therefore its ability to predict outcome in trauma patients in the ICU is questionable (Bouch and Thompson, 2008).

The Simplified Acute Physiology Score (SAPS) was developed in 1984 and consisted of the evaluation of 14 physiological variables. The SAPS was subsequently upgraded to SAPS II and SAPS III, both of which evaluate 12 physiological variables and include data related to pre-exisitng health status and age. Similar to the APACHE II, the SAPS III is calculated within the first 24 hours of ICU admission (Bouch and Thompson, 2008).

1.6.1.2. *Anatomic and physiologic scores*

Various anatomic scores, such as the abbreviated injury score (AIS) and the injury severity score (ISS), were developed to predict mortality in patients who suffered traumatic injury. The AIS was a complex scoring system and formed the basis for the development of the less complex ISS. Various physiologic scores were also developed, such as the revised trauma score (RTS) and the SIRS score (Table 1.2). These scores use physiologic parameters to assess patient outcome. A SIRS score equal to or greater than two has been shown to be predictive of ICU admission and greater risk of mortality than a score less than two (Malone *et al.*, 2001). Some limitations to the effectiveness of the RTS have been documented, especially in relation to accurate assessment of the Glasgow coma scale (GCS) component in patients who are intubated and mechanically ventilated.

Table 1.2: Systemic inflammatory response syndrome score.

Each component is assigned 1 point.

- Fever or hypothermia (temperature >38°C or <36°C)
- Tachypnoea (respiratory rate >20 breaths/minute or $PaCO_2$ <32 mmHg)
- Tachycardia (heart rate >90 beats/minute)
- Leukocytosis or leukopenia (white cell count >12,000/mm^3 or <4000/mm^3)

SIRS score can range from 0–4.

Table 1.3: Trauma and injury severity score (TRISS).

ISS calculator (AIS scores)		RTS calculator		TRISS	
Head	□	Systolic BP	□	Age	□
Face	□	Respiratory rate	□	Probability of survival:	
Chest	□	GCS	□	Blunt injury	□
Abdomen	□			Penetrating injury	□
Extremity	□				
External	□				
	ISS:		**RTS:**		
	□		□		

Online TRISS calculator can be accessed at http://www.trauma.org/js/trisscalc.html

1.6.1.3. *TRISS and ASCOT scores*

Combined scores were subsequently developed for more accurate assessment of injury severity and outcome after trauma, and these scores incorporate existant anatomic and physiologic scores. The Trauma and Injury Severity Score (TRISS) is the most commonly used tool to assess outcome from traumatic injury over time. It was developed in 1983 and a patient's probability to survive traumatic injury is determined through a weighted combination of patient age, ISS and RTS (Schluter, 2011). The advantage of this score is that it takes into account whether the patient suffered from blunt or penetrating trauma (Table 1.3). There are some limitations associated to the use of this score and, in order to address these limitations, another score was developed, namely A Severity Characterisation of Trauma (ASCOT) score. This score, however, was found to be much more cumbersome to administer by clinicians and researchers alike, and was not widely accepted for use. Therefore the

TRISS score remains the most widely used combined classification score for patients with traumatic injuries, despite its documented limitations (Schluter, 2011).

1.6.2. *Morbidity scoring systems*

1.6.2.1. *SOFA score*

The Sepsis-related Organ Failure Assessment (SOFA) score was developed in 1994 during a consensus conference organised by the European Society of Intensive Care Medicine. This scoring system was developed to assess the degree of organ dysfunction that critically ill patients developed over time. The SOFA score was designed to be used in various patient populations and was renamed the Sequential Organ Failure Assessment (Vincent *et al*., 1996; Vincent *et al*., 1998). It consists of scores for six organ systems (brain, cardiovascular, coagulation, renal, hepatic and respiratory), and organ function is scored from zero (normal) to four (extremely abnormal) on a daily basis (Antonelli *et al*., 1999) (Table 1.4). The nature of the SOFA scoring system gives insight into the degree of organ failure and the morbidity of the critically ill patient. The higher the score, the greater the risk of mortality. This system was not designed to compete with existent severity scores that predict mortality, but to complement them.

A comparison between the SOFA, APACHE II and TRISS methods for predicting outcomes in trauma patients in the ICU was recently conducted. The results showed that all three scoring systems were effective in predicting outcome in this patient population, but that the SOFA was simpler to use than APACHE II and TRISS (Hwang *et al*., 2012).

1.6.3. *Paediatric scoring systems*

In children, a number of trauma scoring systems are used, including the paediatric GCS, AIS, paediatric age-adjusted TRISS, RTS, ISS, Penetrating Abdominal Trauma Index (PATI), Paediatric Risk Index (PRI) and Paediatric Trauma Score (PTS) (Marcin and Pollack, 2002). There are also specific scores for individual organs and trauma types (Narci *et al*.,

Table 1.4: SOFA scoring system.

Respiratory system	
PaO_2/FiO_2 (mmHg)	SOFA score
<400	1
<300	2
<200 and mechanically ventilated	3
<100 and mechanically ventilated	4
Central nervous system	
GCS	SOFA score
13–14	1
10–12	2
6–9	3
<6	4
Cardiovascular system	
Mean arterial pressure OR administration of vasopressors required	SOFA score
MAP <70 mmHg	1
Dopamine ≤5 OR dobutrex (any dose)	2
Dopamine >5 OR epinephrine ≤0.1 OR noradrenaline ≤0.1	3
Dopamine >15 OR epinephrine >0.1 OR noradrenaline >0.1	4
*vasopressor drug doses are mcg/kg/min	
Hepatic system	
Bilirubin (mg/dl) [μmol/L]	SOFA score
1.2–1.9 [>20.5–32.5]	1
2.0–5.9 [34.2–100.9]	2
6.0–11.9 [102.6–203]	3
>12.0 [>205]	4
Coagulation	
Platelets x 10^3/mcl	SOFA score
<150	1
<100	2
<50	3
<20	4
Renal system	
Creatinine (mg/dl) [μmol/L] (or urine output)	SOFA score
1.2–1.9 [92–145]	1
2.0–3.4 [152–259]	2
3.5–4.9 [267–374] (or <500 ml/d)	3
>5.0 [>382] (or <200 ml/d)	4

Where a patient's physiological parameters do not match any row, a score of zero is given. If the patient's physiological parameters match more than one row, the row with the most points is picked. Online SOFA calculator can be accessed at http://clincalc.com/IcuMortality/SOFA.aspx

2009) and paediatric risk of mortality scores for use on admission to a paediatric ICU. The ISS has been found to be one of the most valuable trauma scoring systems for use in paediatric patients in two studies (Öztürk *et al.*, 2002; Narci *et al.*, 2009).

1.7. Conclusion

The information provided in this chapter should assist physiotherapists who work in the acute care setting to perform evidence-based clinical reasoning in their management approach to patients who suffer from critical illness as a result of trauma-related injuries sustained.

Key Messages

- An appropriate patient management plan that addresses muscle weakness, joint range of motion and mobilisation is essential to the care of a patient who has suffered critical illness as a result of trauma in order to overcome the complications related to cytokine imbalances.
- The critically ill trauma patient may present with hypoxaemia due to injuries sustained, critical illness itself and various ICU-related procedures.
- Regular assessment of the critically ill trauma patient for the presence of deep venous thrombosis is an important role of the physiotherapist in ICU.

Bibliography

Antonelli, M., Moreno, R., Vincent, J.-L., *et al.* (1999). Application of SOFA score to trauma patients, *Intensive Care Med.,* **25**, 389–394.

Bouch, D.C., and Thompson, J.P. (2008). Severity scoring systems in the critically ill, *Cont. Edu. Anaesth Crit. Care and Pain,* **8**, 181–185.

Callahan, L.A., and Supinski, G.S. (2009). Sepsis-induced myopathy, *Crit. Care Med.,* **37** [Suppl], S354–S367.

Chan, A.K.C., and Paredes, N. (2013). 'The coagulation system in humans', in Monagle, P. (ed), *Haemostasis: Methods and Protocols*, Springer Protocols

Series: Methods in Molecular Biology, Humana Press, New York, vol. 992, pp. 3–12.

Clarke, G.M. (2003). 'Severe sepsis', in Bersten, A.D., and Soni, N. (eds), *Oh's Intensive Care Manual*, 5th edn., Butterworth Heinemann, Edinburgh, pp. 637–643.

Costa, E.L.V., and Amato, M.B.P. (2013). The new definition for acute lung injury and acute respiratory distress syndrome: is there room for improvement?, *Curr. Opin. Crit. Care,* **19**, 16–23.

Eakins, J. (2009). Blood glucose control in the trauma patient, *J. Diabetes Sci. Technol.,* **3**, 1373–1376.

Gale, S.C., Sicoutris, C., Reilly, P.M., *et al.* (2007). Poor glycemic control is associated with increased mortality in critically ill trauma patients, *Am. Surg.,* **73**, 454–460.

Garrioch, M.A. (2004). The body's response to blood loss, *Vox Sang.,* **87** [Suppl 1], S74–S76.

Hietbrink, F., Koenderman, L., Rijkers, G.T., *et al.* (2006). Trauma: the role of the innate immune system, *World J. Emerg. Surg.,* **1**, 1–15.

Hwang, S.Y., Lee, J.H., Lee, Y.H., *et al.* (2012). Comparison of the Sequential Organ Failure Assessment, Acute Physiology And Chronic Health Evaluation II scoring system and Trauma and Injury Severity Score method for predicting the outcomes of intensive care unit trauma patients, *Am. J. Emerg. Med.,* **30**, 749–753.

Jawa, R.S., Anillo, S., Huntoon, K., *et al.* (2011). Interleukin-6 in surgery, trauma and critical care part II: clinical implications, *J. Intensive Care Med.,* **26**, 73–87.

Kapasi, Z.F. (2006). 'The immune system and infectious diseases and disorders', in Malone, D.J., and Lindsay, K.L.B. (eds), *Physical Therapy in Acute Care: A Clinician's Guide*, Slack Incorporated, Thorofare, NJ, pp. 111–116.

Malone, D.L., Kuhls, D., Napolitano, L.M., *et al.* (2001). Back to basics: validation of the admission systemic inflammatory response syndrome score in predicting outcome in trauma, *J. Trauma,* **51**, 458–463.

Marcin, J.P., and Pollack, M.M. (2002). Triage scoring systems, severity of illness measures, and mortality prediction models in pediatric trauma, *Crit. Care Med.,* **30** [Suppl], S457–S467.

McLuckie, A. (2003). 'Shock: an overview', in Bersten, A.D., and Soni, N. (eds), *Oh's Intensive Care Manual*, 5th edn., Butterworth Heinemann, Edinburgh, pp. 71–77.

Mukhopadhyay, S., Hoidal, J.R., and Mukherjee, T.K. (2006). Role of TNF-α in pulmonary pathophysiology, *Respir. Res.,* **7**, 125–134.

Narci, A., Solak, O., Turhan-Haktanir, N., *et al.* (2009). The prognostic importance of trauma scoring systems in pediatric patients, *Pediatr. Surg.,* **25**, 25–30.

Nguyen, H.B., Rivers, E.P., Abrahamian, F.M., *et al.* (2006). Severe sepsis and septic shock: review of the literature and emergency department management guidelines, *Ann. Emerg. Med.,* **48**, 28–54.

Nguyen, H.B., and Smith, D. (2007). Sepsis in the 21st century: recent definitions and therapeutic advances, *Am. J. Emerg. Med.,* **25**, 564–571.

Osuchowski, M.F., Welch, K., Siddiqui, J., *et al.* (2006). Circulating cytokine/inhibitor profiles reshape the understanding of the SIRS/CARS continuum in sepsis and predict mortality, *J. Immunol.,* **177**, 1967–1974.

Öztürk, H., Dokucu, A.I., Otcu, S., *et al.* (2002). The prognostic importance of trauma scoring systems for morbidity in children with penetrating abdominal wounds: 17 years of experience, *J. Pediatr. Surg.,* **37**, 93–98.

Parrillo, J.E., and Dellinger, R.P. (2008). *Critical Care Medicine: Principles of Diagnosis and Management in the Adult,* 3rd edn., Mosby Elsevier, Philadelphia, PA.

Pittas, A.G., Siegel, R.D., and Lau, J. (2004). Insulin therapy for critically ill hospitalised patients: a meta-analysis of randomized controlled trials, *Arch. Intern. Med. 164*, **18**, 2005–2011.

Scharte, M., and Fink, M.P. (2003). Red blood cell physiology in critical illness, *Crit. Care Med.,* **31** [Suppl], S651–S657.

Schluter, P.J. (2011). The Trauma and Injury Severity Score (TRISS) revised, *Injury,* **42**, 90–96.

Schroeder, J.E., Weiss, Y.G., and Mosheiff, R. (2009). The current state in the evaluation and treatment of ARDS and SIRS, *Injury,* **40** [Suppl], S82–S89.

Thomson, S.R. (2003). 'Trauma of the abdomen: blunt and penetrating', in Mieny, C.J., and Mennen, U. (eds), *Principles of Surgical Patient Care*, 2nd edn., New Africa Books, Claremont, Cape Town, pp. 863–865.

Van Dyk, A. (2008). *HIV/AIDS Care and Counselling: A Multidisciplinary Approach*, 4th edn., Pearson Education, Cape Town.

Vincent, J.-L., Moreno, R., Takala, J., *et al.* (1996). The SOFA (Sepsis-related Organ Failure Assessment) score to describe organ dysfunction/failure, *Intensive Care Med.,* **22**, 707–710.

Vincent, J.-L., De Mendonça, A., Cantraine, F., *et al.* (1998). Use of the SOFA score to assess the incidence of organ dysfunction/failure in intensive care units: results of a multicenter, prospective study, *Crit. Care Med.,* **26**, 1793–1800.

Winkelman, C. (2004). Inactivity and inflammation: selected cytokines as biologic mediators in muscle dysfunction during critical illness, *AACN Clin. Issues,* **15**, 74–82.

Winkelman, C., Higgins, P.A., Chen, Y.J.K., *et al.* (2007). Cytokines in chronically critically ill patients after activity and rest, *Biol. Res. Nurs.,* **8,** 261–271.

Wong, D.T., and Knaus, W.A. (1991). Predicting outcome in critical care: the current status of the APACHE prognostic scoring system, *Can. J. Anaesth.,* **38**, 374–383.

Chapter 2

Not Just 'Small Adults': Paediatric Anatomy and Physiology in Relation to Trauma

Written by B.M. Morrow

Children cannot be considered merely as 'small adults'. Children are fundamentally different in terms of cognitive, physical and psychological development, anatomy and physiology. For the purposes of this textbook, the term 'paediatric' includes infants, children and adolescents up to the age of 16 years.

In this chapter information is shared about:

- The anatomical and physiological differences between the adult and child in relation to:
  - The airway.
  - The chest, lungs and breathing.
  - The heart and circulation.
  - The head, neck and central nervous system.
  - The abdomen.
  - The musculoskeletal system.
  - Temperature regulation.

2.1. Introduction

Trauma is a significant contributor to childhood mortality and morbidity. In most developed countries, in which less than 20% of the population is under 15 years of age, trauma is the main cause of childhood mortality (Bayreuther *et al.*, 2009). In developing countries, in which children represent almost half the population, trauma has an even bigger impact on child health (Van As and Rode, 2006). It is estimated that more than 95% of all injury-related deaths in children occur in low and middle-income countries. This is at least partly explained by inadequate adult supervision and exposure to hazardous environments (e.g. traffic, unsafe play areas, cramped living conditions with open fires and unprotected windows (absence of burglar bars or mesh covered windows)).

The nature of activities at different maturation and neuro-developmental stages (with changing levels of independence) predispose infants, children and adolescents to different patterns of injury to those of adults. Children inhabit a different physical zone to adults; they are closer to the ground, and potentially also closer to a number of associated hazards which are not a problem to the taller adult. Young children are inquisitive and know no fear; they climb, squeeze into small spaces and pull things down from high surfaces to investigate them (WHO, 2008a).

Pre-ambulatory children (toddlers) cannot remove themselves from a dangerous situation or environment; such youngsters do not have sufficient judgement to recognise potentially dangerous situations. Additionally, pre-reading children cannot read warning signs to alert them to possible hazards, and pre-adolescent and adolescent children may take unreasonable risks due to cognitive immaturity and normal 'risk-taking' behaviours. Boys tend to have more frequent and more severe injuries than girls, possibly due to greater risk-taking activities, higher activity levels, more impulsive behaviour and less social restriction than girls (Miller *et al.*, 2002; WHO, 2008a).

Whilst adults are frequently involved in industrial or other work-related accidents and motor vehicle accidents, common injuries in children relate to falls and playground accidents. Even when experiencing the same accident as their adult counterparts, infants and children may present with substantially different injuries. For example, a pedestrian vehicle accident involving an adult will frequently result in fractured long bones (because of the taller stature), whereas a child may present with abdominal or thoracic injuries (Crameri, 2010).

Being dependent on adults unfortunately also puts infants and children at risk of abuse. Physiotherapists treating young children should be aware of the potential for non-accidental injury (NAI), and report it promptly should the child or caregiver disclose any suspicious circumstances or if the examination yields concerning findings. Care should be taken that physiotherapy intervention is not seen as a perpetuation of physical abuse.

2.2. Anatomical and Physiological Differences between the Adult and Child

2.2.1. *General*

The smaller the child, the greater the likelihood that a single traumatic impact will injure multiple organ systems. When exposed to intense heat, delicate infant skin burns more quickly and to a greater depth than the thicker skin of adults (WHO, 2008b).

2.2.2. *The airway*

Children are significantly different to adults in their upper airways (Fig. 2.1). The tongue is relatively larger in a child than in an adult and the oral cavity is relatively smaller. The tongue is therefore more likely to obstruct the airway than in an adult. Correct positioning of the head and jaw is therefore imperative to ensure airway patency during resuscitation (Fig. 2.2) (Santillanes and Gausche-Hill, 2008; Crameri, 2010; Harless *et al.*, 2014).

Infants are obligatory nose breathers for the first four to six months of age, in order to allow them to suck and breathe simultaneously. They are therefore more prone to experiencing respiratory compromise if the nose is blocked (by blood or mucus for example). By five to six months of age, infants can take occasional effective oral breaths, and by eight months they are able to breathe normally through the mouth (Santillanes and Gausche-Hill, 2008; Crameri, 2010).

The paediatric airway has a smaller diameter than that of an adult and is very compliant with poor support by surrounding structures. This predisposes the infant to airway obstruction. By Poiseuille's Law, resistance

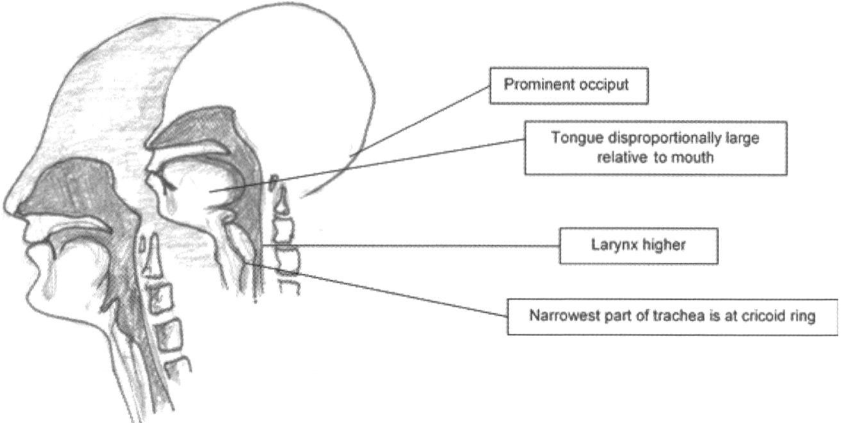

Fig. 2.1: Some differences between adult and paediatric upper airways.

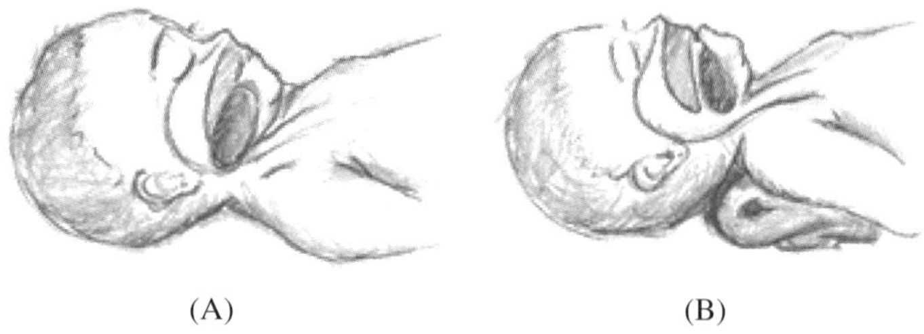

Fig. 2.2: Airway opening (sniffing position) in an infant. The large occiput in image (A) causes head flexion, which leads to obstruction of the upper airway by the base of the tongue. In image (B) placing a towel roll under the shoulders has increased neck extension, thus relieving the obstruction.

is inversely proportional to the fourth power of the radius. Therefore, a small change in airway diameter has a large impact on overall airway resistance (Fig. 2.3). A small amount of swelling can cause significant obstruction, with resulting increases in airway resistance and work of breathing. If the radius is halved, then resistance increases 16 times. Only by the age of eight does the paediatric airway function in a similar manner to the adult airway (Santillanes and Gausche-Hill, 2008; Crameri, 2010).

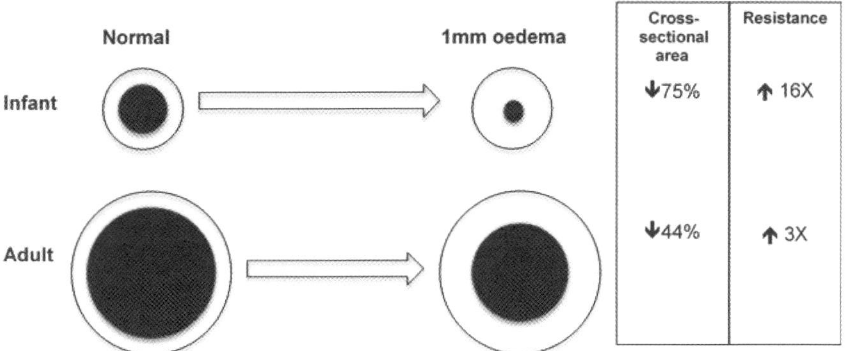

Fig. 2.3: Airway obstruction in infants compared to adults.

Foreign body aspiration is common in children, particularly those with loose deciduous teeth. Aspiration of a small object can lead to significant airway compromise due to the small diameter of the central airways (Crameri, 2010).

The trachea is cartilaginous and more pliable than in an adult, making it easy to collapse and obstruct. The paediatric trachea is also comparatively shorter than that of the adult, which increases the risk of accidental extubation. Large tonsils in young children may also contribute to airway obstruction and make intubation difficult (Santillanes and Gausche-Hill, 2008).

The larynx is higher and more anterior (at the level of the 2nd–3rd cervical vertebrae) in the young child, compared with the 6th–7th cervical vertebrae in the adult (Fig. 2.1). This makes visualisation of the larynx more difficult in the paediatric airway, which also has implications for intubation (Crameri, 2010).

The epiglottis of the young child is horseshoe-shaped and projects posteriorly at 45°. Again, this makes intubation more difficult.

The cricoid ring is the narrowest point in the airway in children and this region is lined with a delicate epithelium which is easily injured, leading to oedema. Therefore, an uncuffed endotracheal tube is usually used in cases of paediatric trauma in order to prevent subglottic stenosis (Santillanes and Gausche-Hill, 2008; Crameri, 2010).

2.2.3. *The chest, lungs and breathing*

The ribs of infants are cartilaginous and are positioned more horizontally than those of adults, with a resulting barrel-shaped chest (Figs 2.4 and 2.5). Although the intercostal muscles are present and functional, the position of the ribs confers a mechanical disadvantage to intercostal contraction and the diaphragm is therefore the main muscle of respiration in infants and young children. The resulting rib excursion is therefore limited, which in turn limits the capacity to increase tidal volumes.

Because the diaphragm is the main respiratory muscle, any increase in abdominal pressure (e.g. abdominal distension) will impact on respiratory function. Decompression of the stomach is important after trauma to prevent a distended abdomen from impinging on diaphragmatic excursion. The paediatric diaphragm also has fewer type 1 (fatigue-resistant) muscle fibres than in adults and is therefore prone to fatigue (Santillanes and Gausche-Hill, 2008; Crameri, 2010).

The chest wall is more compliant than adults, but the lungs are relatively less compliant. As a result of this increased elasticity of the chest wall, blunt chest trauma may not result in rib fractures in the infant and young child. However, the force may be transmitted through the cartilaginous ribs to the underlying structures, potentially causing significant internal injuries. Small children are more susceptible to pneumothoraces

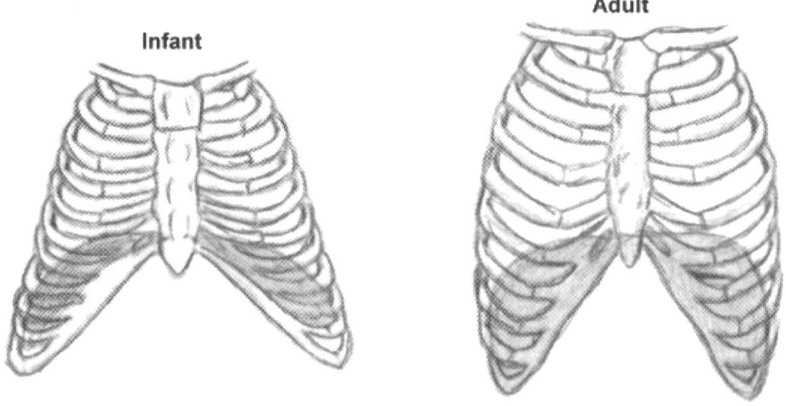

Fig. 2.4: Position of ribs and diaphragm in paediatric versus adult thorax.

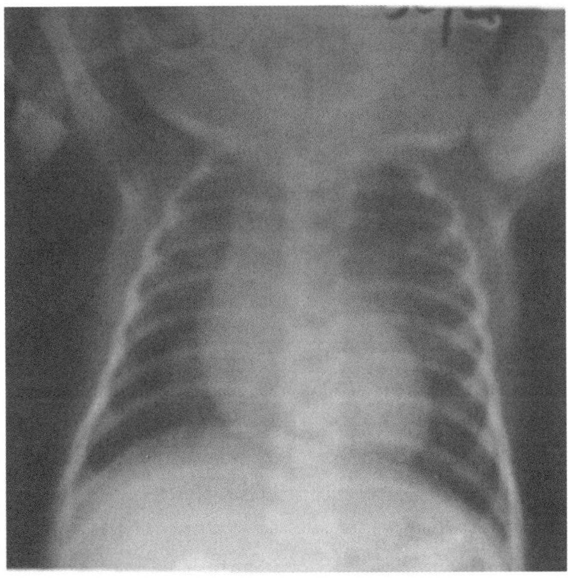

Fig. 2.5: Chest x-ray of a three-week-old infant, showing horizontal ribs and relatively flatter diaphragm.

on the application of positive pressure. Infants tire quicker and more easily than adults, so early aggressive intervention may be needed to protect the airways and maintain ventilation. Early signs of respiratory distress can deteriorate very rapidly, so close observation is required (Kadish, 2006; Escobar and Caty, 2011).

The highly compliant chest wall provides little support for the lungs, thus the negative intrathoracic pressure is poorly maintained and the work of breathing can increase to approximately three times that of the adult.

The number and size of alveoli increase from 20–50 million alveoli at birth until about 300 million alveoli at eight years of age. Young children therefore have less surface area for gaseous exchange than adults. The collateral ventilatory channels are also poorly developed in young children, predisposing them to atelectasis (Charnock and Doershuk, 1973; WHO, 2008a) (Fig. 2.6).

It has long been taught that children have a different pattern of ventilation to adults: whereas adults uniformly preferentially ventilate the dependent lung, children were thought to preferentially ventilate the non-dependent lung, and this pattern was said to continue well into the second decade of

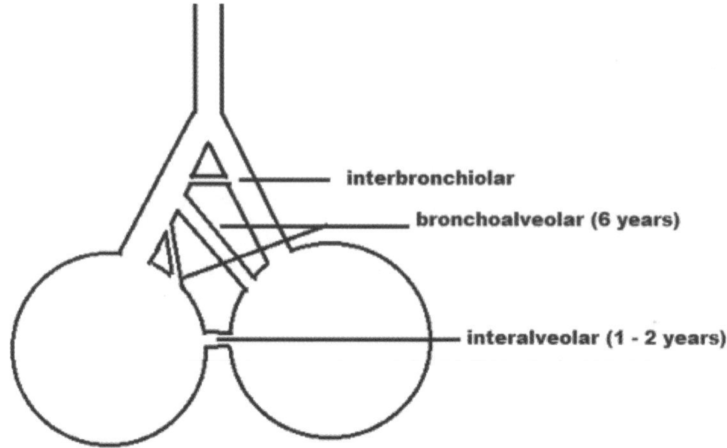

Fig. 2.6: Development of collateral ventilation channels (interbronchiolar channels of Martin; bronchoalveolar channels of Lambert; interalveolar pores of Kohn).

life (Davies *et al.*, 1985; Bhuyan *et al.*, 1989; Davies *et al.*, 1992). More recent studies using electrical impedance tomography in infants under six months of age (Frerichs *et al.*, 2003; Schibler *et al.*, 2009) and older infants and children (Lupton-Smith *et al.*, 2014) have refuted this hypothesis. Neonates appear to have a similar pattern of ventilation to adults, while the distribution of ventilation in both spontaneously breathing and mechanically ventilated older infants and children is highly variable (Lupton-Smith *et al.*, 2014; Lupton-Smith *et al.*, unpublished data). Further studies are required to determine what factors influence the pattern of ventilation in children, but individual assessment of response to treatment is recommended, rather than prescribing standard positions for specific lung zones.

Children have higher metabolic rates than adults and therefore they also have higher oxygen demand (6 ml/kg/min in a child vs. 3 ml/kg/min in an adult) (Fig. 2.7). This results in higher respiratory rates, which vary by age (WHO, 2008a) (Table 2.1).

Tidal volume remains relatively constant throughout life, at about 7 ml/kg (Fig. 2.8). As mentioned previously, the position of the ribs makes it difficult for young children to lower intrapleural pressures in order to increase inspiratory volume effectively. Consequently, maintaining or increasing ventilation is dependent on increasing the respiratory rate in infants and children, whereas adults tend to first increase the depth of breathing.

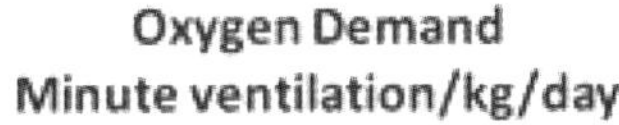

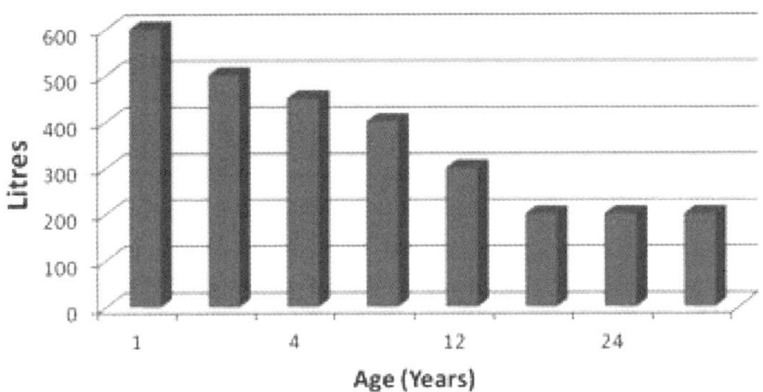

Fig. 2.7: Changes in oxygen demand with chronological age (adapted from WHO, 2008a).

Table 2.1: Normal paediatric vital signs by age group.

Age	Respiratory rate (breaths per minute)	Heart rate (beats per minute)	Minimum systolic blood pressure (mmHg)
Term neonate	40–60	100–170	50
3 months	30–50	100–170	50
6 months	30–50	100–170	60
1 year	30–40	110–160	70–90
1–2 years	25–35	100–150	80–95
2–5 years	25–30	95–140	80–100
5–12 years	20–25	80–120	90–110
>12 years	15–20	60–100	100–120

Key Message

The combination in young children of being respiratory-rate dependent and having higher oxygen utilisation means that decompensation occurs more rapidly once the respiratory muscles (especially the diaphragm) fatigue.

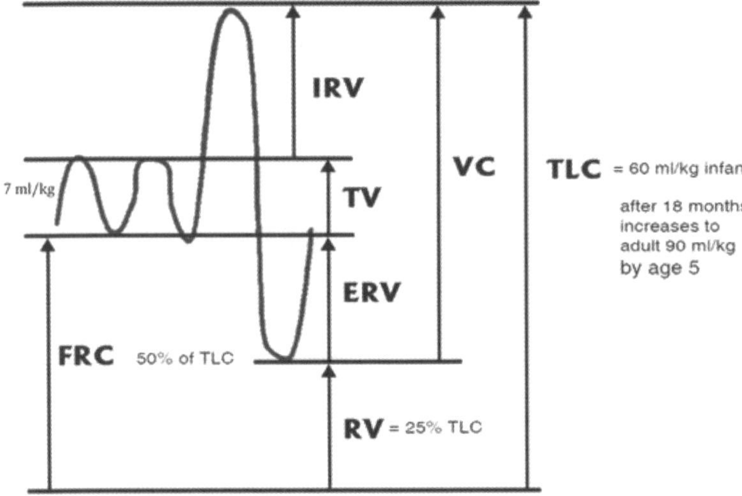

Fig. 2.8: Normal lung volumes and capacities in the child. Tidal volume (TV); inspiratory reserve volume (IRV); expiratory reserve volume (ERV); vital capacity (VC); total lung capacity (TLC); residual volume (RV).

The functional residual capacity (FRC) of an infant that is awake is similar to an adult when normalised to body weight; however, it may decrease to less than 15% of total lung capacity in states of complete relaxation. This low FRC is close to the closing capacity of the airways, resulting in atelectasis, ventilation/perfusion mismatching and desaturation (Bhuyan *et al.*, 1989).

2.2.3.1. *Signs of paediatric respiratory distress*

It is essential that physiotherapists are able to recognise the signs of respiratory distress in infants and children who have suffered traumatic injury. Early recognition and prompt management of respiratory compromise is essential to ensure optimal outcome and to prevent respiratory failure. Signs of paediatric respiratory distress are discussed below in order of significance.

- Tachypnoea is one of the first signs of respiratory distress; infants and young children first increase the rate rather than the depth of breathing.

This must be recognised early, as, regardless of cause, rapidly breathing children will eventually tire, leading to respiratory arrest.

Key Message

Slow respiratory rate in acutely ill or injured children is sometimes associated with an altered level of consciousness and is an ominous sign. Do not assume slowing respiratory rates means clinical improvement.

- Nasal or alar flaring is the excessive opening of the nostrils during respiratory distress and is a subconscious attempt by the infant or child to decrease airway resistance (Santillanes and Gausche-Hill, 2008).
- Grunting is a sound heard during expiration as air passes through a partially closed glottis. This is an automatic reaction to respiratory insufficiency, providing the lungs with increased expiratory pressures in order to optimise gaseous exchange by splinting airways open.
- Recessions or retractions are an indrawing of the thoracic soft tissues during inspiration due to the very compliant chest wall. They may be subcostal, intercostal, supracostal, suprasternal or substernal (Fig. 2.9). A sign of imminent respiratory failure is 'seesaw' breathing. This is a combination of paradoxical and abdominal breathing as defined by the chest wall moving inwards during inspiration and the abdomen bulging outwards with the opposite occurring during expiration (Santillanes and Gausche-Hill, 2008).

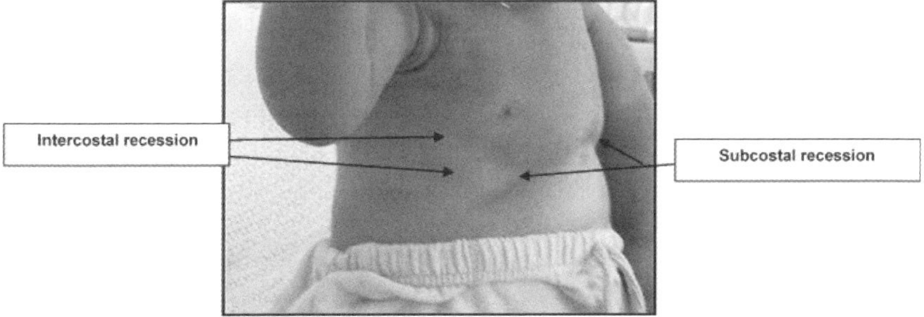

Fig. 2.9: Subcostal and intercostal recessions in an eight-month-old child.

- Head bobbing may occur in infants, indicating the use of the accessory muscles of respiration. The neck is extended on inspiration and relaxed during expiration in an attempt to increase inspiratory pressure (Santillanes and Gausche-Hill, 2008).
- Abnormal positioning includes a refusal to lie down and the child assuming the 'tripod' or 'sniffing' position to instinctively open the airways and use the accessory muscles of ventilation most effectively. Respiratory opisthotunus (extensor posturing of the neck) should not be corrected, as opposed to neurological extensor posturing, which may be inhibited during physiotherapy treatment and positioning (Santillanes and Gausche-Hill, 2008).
- Expiratory wheeze or prolonged expiration may indicate an inhaled foreign body.

Key Message

Symptoms or signs of respiratory distress should not be ignored or discounted in a child simply because the oxygen saturation reading is greater than 94%. Children in respiratory distress or failure can maintain acceptable oxygen saturation levels by increasing the work of breathing and respiratory rate until the point of respiratory arrest, particularly if they are receiving supplementary oxygen.

2.2.3.2. *Signs of inadequate respiratory effort*

Table 2.2 lists the signs of impending respiratory failure (alarm bells), and prompt action should be taken when paediatric patients exhibit any of these signs.

Table 2.2: Signs of impending respiratory failure.

- Decreasing respiratory rate or gasping
- Poor chest excursion and air entry
- Cyanosis or hypoxia (low saturation of oxygen of arterial blood (SaO2))
- Hypoxaemia and/or hypercapnoea with acidosis on arterial blood gas
- Tachycardia followed by bradycardia
- Altered level of consciousness and hypotonia

Appendix 1 lists the normal values for paediatric arterial blood gas results according to age.

2.2.4. *The heart and circulation*

Generally, the cardiovascular system in children is healthy (not having experienced exposure to as much environmental hazard as adults), and therefore pre-existing cardiac disease is less prevalent.

Cardiac output at birth is 200 ml/kg/min, which progressively decreases to 100 ml/kg/min by adolescence. Children are not able to increase stroke volume (due to a noncompliant and poorly developed left ventricle), therefore they increase heart rate in order to increase cardiac output. Normal age-related heart rate ranges are provided in Table 2.1.

Vascular access may be very difficult in small children as they have smaller blood vessels and relatively more subcutaneous tissue than adults.

The sympathetic nervous system is not well developed in infants, predisposing them to bradycardia. Therefore, bradycardia can lead to a marked drop in blood pressure. Heart rate is influenced by respiratory insufficiency, with infants rapidly becoming bradycardic with hypoxia (Crameri, 2010).

It is important to remember that the majority of paediatric cardiopulmonary arrests are secondary to respiratory failure (Zideman and Hazinski, 2008). Therefore, the prevention of hypoxia and maintenance of respiratory function is the focus of resuscitation in young children (see Chapter 5 for 'ABC' or 'CAB' emergency response approaches in children compared to adults). Children have a high metabolic rate (higher oxygen consumption) at rest and very little reserve (low FRC), thus any additional stress such as hypothermia is very poorly tolerated and may result in rapid, severe hypoxia. Young children and infants are very sensitive to hypoxia and may develop reflex bradycardia and asystole as a result (Kadish, 2006).

Key Message

Circulatory compromise in the infant is usually as a result of respiratory failure.

The blood volume in a child is relatively larger, but the absolute blood volume is smaller than in adults (80–90 ml/kg vs. 65–70 ml/kg). Therefore, relatively small volumes of blood constitute significant blood loss in small children. For example, 100 ml blood loss in a 5 kg baby represents about 28.5% of total blood volume lost, whereas the same amount of blood loss in a 70 kg adult constitutes 1.5% of total blood volume lost.

In children, systemic vascular resistance is lower than in adults, increasing from birth throughout childhood. The normal systolic blood pressure values for different ages are provided in Table 2.1. Hypotension is a late sign of blood loss, as children are able to compensate with normal blood pressure until intravascular volumes of up to 25% are lost; thus one cannot wait for hypotension to diagnose shock: hypotension is a sign of severe hypovolaemia (Bliss and Silen, 2002). Therefore, urine output is often used to assess circulation in children (1–2 ml/kg/hour in children or infants compared to 0.5–1 ml/kg/hour in adults) (Crameri, 2010). Signs of shock in children include a capillary refill time greater than 2–3 seconds, cool skin, low urine output, changes in mental status, elevated heart rate, narrowed pulse pressure and elevated lactate.

The increased mobility of the mediastinum in childhood increases the risk of a tension pneumothorax developing from a simple pneumothorax (refer to Chapter 5 for definitions of simple and tension pneumothoraces).

The circulatory assessment establishes the adequacy of cardiac output and perfusion to vital organs. When determining the circulatory status of an adult, heart rate and blood pressure are the most valuable indicators. In children, however, those vital signs can be deferred until later in the initial assessment. In children, skin appearance is a reliable initial indication that something may be wrong with their circulation (Santillanes and Gausche-Hill, 2008).

When perfusion to the skin or mucus membranes is poor, pallor is usually the first observable sign. This is due to neuromuscular regulation of blood flow as the body attempts to maintain core perfusion. As the blood vessels to the skin constrict, mottling may also appear. Cyanosis is a late sign of hypoxia in children. Generally, the child will have shown pallor, mottling or other signs before becoming cyanotic. Also, it is important to distinguish between acrocyanosis and true cyanosis. Acrocyanosis occurs in infants younger than two months old when they are exposed to the cold and presents as blue discolouration of the extremities only. True cyanosis (central cyanosis) is present throughout the body and occurs with severe oxygen deprivation (Steinhorn, 2008). Appendix 1 lists normal paediatric values for haemoglobin levels according to age.

2.2.5. *Head, neck and central nervous system*

Infants have a relatively larger occiput and it may be more difficult to perform airway opening manoeuvres (Fig. 2.2). The large head to body ratio results in a higher centre of gravity in the child, contributing to the higher incidence of head trauma in this age group (Crameri, 2010). The larger head in children, combined with relatively lax spinal ligaments, also increases the likelihood of vertebral movement during trauma, with resulting injury to a normal spinal cord. Spinal cord injury without radiological anomaly (SCIWORA) is an important entity in childhood, as significant spinal cord oedema may occur without obvious radiological changes. Careful assessment of all systems is required in order to avoid missing cases of SCIWORA (Pang and Wilberger, 2012).

The spinal fulcrum is at C1–2 in young children, as opposed to C6–7 in adults. Therefore, cervical spine injuries in children under the age of eight years most commonly occur in the first three vertebrae; whereas, in the adult, injuries tend to be lower in the vertebral column (Crameri, 2010).

The cranial sutures in young children remain open and therefore present a vulnerable area for head injury, but also a useful assessment tool. The anterior fontanelle may be palpable until 18 months of age and the posterior fontanelle is usually palpable until two months of age. In the context of trauma, bulging fontanelles suggest an increased intracranial pressure, possibly due to intracranial bleeding. Conversely, a sunken fontanelle may indicate significant blood loss (Crameri, 2010).

Considering that the cranial sutures only fuse when the head reaches adult proportions, the brain in young children is relatively protected from injury by allowing some expansion in the presence of swelling or intracranial bleeding. However, the thinner cranial bones in children afford less protection from direct head injury than the thicker adult skull (Coates and Margulies, 2006).

Key Message

Signs of exhaustion or falling conscious levels in children are ominous.

A quick general impression of appearance and function can provide an accurate gross assessment of ventilation, oxygenation, brain perfusion and central nervous system function. Loud, boisterous crying is the best sound anyone can hear going into an unknown paediatric emergency. An unresponsive, limp child with a fixed gaze should be considered seriously ill or injured, requiring immediate emergency care to ensure adequate ventilation and oxygenation.

2.2.6. *The abdomen*

The abdominal wall in children is relatively thin, with less muscle and subcutaneous fat than in adults, thereby affording less protection to abdominal organs. The flatter diaphragm in children pushes the liver and spleen lower below the rib cage than in adults and these organs are therefore more prone to injury during abdominal trauma. The bladder in infants is also an intra-abdominal organ, increasing the risk of bladder damage in abdominal trauma (Crameri, 2010).

2.2.7. *Musculoskeletal system*

Before the ossification of long bones, even significant injury may not result in fractures. The absence of a fracture, however, does not equate to absence of injury, as the force of the injury can result in significant injury to surrounding tissues and organs. Growth or epiphyseal plates only fuse when children reach skeletal maturity after puberty. A fracture through the growth plate can seriously affect the future growth of the fractured bone (Dandy and Edwards, 2009; Crameri, 2010).

2.2.8. *Temperature regulation*

The infant is particularly vulnerable to hypothermia because of both the large ratio of body surface area to weight and a limited ability to cope with cold stress (e.g. a young infant cannot shiver). Oxygen consumption increases in direct relation to the increasing differences between skin and environmental temperature. Thus all steps should be undertaken to minimise heat loss in an unwell or injured child (Kadish, 2006). Appendix 1 lists normal values for paediatric body temperature.

2.3. Conclusion

Children and infants differ substantially from adults in almost all respects of cardio-respiratory physiology. These differences impact all phases of care (emergency response, acute, sub-acute and chronic) for the paediatric trauma victim. It is, however, important to recognise that the basic principles of trauma management are the same, regardless of the age of the patient.

Bibliography

Bayreuther, J., Wagener, S., Woodford, M., *et al.* (2009). Paediatric trauma: injury pattern and mortality in the UK, *Arch. Dis. Child. Education and Practice Edition,* **94**, 37–41.

Bhuyan, U., Peters, A.M., Gordon, I., *et al.* (1989). Effects of posture on the distribution of pulmonary ventilation and perfusion in children and adults, *Thorax,* **44**, 480–484.

Bliss, D., and Silen, M. (2002). Pediatric thoracic trauma, *Crit. Care Med.*, **30**[Suppl], S409–S415.

Charnock, E.L., and Doershuk, C.F. (1973). Developmental aspects of the human lung, *Pediatr. Clin. North Am.,* **20**, 275–292.

Coates, B., and Margulies, S.S. (2006). Material properties of human infant skull and suture at high rates, *J. Neurotrauma,* **23**, 1222–1232.

Crameri, J. (2010). *Trauma: 11 How are Children Different?* The Royal Children's Hospital Melbourne. [Online] Available at: http://www.rch.org.au/paed_trauma/manual.cfm?doc_id=12411 [Accessed 1 April 2013].

Dandy, D.J., and Edwards, D.J. (2009). *Essential Orthopaedics and Trauma*, 5th edn., Churchill Livingstone Elsevier, Edinburgh.

Davies, H., Kitchman, R., Gordon, I., *et al.* (1985). Regional ventilation in infancy: reversal of adult pattern, *N. Engl. J. Med.,* **313**, 1626–1628.

Davies, H., Helms, P., and Gordon, I. (1992). Effect of posture on regional ventilation in children, *Pediatr. Pulmonol.,* **12**, 227–232.

Escobar, M.A., and Caty, M.G. (2011). 'Thoracic injuries in children', in Fuhrman, B.P., and Zimmerman, J.J. (eds), *Pediatric Critical Care*, 4th edn., Elsevier Saunders, Philadelphia, PA, pp. 1520–1527.

Frerichs, I., Shiffmann, H., Oehler, R., *et al.* (2003). Distribution of lung ventilation in spontaneously breathing neonates lying in different positions, *Intensive Care Med.,* **29**, 787–794.

Harless, J., Ramaiah, R., and Bhananker, S.M. (2014). Pediatric airway management, *Int. J. Crit. Illn. Inj. Sci.,* **4**, 65–70.

Kadish, H.A. (2006). 'Thoracic trauma', in Fleisher, G.R., Ludwig, S., Henretig, F.M. *et al.* (eds), *Textbook of Pediatric Emergency Medicine*, 5th edn., Lippincott Williams & Wilkins, Baltimore, MD, pp. 1433–1452.

Lupton-Smith, A., Argent, A.C., Rimensberger, P., *et al.* (2014). Challenging a paradigm: positional changes in ventilation distribution are highly variable in healthy infants and children, *Pediatr. Pulmonol.*, **49**, 764–771.

Miller, M.D., Marty, M.A., Arcus, A., *et al.* (2002). Differences between children and adults: implications for risk assessment at California EPA, *Int. J. Toxicol.*, **21**, 403–418.

Pang, D., and Wilberger, J.E. (2012). Spinal cord injury without radiological abnormalities in children, *J. Neurosurg.,* **116**, 114–129.

Santillanes, G., and Gausche-Hill, M. (2008). Pediatric airway management, *Emerg. Med. Clin. N. Am.,* **26**, 961–975.

Schibler, A., Yuill, M., Parsley, C., *et al.* (2009). Regional ventilation distribution in non-sedated spontaneously breathing newborns and adults is not different, *Pediatr. Pulmonol.,* **44**, 851–858.

Steinhorn, R.H. (2008). Evaluation and management of the cyanotic neonate, *Clin. Pediatr. Emerg. Med.,* **9**, 169–175.

Van As, A.B., and Rode, H. (2006). The history of paediatric trauma care in Cape Town, *S. Afr. Med. J.,* **96**, 874–876.

World Health Organisation (WHO). (2008a). *Children are not Little Adults. Children's Health and the Environment WHO Training Package for the Health Sector*. World Health Organisation. [Online] Available at: http://www.who.int/ceh/capacity/Children_are_not_little_adults.pdf [Accessed 1 June 2012].

World Health Organisation (WHO). (2008b). *World Report on Child Injury Prevention*, WHO Press, Geneva.

Zideman, D.A., and Hazinski, M.F. (2008). Background and epidemiology of pediatric cardiac arrest, *Pediatr. Clin. N. Am.,* **55**, 847–859.

Chapter 3

Trauma and Immunosuppressive Diseases

Written by H. van Aswegen and B.M. Morrow

Nobody is exempt of the risk from being involved in a traumatic event. The result is that people who suffer from chronic health problems may end up in hospital due to traumatic injury and not due to exacerbation of their disease. A group of people at particular risk after traumatic injury are those who have immunosuppressive diseases such as human immunodeficiency virus (HIV) or acquired immunodeficiency syndrome (AIDS), as they may have an altered response to injury.

This chapter provides the physiotherapist with information about:

- The pathogenesis of HIV and AIDS.
- Pulmonary diseases that may develop as a result of HIV and AIDS.
- Pulmonary complications associated with antiretroviral therapy.
- Extrapulmonary complications associated with HIV and antiretroviral therapy.

3.1. Introduction

Despite the decline in new HIV infections (about 20% globally between 1999 and 2009; 25% in 33 countries including sub-Saharan Africa), as a result of both HIV prevention strategies and the natural course of the epidemic (UNAIDS, 2010), HIV remains a serious public health concern in some areas of the world. The resurgence of HIV in eastern Europe and central Asia is cause for concern, as the incidence of HIV in these countries has tripled since 2000 (UNAIDS, 2010). In regions with high HIV prevalence, knowledge of underlying obstructive and restrictive respiratory conditions and the effects of HIV and antiretroviral therapy (ART) on other organ systems are essential to assist physiotherapy clinicians in understanding the clinical presentation of an HIV-infected patient who has suffered traumatic injury.

3.2. Pathogenesis of HIV and AIDS

AIDS is a syndrome of opportunistic diseases caused by HIV. HIV is a retrovirus which attacks the immune system by transporting its own genetic material, namely ribonucleic acid (RNA), into body cells via cell surface receptors and, particularly, the CD4 receptors. HIV uses the enzyme reverse transcriptase to copy itself inside the infiltrated cells and forms deoxyribonucleic acid (DNA) which is earmarked as proviral DNA. The proviral DNA lies dormant until the cell is activated and then the proviral DNA forms RNA, which forms the basis for the production of new HIV under the control of enzymes such as proteases. The young HIV leaves the infiltrated cells, matures and goes off to invade more cells via their CD4 receptors (Wesselingh and French, 2003; Van Dyk, 2008). Perinatally infected children progress to symptomatic disease (AIDS) more rapidly than HIV-infected adults. Death (apoptosis) of CD4 lymphocytes and abnormalities in the T-lymphocyte helper maturation, along with other defects, lead to susceptibilities to viral and intracellular organisms. HIV-infected children are further predisposed to bacterial sepsis as a result of defects in B-lymphocytic function, natural killer cell activity, neutrophil bactericidal activity and defective antigen-specific immunoglobulin production, all despite an increase in total globulin fraction. Encapsulated bacteria such as *Streptococcus pneumonia* are particular problems in children due to greater antibiotic resistance (Madhi *et al.*, 2000; Musiime *et al.*, 2013). HIV-infected children may also present with cardiac dysfunction (including dysrhythmia, left ventricular systolic function, increased left ventricular mass and pericardial effusion), anaemia and encephalopathy (Harmon *et al.*, 2002; Okoromah *et al.*, 2012; Walker *et al.*, 2013).

3.3. HIV and AIDS and the Pulmonary System

People with HIV infection seem to be at increased risk of developing pulmonary diseases such as chronic obstructive pulmonary disease (COPD), changes in lung parenchyma that lead to restrictive disease and infective diseases (Morris *et al.*, 2011). The antiretroviral medication that many people with HIV take on a daily basis has also been associated with changes observed in the pulmonary system (Morris *et al.*, 2011). A short discussion of these pulmonary complications and the diseases that occur in adults and children living with HIV or AIDS follows below. Table 3.1 summarises the common pulmonary complications encountered in adults and children living with HIV or AIDS.

3.3.1. *Chronic obstructive pulmonary disease*

3.3.1.1. *Emphysema*

People who live with HIV are at particular risk of developing COPD due to the high prevalence of smoking and intravenous drug use observed in this population (Raynaud *et al.*, 2011). Evidence of small airways disease in the form of early emphysema observed through high resolution computed tomography (CT) scans taken in people with HIV has been reported by various researchers. Lung function abnormalities in people with HIV

Table 3.1: Summary of common pulmonary complications or diseases associated with HIV or AIDS and antiretroviral therapy in adults and children.

- Chronic obstructive pulmonary disease (emphysema, bronchiectasis)
- Tuberculosis (pleural, pulmonary, upper airways)
- Pneumonia (pneumocystic, bacterial)
- Decreased diffusion capacity
- Pulmonary fibrosis
- Repeated respiratory tract infections

(prior to the onset of AIDS) such as impaired diffusion capacity of carbon monoxide (D_{LCO}), lowered forced expiratory volume in one second and lower forced expiratory flow have also been reported by several authors (King *et al.*, 1997; Diaz *et al.*, 1999; Gelman *et al.*, 1999; Morris *et al.*, 2011; Raynaud *et al.*, 2011). HIV has also been linked to an acceleration of the onset of smoking-related emphysema, likely due to cytotoxic lymphocyte activity. Pulmonary function abnormalities continue to be present even in people with HIV who are on ART. A possible reason for this finding is that HIV-infected individuals on ART have a longer life expectancy and therefore are exposed to the detrimental effects of smoking for a longer time period (Rosen, 2008; Gingo *et al.*, 2010; Morris *et al.*, 2011; Raynaud *et al.*, 2011).

Presenting symptoms of emphysema include breathlessness on exertion, chest tightness, cough and wheeze as a result of airflow limitation due to peripheral airway remodelling, hypoxaemia and hypercapnia. As the disease progresses, chest configuration changes to that of a barrel-shaped appearance and pursed lip breathing is used in an attempt to splint open airways that collapse prematurely on expiration to allow for improved expiratory flow and less air trapping (McKenzie *et al.*, 2003). Radiological features of emphysema are characterised by dark hyperinflated lung fields, flattened hemidiaphragms and an elongated heart shadow (Fig. 3.1). Bullae may be visible on chest x-rays and CT scans in the advanced phase of emphysema (Corne and Pointon, 2010) (Fig. 3.2).

3.3.1.2. *Bronchiectasis*

People with HIV have a high tendency to develop airway diseases such as bronchiectasis even if they do not smoke. Asymptomatic people may complain of a dry non-productive cough. Symptomatic people present with dyspnoea, wheezing and increased amounts of purulent sputum production, especially during periods of exacerbation (Tino and Weinberger, 2010). Radiological features of bronchiectasis include increased density of affected lobes with tramline shadows (diseased bronchi seen side on) towards the lung periphery. Ring shadows (diseased bronchi seen end on) may also be visible (Corne and Pointon, 2010) (Fig. 3.3).

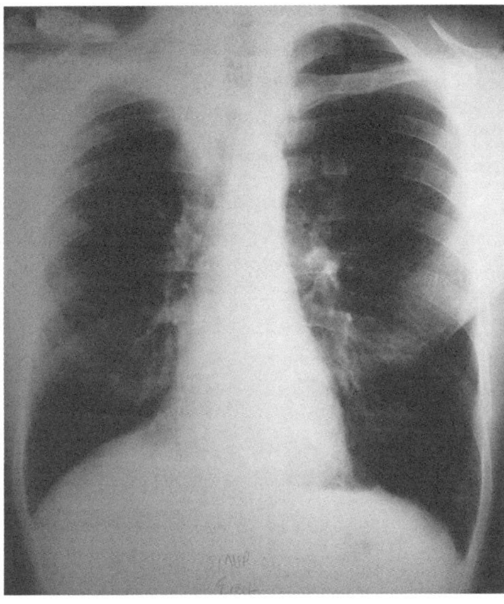

Fig. 3.1: Chest x-ray of a patient with early signs of emphysema and right upper lobe collapse. Note the hyperinflation of the left lung with flattened hemidiaphragm and elongated heart shadow. The shape of the right hemidiaphragm appears normal due to the volume loss in the upper lobe.

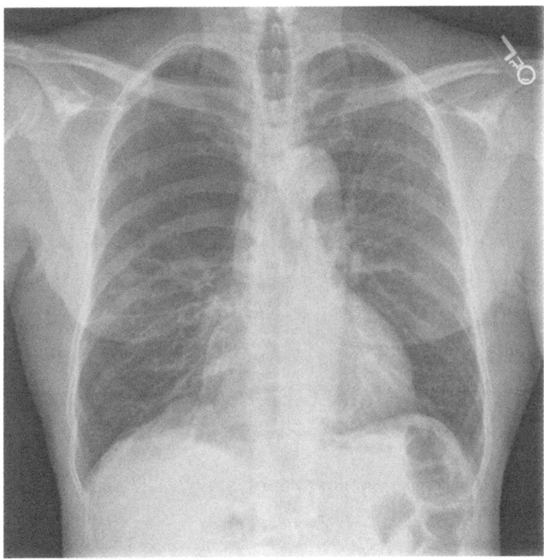

Fig. 3.2: Chest x-ray of a patient with a large right upper lung bulla due to paraseptal emphysema. Published with permission from Jeffrey L. Koning MD, www.radiologypics.com.

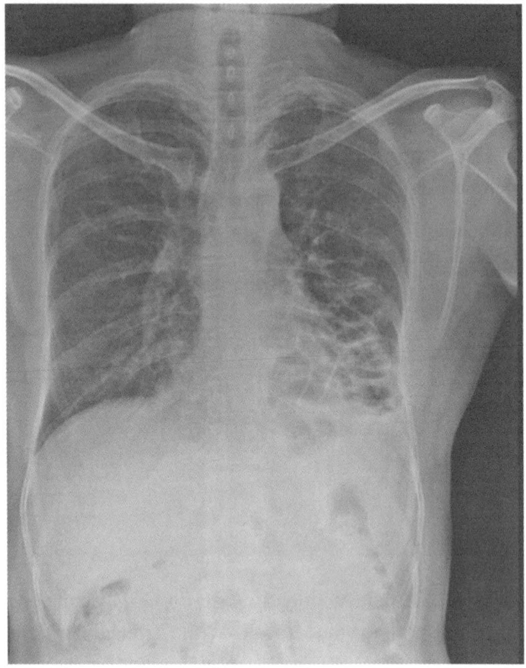

Fig. 3.3: Chest x-ray of a male patient with bronchiectatic changes in the left basal lung segments. Published with permission from Radiopaedia.org.

3.3.1.3. *Implications for physiotherapy*

It is important that physiotherapists remember to include education on management of episodes of breathlessness, the correct usage of prescribed symptom-relieving pulmonary medication, especially those administered through an inhaler device and effective methods of self-management of pulmonary hygiene in their management of a patient with HIV or AIDS and COPD in the trauma intensive care unit (ICU) and ward settings. Referral to a pulmonary rehabilitation programme, if the patient is not involved with one already, after discharge from hospital is also recommended.

3.3.2. *Mycobacterium infections*

3.3.2.1. *Mycobacterium tuberculosis*

The highest risk factor for the development of *Mycobacterium tuberculosis* is HIV infection (Boyton, 2005; Rosen, 2008). Tuberculosis (TB) recurrence is higher in people with HIV who are not on ART than in those on therapy. Tuberculosis may accelerate the progression of HIV infection due to suppressed cell immunity that leads to increased HIV replication and mutation in the lung, and may therefore be associated with higher mortality in HIV infection (Boyton, 2005; Rosen, 2008).

Presenting symptoms of post-primary pulmonary TB are non-specific and include: fever and night sweats, weight loss, anorexia, malaise and general weakness. The cough that develops starts out as a dry cough and eventually becomes productive of purulent secretions, with or without streaks of blood, or even massive haemoptysis. Subpleural parenchymal lesions may lead to the development of chest pain and dyspnoea may develop in extensive disease (Raviglione and O'Brien, 2010). Post-primary TB on chest x-rays is characterised by an increased density of the affected lobes due to fibrotic changes in the lung parenchyma as a result of the reactivation of latent infection (Fig. 3.4). Small infiltrations on chest x-rays indicate limited parenchymal infection, whereas large cavity formation is indicative of massive parenchymal infection (Raviglione and O'Brien, 2010). Classic radiological features of miliary TB include a 'ground glass appearance' throughout both lungs. Despite this ground glass appearance the normal anatomy of the lung is still visible (Corne and Pointon, 2010).

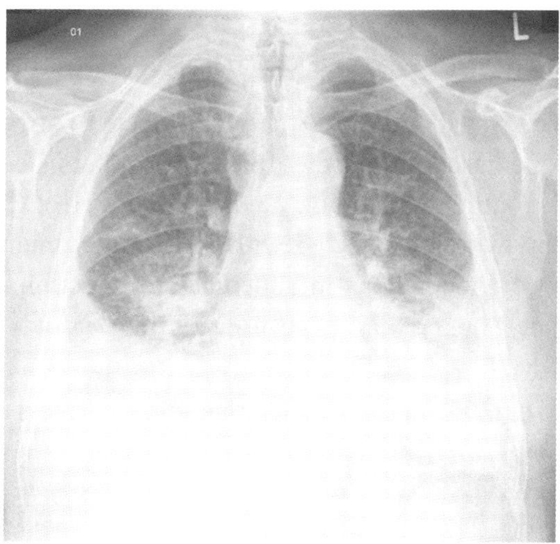

Fig. 3.4: Chest x-ray of a patient with post-primary TB in the lower lung regions. Published with permission from Radiopaedia.org.

3.3.2.2. *Mycobacterium xenopi*

A less common respiratory disease, caused by *Mycobacterium xenopi* in people with HIV infection, has also been reported. *Mycobacterium xenopi* is an opportunistic pathogen which leads to the development of pneumonia and other lower respiratory tract diseases. Presenting symptoms include long-lasting low-level fever, weight loss, night sweats, diffuse lymphadenopathy, mild chest pain and cough, and it is often misdiagnosed as TB. However, mortality associated with *Mycobacterium xenopi* remains low (Manfredi *et al*., 2003).

3.3.2.3. *Extrapulmonary tuberculosis*

Extrapulmonary TB is common in HIV-infected patients. If the upper airways are infected with *Mycobacterium tuberculosis* the patient may present with chronic productive cough, hoarseness of the voice, dysphonia and dysphagia. Patients with pleural TB may present with pleuritic chest pain, dyspnoea and fever if the effusion is large. Extrapulmonary TB often includes infection of the lymphatic system and the pericardium (Raviglione and O'Brien, 2010).

Mycobacterium xenopi may affect extrapulmonary sites such as the skin, bone and joints, endocardium and genitourinary tract (Manfredi *et al*., 2003).

3.3.2.4. *Implications for physiotherapy*

It is often difficult to diagnose TB in HIV-infected patients in a timely manner due to increased frequency of negative sputum smears and atypical radiographic findings (Raviglione and O'Brien, 2010). Physiotherapists that treat patients who are infected with HIV in the trauma ICU setting should therefore be meticulous in adherence to infection control principles to reduce their own risk of exposure to TB.

3.3.3. *Pulmonary complications associated with antiretroviral therapy*

The morbidity and mortality associated with HIV infection has changed dramatically worldwide due to the use of combination ART. Some clinical problems that relate to the use of ART in critically ill patients have, however, been reported (Huang *et al.*, 2006). Intensive care unit admission for people with HIV has mostly centred on the development of respiratory failure due to *Pneumocystis pneumonia*, bacterial pneumonia and TB. However, respiratory failure can also result from immune reconstitution syndromes to TB, pneumocystic pneumonia and other bacterial diseases after the initiation of ART (Boyton, 2005; Huang *et al.*, 2006). The development of acute respiratory distress syndrome (ARDS) in patients with HIV infection who are critically ill necessitates lung protective ventilation strategies according to guidelines produced by the ARDS network. Lung protective ventilation strategies are recommended in order to minimise the risk for the development of a spontaneous pneumothorax (due to decreased lung compliance) while the patient receives mechanical ventilation (Huang *et al.*, 2006). Lung protective ventilation strategies are not only recommended for patients with HIV but also for all patients with ARDS in order to minimise the risk of ventilator-induced lung injury.

3.3.4. *Restrictive pulmonary disease*

Impairment in D_{LCO} in the lungs of people living with HIV (regardless of CD4 count) has been reported in the literature. Parenchymal lung damage secondary to HIV-related inflammatory events has been proposed as a cause for this abnormality (Diaz *et al.*, 1999). People infected with HIV seem to be at higher risk of the development of lung cancer and pulmonary fibrosis compared to their non-infected counterparts (Crothers *et al.*, 2011). Patients with restrictive pulmonary disease present with a dry cough and progressive shortness of breath during activities of daily living as the disease progresses.

3.3.4.1. *Implications for physiotherapy*

Physiotherapy management of patients with HIV and impairments in D_{LCO} in the trauma ICU and ward setting includes adequate provision of supplemental oxygen and close monitoring of changes in vital signs when patient activity levels are increased. Long-term goals of management should include education of the patient on the management of episodes of breathlessness if the patient complains of frequent episodes of dyspnoea during activities of daily living.

3.3.5. *Paediatric pulmonary disease*

In children, HIV infection is also associated with severe opportunistic infections such as *Pneumocystis pneumonia*, which continues to be a significant problem in some parts of the world, with high morbidity and mortality, despite the availability of ART and the prevention of mother-to-child transmission programmes (Morrow *et al.*, 2010). Tuberculosis is the cause of death in 13% of people with AIDS (Ackerman and Singhi, 2010), and pulmonary TB is frequently diagnosed in HIV-infected children. Those who are started on ART are at particular risk of the development of pulmonary TB due to drug-induced immune reconstitution (Zampoli *et al.*, 2007; Walters *et al.*, 2008). Bacterial and viral respiratory tract infections are also more common and often more severe than in HIV-negative children (Morrow *et al.*, 2006). Such repeated infections in HIV-positive children (not on ART) lead to irreversible airway damage, which may be a precursor for the development of COPD in later life. Children with immune compromise are also more likely to be at risk of nosocomal infections (both bacterial and viral) whilst in hospital, which in turn is associated with significant morbidity and mortality (Foglia *et al.*, 2007; Morrow and Argent, 2009). Therefore, special care with regard to infection control and prophylactic measures has to be taken in all HIV-infected or HIV-exposed paediatric trauma victims.

Key Messages

Respiratory signs and symptoms that may be evident in patients who live with HIV/AIDS and pulmonary disease:

- Chest pain (pleuritis due to pneumonia, pleural effusion due to TB, pulmonary TB).
- Decreased tidal volumes (pulmonary fibrosis, pulmonary TB).
- Decreased lung compliance (pulmonary fibrosis, pulmonary TB).
- Dry cough (pulmonary fibrosis, pulmonary TB).
- Excessive secretion production (bronchiectasis, emphysema).
- Shortness of breath (large pleural effusion, pneumonia, pulmonary TB, pulmonary fibrosis).

3.4. Extrapulmonary Complications Associated with HIV and Antiretroviral Therapy

Even though the use of combination ART has reduced the morbidity and mortality associated with HIV or AIDS, associated drug interactions lead to complications related to other bodily systems of people living with HIV. Table 3.2 provides a summary of the common extrapulmonary complications observed in adults and children living with HIV or AIDS.

3.4.1. *Allergic skin reactions*

Non-nucleoside reverse transcriptase inhibitors such as nevirapine have been associated with the development of skin rashes and may lead to severe syndromes such as Stevens–Johnson Syndrome (SJS) and toxic epidermal necrolysis (TEN) (Wesselingh and French, 2003; Khalili and Bahna, 2006; Mockenhaupt *et al.*, 2007). In both of these conditions keratinocyte apoptosis occurs, which leads to the separation of the epidermis from the dermis. Presenting signs and symptoms include fever, malaise, erosion of mucous membranes and blister formation (Khalili and Bahna, 2006; Mockenhaupt *et al.*, 2007). The extent of skin detachment differs between these conditions, with reported 10% or less in SJS and more than 30% in TEN (Khalili and Bahna, 2006). Mortality associated with these conditions increases significantly in the presence of HIV seropositivity.

Table 3.2: Summary of common extrapulmonary complications associated with HIV or AIDS and antiretroviral therapy.

- Allergic skin reactions
- Lipodystrophy
- Diabetes
- Hypertension
- Ischaemic heart disease
- Peripheral neuropathy
- Fatigue
- Surgical site infections

3.4.2. *Lipodystrophy syndrome*

Lipodystrophy is often referred to as loss of subcutaneous fat. HIV infection alone was thought to lead to the development of lipodystrophy; however, evidence exists to also support the role of combination ART in the development of lipodysthropy. HIV-associated lipodystrophy is characterised by facial and peripheral fat atrophy with visceral fat accumulation (Wesselingh and French, 2003; Guimaraes *et al.*, 2007; Anuurad *et al.*, 2009). Metabolic alterations that occur as a result of HIV-associated lipodystrophy include diabetes, hypertension, glucose intolerance, dyslipidaemia, endothelial dysfunction and atherosclerosis (Loonam and Mullen, 2012). HIV and lipodystrophy have been associated with an increased risk for the development of ischaemic heart disease (Islam *et al.*, 2012).

3.4.3. *Peripheral neuropathy*

Distal sensory peripheral neuropathy has been reported in HIV positive individuals not on ART as well as in those who are on such therapy. It consists of two types; namely primary HIV-associated distal sensory polyneuropathy and antiretroviral toxic neuropathy. Antiretroviral toxic neuropathy is the most frequently observed ART-related toxicity in sub-Saharan Africa. These neuropathies together involve approximately 30–67% of patients with advanced HIV (Evans *et al.*, 2011; Luma *et al.*, 2012). Small and large peripheral nerve fibres are affected length-wise in sensory peripheral neuropathy and result in reduced or absent ankle reflexes compared to patellar reflexes, reduced or absent vibration sensation in the toes and decreased pin and temperature sensation in a glove or stocking distribution pattern. Numbness, paraesthesia, burning sensation and stabbing pain are among the most commonly reported symptoms (Evans *et al.*, 2011). Peripheral neuropathy tends to persist in patients with nerve damage obtained from HIV or medication use, despite the reduction in use of neurotoxic ART in developed countries. Interestingly, protease inhibitor medication seems not to be associated with the development of peripheral neuropathy. Increasing age, alcohol intake, diagnosis of diabetes, history of treatment with anti-TB drug isoniazid and low CD4 count are some of the important factors identified as posing an increased risk for the development of sensory peripheral neuropathy (Evans *et al.*, 2011; Luma *et al.*, 2012).

3.4.4. *Other antiretroviral therapy-related complications*

Nucleoside reverse transcriptase inhibitors have been associated with the development of fatigue and fat wasting. Other reported ART-related consequences include cachexia related to weight loss, chronic weakness and diarrhoea, increased tumour necrosis factor-alpha (TNF-α) activity, osteoporosis and changes in glucose homeostasis as well as in the immune and cytokine systems (Anuurad *et al.*, 2009). Osteoporosis has been reported in adults and children as part of the metabolic syndrome relating to HIV infection itself and ART (Fortuny *et al.*, 2008; Schafer *et al.*, 2013). This is associated with increased fracture rates in the HIV-infected population (McComsey *et al.*, 2010; Schafer *et al.*, 2013).

3.4.5. *Surgical site infection*

People who live with HIV or AIDS have a two-fold higher risk of the development of surgical site infections than those who are HIV negative (Drapeau *et al.*, 2009). Surgical site infections in the HIV population tend to be more severe than those in the general population, with a post-discharge sepsis incidence rate of 10%. Surgical site infections for people with HIV who underwent orthopaedic surgery due to trauma-related injuries has been reported to be 16.7%. The incidence of surgical site infection in those with HIV who had open reduction of fractures is reported to be as high as 71.4% (Drapeau *et al.*, 2009). Surgical site infection in people with HIV who underwent abdominal surgery is reported to be as high as 37.9% (Zhang *et al.*, 2012). The presence of Hepatitis-C virus and a low CD4 count (< 200 cells/μL) are the most commonly reported risk factors for the development of surgical site infections in people living with HIV or AIDS (Drapeau *et al.*, 2009; Zhang *et al.*, 2012).

3.4.6. *Implications for physiotherapy*

It is important that physiotherapists who treat patients in the ICU and on the wards who live with HIV or AIDS and have suffered trauma-related injuries adhere to strict infection control principles in an attempt to reduce the incidence of surgical site infection. Adherence to infection control principles during the management of patients with allergic skin reactions such as SJS and TEN is of utmost importance in order to prevent infection of the open wounds of the skin.

Physiotherapists should also remember that rehabilitation of trauma patients who live with HIV or AIDS and receive ART might be affected by the sensory deficits associated with peripheral neuropathy, especially in relation to the re-education of gait, balance and pain sensation. Rehabilitation may also be affected by the chronic inflammatory state of the patient as a result of increased TNF-α activity as well as cachexia, which will impact on muscle function. Fatigue associated with ART may impact on the patient's level of endurance. The duration of rehabilitation of such patients might be prolonged in comparison to that of HIV-negative patients who have suffered traumatic injury, due to the factors mentioned above.

Patients who live with HIV/AIDS, have suffered traumatic injury and have been diagnosed with lipodystrophy may benefit from education on regular cardiovascular and resistance exercise training, of appropriate intensity and frequency, that becomes part of their weekly routine after discharge from the hospital, in order to reduce their risk of development of ischaemic heart disease.

Lastly, physiotherapists should be aware that people who live with HIV or AIDS may suffer from mental illnesses such as depression, anxiety, panic attacks and post-traumatic stress disorder as a result of their HIV or AIDS diagnosis. Researchers report that up to 50% of HIV or AIDS sufferers present with the aforementioned mental illnesses (Kelly *et al.*, 1998; Whetten *et al.*, 2008; Adewuya *et al.*, 2009). Mental illness in a trauma patient who lives with HIV or AIDS may impact her/his concordance with therapy, the rehabilitation process and, consequently, outcomes from therapy.

3.5. Conclusion

This chapter provides the physiotherapist with background knowledge on HIV and AIDS, the complications associated with these diseases and its pharmaceutical management. Physiotherapists who work in the acute care setting in developing or developed countries should therefore be able to modify their management approach to trauma survivors who live with HIV or AIDS accordingly, to provide the highest quality of care for these patients.

Bibliography

Ackerman, A.D., and Singhi, S. (2010). Pediatric infectious diseases: 2009 update for *Rogers' Textbook of Pediatric Intensive Care*, *Pediatr. Crit. Care Med.,* **11**, 117–123.

Adewuya, A.O., Afolabi, M.O., Ola, B.A., *et al.* (2009). Post-traumatic stress disorder (PTSD) after stigma related events in HIV infected individuals in Nigeria, *Soc. Psychiatry Psychiatr. Epidemiol.,* **44**, 761–766.

Anuurad, E., Semrad, A., and Berglund, L. (2009). Human immunodeficiency virus and highly active antiretroviral therapy-associated metabolic disorders and risk factors for cardiovascular disease, *Metab. Syndr. Relat. Disord.,* **7**, 401–410.

Boyton, R. (2005). Infectious lung complications in patients with HIV/AIDS, *Curr. Opin. Pulmon. Med.,* **11**, 203–207.

Corne, J., and Pointon, K. (2010). *Chest X-Ray Made Easy*, 3rd edn., Churchill Livingstone Elsevier, Edinburgh.

Crothers, K., Huang, L., Goulet, J.L., *et al.* (2011). HIV infection and risk for incident pulmonary diseases in the combination antiretroviral therapy era, *Am. J. Respir. Crit. Care Med.,* **183**, 388–395.

Diaz, P.T., King, M.A., Pacht, E.R., *et al.* (1999). The pathophysiology of pulmonary diffusion impairment in human immunodeficiency virus infection, *Am. J. Respir. Crit. Care Med.,* **160**, 272–277.

Drapeau, C.M.J., Pan, A., Bellacosa, C., *et al.* (2009). Surgical site infections in HIV-infected patients: results from an Italian prospective multicenter observational study, *Infection,* **37**, 455–460.

Evans, S.R., Ellis, R.J., Chen, H., *et al.* (2011). Peripheral neuropathy in HIV: prevalence and risk factors, *AIDS,* **25**, 919–992.

Foglia, E., Meier, M.D., and Elward, A. (2007). Ventilator-associated pneumonia in neonatal and pediatric intensive care unit patients, *Clin. Microbiol. Rev.,* **20**, 409–425.

Fortuny, C., Noguera, A., Alsina, L., *et al.* (2008). Long-term use of bisphosphonates in the treatment of HIV-related bone pain in perinatally infected pediatric patients, *AIDS,* **22**, 1888–1890.

Gelman, M., King, M.A., Neal, D.E., *et al.* (1999). Focal air trapping in patients with HIV infection: CT evaluation and correlation with pulmonary function test results, *Am. J. Radiol.,* **172**, 1033–1038.

Gingo, M.R., George, M.P., Kessinger, C.J., *et al.* (2010). Pulmonary function abnormalities in HIV-infected patients during the current antiretroviral therapy era, *Am. J. Respir. Crit. Care Med.,* **182**, 790–796.

Guimaraes, M.M., de Oliveira, A.R., Jr, Penido, M.G., *et al.* (2007). Ultrasonographic measurement of intra-abdominal fat thickness in HIV-infected patients treated or not with ARV and its correlation to lipid and glycemic profiles, *Ann. Nutr. Metab.,* **51**, 35–41.

Harmon, W.G., Dadlani, G.H., Fisher, S.D., *et al.* (2002). Myocardial and pericardial disease in HIV, *Curr. Treat. Options Cardiovasc. Med.,* **4**, 497–509.

Huang, L., Quartin, A., Jones, D., *et al.* (2006). Intensive care of patients with HIV infection, *N. Engl. J. Med.,* **355**, 173–181.

Islam, F.M., Wu, J., Jansson, J., *et al.* (2012). Relative risk of cardiovascular disease among people living with HIV: a systematic review and meta-analysis, *HIV Med.,* **13**, 453–468.

Kelly, B., Raphael, B., Judd, F., *et al.* (1998). Posttraumatic stress disorder in response to HIV infection, *Gen. Hosp. Psychiatry,* **20**, 345–352.

Khalili, B., and Bahna, S.L. (2006). Pathogenesis and recent therapeutic trends in Stevens-Johnson syndrome and toxic epidermal necrolysis, *Ann. Allergy Asthma Immunol.,* **97**, 272–281.

King, M.A., Neal, D.E., St John, R., *et al.* (1997). Bronchial dilatation in patients with HIV infection: CT assessment and correlation with pulmonary function tests and findings at bronchoalveolar lavage, *Am. J. Radiol.,* **168**, 1535–1540.

Loonam, C.R., and Mullen, A. (2012). Nutrition and the HIV-associated lipodystrophy syndrome, *Nutr. Res. Rev.,* **25**, 267–287.

Luma, H.N., Tchaleu, B.C.N., Doualla, M.S., *et al.* (2012). HIV-associated sensory neuropathy in HIV-1 infected patients at the Douala General Hospital in Cameroon: a cross-sectional study, *AIDS Res. Ther.,* **9**, 35. [Online] Available at: http://www.aidsrestherapy.com/content/9/1/35 [Accessed 13 November 2014].

Madhi, S.A., Petersen, K., Madhi, A., *et al.* (2000). Impact of human immunodeficiency virus type 1 on the disease spectrum of *Streptococcus pneumoniae* in South African children, *Pediatr. Infect. Dis. J.,* **19,** 1141–1147.

Manfredi, R., Nanetti, A., Tadolini, M., *et al.* (2003). Role of *Mycobacterium xenopi* disease in patients with HIV infection at the time of highly active antiretroviral therapy (HAART). Comparison with pre-HAART period, *Tuberculosis,* **83**, 319–328.

McComsey, G.A., Tebas, P., Shane, E., *et al.* (2010). Bone disease in HIV infection: a practical review and recommendations for HIV care providers, *Clin. Infect. Dis.,* **51**, 937–946.

McKenzie, D.K., Frith, P.A., Burdon, J.G.W., *et al.* (2003). The COPDX plan: Australian and New Zealand guidelines for the management of chronic obstructive pulmonary disease, *Med. J. Aust.,* **178** [Suppl], S1–S39. Mockenhaupt, M., Viboud, C., Dunant, A., *et al.* (2007). Stevens-Johnson syndrome and toxic epidermal necrolysis: assessment of medication risks with emphasis on recently marketed drugs. The EuroSCAR-study. *J. Invest. Dermatol.,* **128**, 35–44.

Morris, A., George, P., Crothers, K., *et al.* (2011). HIV and chronic obstructive pulmonary disease: is it worse and why? *Proc. Am. Thorac. Soc.,* **8**, 320–325.

Morrow, B.M., and Argent, A.C. (2009). Ventilator-associated pneumonia in a paediatric intensive care unit in a developing country with high HIV-prevalence. A retrospective survey, *J. Pediatr. Child Health,* **45**, 104–111.

Morrow, B.M., Hatherill, M., Smuts, H.E.M., *et al.* (2006). A comparison of the clinical course of hospitalised children infected with human metapneumovirus and human respiratory syncytial virus, *J. Pediatr. Child Health,* **42**, 174–178.

Morrow, B.M., Hsaio, N-Y., Zampoli, M., *et al.* (2010). Pneumocystis pneumonia in South African children with and without human immunodeficiency virus infection in the era of highly active antiretroviral therapy, *Pediatr. Infect. Dis. J.,* **29**, 535–539.

Musiime, V., Cook, A., Bakeera-Kitaka, S., *et al.* (2013). Bacteraemia, causative agents and antimicrobial susceptibility among HIV-1 infected children on antiretroviral therapy in Uganda and Zimbabwe, *Pediatr. Infect. Dis. J.,* **32**, 856–862.

Okoromah, C.A., Ojo, O.O., and Ogunkule, O.O. (2012). Cardiovascular dysfunction in HIV-infected children in a sub-Saharan African country: comparative cross-sectional observational study, *J. Trop. Pediatr.,* **58**, 3–11.

Raviglione, M.C., and O'Brien, R.J. (2010). 'Tuberculosis', in Loscalzo, J. (ed.), *Harrison's Pulmonary and Critical Care Medicine*, McGraw Hill, New York, pp. 121–134.

Raynaud, C., Roche, N., and Chouaid, U. (2011). Interactions between HIV infection and chronic obstructive pulmonary disease: clinical and epidemiological aspects, *Respir. Res.,* **12**, 117. [Online] Available at: http://respiratory-research.com/content/12/1/117 [Accessed 13 November 2014].

Rosen, M.J. (2008). Pulmonary complications of HIV infection, *Respirology,* **13**, 181–190.

Schafer, J.J., Manlangit, K., and Squires, K.E. (2013). Bone health and human immunodeficiency virus infection, *Pharmacotherapy,* **33**, 665–682.

Tino, G., and Weinberger, S.E. (2010). 'Bronchiectasis and lung abscess', in Loscalzo, J. (ed.), *Harrison's Pulmonary and Critical Care Medicine*, McGraw Hill, New York, pp. 166–168.

UNAIDS. 2010. *Epidemic Update. UNAIDS Report on the Global AIDS Epidemic*. Global Report. [Online] Available at: http://www.unaids.org/documents/20101123_GlobalReport_Chap2_em.pdf [Accessed 1 August 2011].

Van Dyk, A. (2008). *HIV/AIDS Care and Counselling: a Multidisciplinary Approach*, 4th edn., Pearson Education, Cape Town.Walker, S.Y., Pierre, R.B.,

Christie, C.D., *et al.* (2013). Neurocognitive function in HIV-positive children in a developing country, *Int. J. Infect. Dis.,* **17**, e862–867.

Walters, E., Cotton, M.F., Rabie, H., *et al.* (2008). Clinical presentation and outcome of tuberculosis in human immunodeficiency virus infected children on antiretroviral therapy, *BMC Pediatr.,* **8**, 1. [Online] Available at: http://www.biomedcentral.com/1471-2431/8/1[Accessed 13 November 2014].

Wesselingh, S., and French, M.A.H. (2003). 'HIV and acquired immunodeficiency syndrome', in Bersten, A.D., and Soni, N. (eds), *Oh's Intensive Care Manual*, 5th edn., Butterworth Heinemann, Edinburgh, pp. 629–636.

Whetten, K., Reif, S., Whetten, R., *et al.* (2008). Trauma, mental health, distrust, and stigma among HIV-positive persons: implications for effective care, *Psychosom. Med.,* **70**, 531–538.

Zampoli, M., Kilborn, T., and Eley, B. (2007). Tuberculosis during early antiretroviral-induced immune reconstitution in HIV-infected children, *Int. J. Tuberc. Lung Dis.,* **11**, 417–423.

Zhang, L., Liu, B.C., Zhang, X.Y., *et al.* (2012). Prevention and treatment of surgical site infection in HIV-infected patients. *BMC Infect. Dis.,* **12**, 115. [Online] Available at: http://www.biomedcentral.com/1471-2334/12/115 [Accessed 13 November 2014].

Chapter 4

Physiotherapy Modalities, Markers and Outcome Measures

Written by B.M. Morrow and H. van Aswegen

This chapter provides information about:

- Early mobilisation and graded exercise therapy.
- Cardiopulmonary physiotherapy techniques, their performance and contraindications and precautions to consider for adult and paediatric patients.
- Subjective and objective markers and outcome measures for the assessment of patient response to treatment interventions.

4.1. Early Mobilisation and Graded Exercise Therapy

'Teach us to live that we may dread
unnecessary time in bed.
Get people up and we may save
our patients from an early grave.'

— RAJ Asher (1957)

People who have sustained traumatic injury are often subjected to a period of bed rest and immobility in the ward or intensive care unit (ICU) setting due to the nature and severity of their injury. The numerous complications of bed rest and immobility, affecting multiple organ systems, have been well described. Complications in both adults and children include muscle weakness and polyneuropathy, deep vein thrombosis, skin ulcers, disuse atrophy of the gut and significant psychological impact on both the patient and their family (Knight *et al.*, 2009a,b,c; Fan, 2012; Dammeyer *et al.*, 2013; Kocan and Lietz, 2013). These complications are exacerbated by inflammation, poor glycaemic control and drugs such as neuromuscular blocking agents administered to the patient (Gosselink *et al.*, 2011). Complications specific to the respiratory system include pneumonia, positional atelectasis, secretion retention, airway obstruction and decreased lung volumes (Knight *et al.*, 2009a; Truong *et al.*, 2009). Survivors of critical illness or injury complain of weakness for months and sometimes even years after discharge from hospital (Fan, 2012).

The general aims of physiotherapy in people following trauma are summarised in Table 4.1 and should be considered alongside the limitations that their injuries will present.

In order to achieve these goals of therapy, physiotherapists must remain cognisant about treating every patient holistically. Specific considerations and applications according to injury type are presented in the relevant chapters of this book.

Table 4.1: General aims of physiotherapy in people who sustained traumatic injury.

- To decrease pain associated with joint stiffness and muscle spasm
- To rehabilitate the patient to the highest level of functional independence as possible
- To restore mobility, normal gait pattern and bodily posture within the limitations posed by each type of injury
- To improve muscle strength
- To maintain or restore full joint range of motion and muscle length
- To facilitate early weaning from mechanical ventilation for those who are intubated and ventilated
- To improve breathing pattern and reduce the work of breathing
- To ensure adequate ventilation of all areas of the lungs
- To assist in the removal of excessive bronchial secretions
- To prevent or resolve pulmonary complications

4.1.1. *Early mobilisation*

During the acute and sub-acute stages after a traumatic injury, the emphasis of physiotherapy management should be on the mobilisation of the patient as soon as their condition has stabilised, appropriate to the:

- age and developmental level of the patient;
- cognitive function of the patient;
- patient's acuity of illness;
- patient's general condition; and
- type, severity and stability of the injury.

Physical activities that may be used even for cooperative intubated and ventilated patients include (Gosselink *et al.*, 2011; Fan, 2012; Stiller, 2013):

- active limb exercises;
- functional bed exercises;
- sitting in bed or in a chair;
- standing and transferring from bed to chair; and
- marching on the spot or walking away from the bedside, using an assistive device if indicated.

The aims of mobilisation include improving thoracic mobility; increasing lung volumes (Zafiropoulos *et al.*, 2004) and functional residual capacity (FRC); improving functional activity, exercise tolerance, muscle strength and cardiovascular fitness (Stiller, 2013), which aid in weaning from mechanical ventilation; preventing postural deformities that could impact on function (including respiratory function); improving bone ossification; improving bladder and bowel function; and providing psychological benefits to the patient (Bailey *et al.*, 2007; Truong *et al.*, 2009).

In adults, mobilisation has been shown to be safe, feasible and effective in the early stage of ICU admission (Bailey *et al.*, 2007; Morris *et al.*, 2008; Schweickert *et al.*, 2009; Truong *et al.*, 2009; Stiller, 2013). Benefits of early rehabilitation include reducing hospital and ICU length of stay, increasing ventilator free days, improving muscle strength and health-related quality of life (QOL) (Kayambu *et al.*, 2013; Stiller, 2013).

Mobilising any patient in the ICU requires a team approach in order to ensure safe and effective graded mobilisation (Dammeyer *et al.*, 2013; Kocan and Lietz, 2013). Note that this area has not been well studied in the paediatric population.

4.1.2. *Exercise therapy*

Exercise therapy is associated with a multitude of beneficial effects on mental and physical health.

4.1.2.1. *Mental health benefits*

Plato stated in the fourth century BC that God provided man with two means in order to lead a successful life: namely education and physical activity. One is for the soul and the other for the body and they are meant to be used together for man to attain perfection (Ströhle, 2009). Physical activity has been shown to have beneficial effects on mood and anxiety levels, life satisfaction, feelings of well-being and cognitive functioning (ACSM, 2014), whereas physical inactivity may be associated with the development of mental disorders such as depression and anxiety (Ströhle, 2009).

4.1.2.2. *Physical health benefits*

Physical fitness involves the cardiovascular, respiratory and musculoskeletal systems. The cardiovascular and respiratory systems are conditioned through aerobic exercise, whereas the musculoskeletal system is conditioned through aerobic, resistance and flexibility exercises (Warburton *et al.*, 2006). Aerobic exercise has various beneficial effects on the cardiopulmonary system and these include decreased blood pressure, increased stroke volume with a resultant decrease in resting heart rate, increased synthesis of high-density lipoproteins and improved insulin sensitivity (ACSM, 2014). As a result of aerobic exercise, muscles develop new capillaries, which increase oxygen extraction ratio. More skeletal muscle cell mitochondria are also produced and therefore maximal oxygen uptake improves and minute ventilation decreases as physical fitness improves. As maximal oxygen uptake increases, less energy is utilised to perform activities of daily living (ADL) and as a result perceived level of QOL improves (ACSM, 2014).

Skeletal muscle mass, strength and aerobic and anaerobic capacity increase with resistance exercise (Kirstensen and Franklyn-Miller, 2012). Several factors influence muscle strength, such as neural control, muscle cross-sectional area and muscle length. Neural control includes the number of motor units that are recruited during a muscle contraction as well as the rate at which the motor units are stimulated (ACSM, 2009; Kirstensen and Franklyn-Miller, 2012). During the first few weeks of resistance training, the brain learns to extract more force from a specific amount of contractile muscle fibres. Muscle cross-sectional area determines the force with which a muscle contracts, whereas maintenance of resting muscle length is important to ensure the greatest strength being generated through that muscle, as actin and myosin are in an optimal position for cross-bridge links to form during muscle contraction (Harman, 2000; ACSM, 2009). New bone formation is stimulated through weight-bearing activities that exceed the minimal essential strain of bone and enhance the osteoblast activity that stimulates bone growth. Examples of such activities are walking, stair climbing and running (Conroy and Earle, 2000; ACSM, 2014).

Recently evidence has come to light that shows that low-level fitness is associated with increased risk of cardiovascular and non-cardiovascular disease mortality for both men and women across short- and long-term follow up periods (Vigen *et al.*, 2012). This information underscores the importance of exercise and its health benefits for all persons, but especially for those recovering from ill health.

4.1.2.3. *Exercise prescription*

Exercise prescription for patients with traumatic injury should follow the same principles as that used for healthy individuals — namely frequency, intensity, time and type (ACSM, 2014) — together with consideration for progression of exercise therapy. Components of a single exercise session are:

- warm up;
- conditioning (aerobic and resistance exercises);
- cool down; and
- stretching and flexibility exercises.

No guidelines for exercise prescription for patients in the acute or sub-acute phases after traumatic injury have been identified in the literature. The recommendations provided in Table 4.2 are based on exercise prescription guidelines for deconditioned adult patients with critical illness or

Table 4.2: Recommendations for exercise prescription in the acute and sub-acute phases after traumatic injury.

Principles of exercise prescription	Recommendations
Frequency	Start with once per day; progress to twice daily or more frequently as indicated
Intensity	Aerobic exercise: • 40–70% of HR_{max}* • 11–13 on Borg rating of perceived exertion scale Resistance exercise: • Low load starting with 45–50% of one repetition maximum (RM); progress to 50–70% of one RM • Repetitions and volume: start with one set of 8–12 repetitions; progress to three sets of 8–12 repetitions before the load is increased • Rest periods: 1–2 minutes between exercise
Type	Aerobic exercise: • Bedside cycle ergometer • Walking, step climbing, stationary bicycle, treadmill walking or running Resistance exercise: • Body weight, free weights, resistance bands, weight machines • Concentric, eccentric and isometric exercises of the trunk, upper and lower limbs • Uni- and bilateral limb exercises • Single- and multiple-joint exercises
Time	Aerobic exercise: • Start with 5–10 minutes; progress to 20 minutes

*Target HR = HR_{max} × % intensity desired; HR_{max} = 220 – age (ACSM, 2014). Patients on cardiac medication such as beta-blockers will present with a blunted HR response to exercise. Clinicians calculate target HR for such patients using the equation (HR_{max} – 50) × % intensity.

untrained individuals (ACSM, 2009; Hanekom *et al.*, 2011; Kirstensen and Franklyn-Miller, 2012; ACSM, 2014).

The study by Berney *et al.* (2012) demonstrated a unique approach to the rehabilitation of survivors of critical illness from ICU admission through to exercise provided for these patients in an outpatient setting. Patients with central nervous system involvement or unstable fractures were excluded from this study. The exercise prescription format that these researchers used with their patients in the ICU and ward setting is summarised in Table 4.3. The progression of aerobic exercise and resistance training was done according to each patient's re-assessment findings (Berney *et al.*, 2012).

Table 4.3: Exercise prescription format for survivors of critical illness in the ICU and ward settings (Berney *et al.*, 2012).

	ICU	Ward environment
Duration of exercise (aerobic, resistance training, functional retraining)	15 minutes to complete: • March on the spot* OR • March on the spot and strength OR • March on the spot and strength and functional retraining OR • Whole body bed exercises	10–15 minutes
Frequency of exercise	Two 15-minute sessions per day; progressed to one 30-minute session per day	Two 30-minute sessions per day; progressed to one 60-minute session per day
Intensity of exercise		
• Aerobic exercise	• Target rate of perceived exertion (RPE) using modified Borg scale 3–5 (moderate to severe exertion)	• Interval training for endurance RPE 4–5 or 60–70% HR_{max}; after two weeks RPE increased to 5–6
• Resistance training	• Until fatigue ○ Started with five repetitions each limb; progressed to three sets of 10 repetitions each limb	• 75% of five RM ○ 1–2 sets of 12–15 repetitions each limb

(*Continued*)

Table 4.3: *(Continued)*

	ICU	Ward environment
Type of exercise		
• Aerobic exercise	• Marching on the spot; progressed to walking away from bedside	• Walking on ward or on treadmill; progressed to stationary bicycle
• Resistance training	• Active to resisted for those with > Grade 3 muscle strength; active-assisted to active for those with < Grade 3 strength	• Resisted limb, pelvis and trunk exercises using own body weight, dumbbells or resistance bands
• Functional retraining	• Sit-to-stand, rolling, supine to sitting, trunk control or balance	• Same activities as in ICU and progressed to stair climbing

*March on spot = three repetitions of 70% of initial physical function in ICU test (PFIT) duration.

The information summarised in Table 4.3 serves as a guide for exercise prescription in the acute care setting and should be modified according to each patient's ability and type of traumatic injury.

No published exercise prescription guidelines for in-hospital rehabilitation could be found for children or adolescents recovering from traumatic injuries or critical illness. In the absence of formal guidelines, clinicians use safe and appropriate fun activities, such as kicking a light ball while sitting in a chair, reaching up to pop bubbles or playing 'Simon Says' in bed or in a chair while carefully monitoring the child's response to these activities. Progression of the duration and intensity of these exercises is performed when appropriate.

We hope that the guidelines shared in this section will provide physiotherapists with a framework within which to tailor exercise prescription in the acute care setting for individual adult and paediatric patients with traumatic injuries based on their pre-injury health status, level of physical fitness and physical ability. The physiotherapist is a member of the interprofessional team that cares for patients with traumatic injury in the acute care setting; therefore decision making regarding the progression of exercise therapy should be done jointly with the team.

Quality of life, exercise therapy and rehabilitation of trauma survivors in the chronic stage following injury (after discharge from hospital) are discussed in Chapter 10.

4.2. Cardiopulmonary Physiotherapy Techniques

A patient who suffered traumatic injury may undergo prolonged periods of immobility due to the severity of injuries sustained, which places them at increased risk for the development of pulmonary complications. Chest physiotherapy, in the form of breathing and exercises, for postoperative and trauma patients was first described in the early 1900s (MacMahon, 1915). Today the term 'chest physiotherapy' or 'respiratory physiotherapy' refers to a large variety of techniques used by cardiopulmonary physiotherapists to prevent the onset of pulmonary complications or manage existing pulmonary complications that have developed in the patients under their care. Despite the widespread use of chest physiotherapy in clinical practice, research evidence to its use remains inconclusive (Stiller, 2013).

Physiotherapists often use multiple techniques in a single treatment session. In the management of critically ill patients it is recommended that routine multimodality chest physiotherapy is no longer appropriate and treatment should be patient-centred and planned based upon careful, thorough clinical and radiographical individual patient assessment and a favourable risk–benefit ratio (Woodward and Jones, 2002; Stiller, 2013). The same approach to patient care for those with traumatic injury is therefore recommended. The frequency of chest physiotherapy treatment should be determined by the needs of each individual patient. Appropriate administration of analgesia is essential to ensure adequate lung ventilation and secretion clearance (Ridley and Heinl-Green, 2002). The precise role of the physiotherapist in managing patients with traumatic injuries is likely to differ among different settings, according to the country, local tradition, staffing levels, training and levels of expertise available.

4.2.1. *Breathing exercises*

In the early 1900s, MacMahon (1915) described using upper extremity exercise, lateral costal expansion exercises and localised thoracic expansion techniques in an attempt to re-expand areas of atelectasis. These techniques are used to this day, in addition to other types of breathing exercises, particularly in non-ventilated patients and those able to obey commands and cooperate voluntarily.

4.2.1.1. *Localised thoracic expansion exercises*

4.2.1.1.1. How to perform the technique

This technique can be performed in adults and children, with the patient positioned either lying or sitting. The therapist's hands are placed over the area of decreased thoracic expansion, providing tactile stimulus, end-expiratory stretch and resistance to the inspiratory muscles (Kigin, 1981). If the patient is alert, verbal commands and encouragement to inhale deeply should be given to ensure optimal thoracic expansion is achieved in the specific area. There is still a lack of standardisation in the technique of performing this type of breathing exercise.

4.2.1.1.2. Contraindications and precautions

- End-expiratory stretch should not be used over the thorax in the presence of rib fractures.
- Pain due to surgical incisions that involve the abdomen or thorax and around insertion sites of intercostal drains will require adaptation of the intensity of an end-expiratory stretch.

4.2.1.2. *Active cycle of breathing technique*

The active cycle of breathing technique (ACBT) is a combination of breathing techniques that were developed for patients with chronic lung diseases such as cystic fibrosis, but have since been adopted by many physiotherapists for patients with a wide range of conditions resulting in secretion retention and lung volume loss. It can be used in children (from as young as three years old) able to understand and follow commands, as well as cognitively intact adults.

The ACBT consists of a cycle of breathing control (diaphragmatic breathing) and thoracic expansion exercises (deep lateral basal breaths), with or without inspiratory holds or inspiratory sniffs, followed by one or two forced expiratory techniques (FET), also known as 'huffs'; FET should always be followed by breathing control to prevent airway or alveolar collapse due to the forced expiration (Lewis *et al.*, 2012) (see Fig. 4.1).

The sequence in which these components are performed may vary in order and number, but all the components must be used during a treatment session (Lewis *et al.*, 2012). The sequence is determined by the needs of each patient, as more emphasis might be placed on thoracic expansion exercises (TEE) in the case of lung volume loss, with less focus on FET.

4.2.1.2.1. How to perform the technique

The patient can perform ACBT in any comfortable position. The effectiveness with which a patient performs ACBT is dependent on the quality of instruction received from the physiotherapist. Table 4.4 summarises the instructions that may be given to patients when performing each component

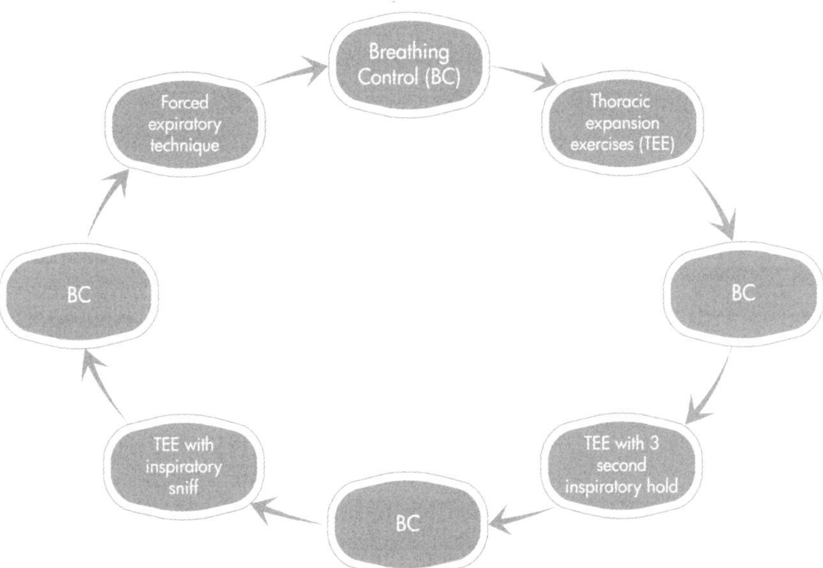

Fig. 4.1: An example of the active cycle of breathing technique. The sequence can be adjusted to place emphasis on a particular component according to the needs of each patient.

Table 4.4: Instructions related to each component of ACBT.

Component	Instructions to the patient
Breathing control	• Breathing control is performed during relaxed normal (tidal volume) breathing. The patient is instructed to place two fingers directly below the breast bone (xiphisternum) and to feel the diaphragm rise and fall during relaxed breathing. Breathing control is the 'recovery phase' of ACBT.
Thoracic expansion exercises:	
• Basic TEE	• Thoracic expansion exercises are performed during the inspiratory phase of deep breathing. The physiotherapist's or patient's hands should be placed over the bottom part of the ribcage on the sides of the chest wall (lateral basal lung segments). The patient is instructed to 'breathe into the hands' during deep inspiration.
• TEE with three-second inspiratory hold	• The same technique is used as described for basic TEE. The patient is instructed to 'hold' the inspiratory breath for three seconds before exhaling. The breath hold aims to improve airflow distribution through the collateral ventilation pathways at bronchiole-alveolar level.
• TEE with inspiratory sniff	• The same technique is used as described for basic TEE. The patient is instructed to breathe in as deeply as possible and then to 'hold' the breath. Immediately after the 'hold' the patient is instructed to sniff in an additional breath through the nose and to then only exhale.
Forced expiratory techniques:	
• Long FET (low volume FET)	• The patient relaxes their arms by the side of the body and is instructed to perform one or two long huffs. This should be done with an open glottis. Huffing is similar to the method used for misting up a mirror or a pair of reading glasses to clean them. Long FET aims to recruit secretions from the periphery of the lungs and move them more centrally for evacuation from the airways.
• Short FET (high volume FET)	• The same technique is used as described for long FET; however, the patient is instructed to perform one or two short, sharp huffs at high lung volume with an open glottis. Short FET assists with evacuating secretions from the central airways.

of ACBT. The physiotherapist should ensure that the patient maintains a steady respiratory rate while performing breathing control (BC) and TEE. The physiotherapist should use their voice to encourage the patient, especially during the TEE and FET components of ACBT.

The number of repetitions of ACBT in one treatment session is determined by the patient's response to the technique; in other words whether the desired results had been obtained. As the patient masters the technique under the guidance and supervision of the physiotherapist, the patient should be encouraged to continue with ACBT unsupervised on a daily basis until the underlying pathology is resolved. The physiotherapist should regularly review the patient's technique and changes in their condition in order to provide adequate instruction for progression of treatment.

4.2.1.2.2. Contraindications and precautions

- There are no contraindications or precautions to using ACBT on awake and cooperative patients with traumatic injury.
- It is important to instruct the patient to breathe away from the physiotherapist's face while performing ACBT for infection control purposes.
- It is important to note that in the presence of pain, general weakness and dyspnoea, these exercises may only be effective if the patient sits with back support (chair or semi-Fowlers position in bed).

Active cycle of breathing technique has been found to be comparable to other airway clearance techniques (conventional chest physiotherapy and oscillatory expiratory pressure devices) for short-term improvements in secretion clearance (Lewis *et al.*, 2012). Forced expiratory technique, specifically, may be a useful technique to clear secretions in patients following thoracic or abdominal injury, where coughing may be extremely painful.

4.2.1.3. *Breath-stacking*

Breath-stacking was described in the late 1980s by Marini and colleagues (1986) as an alternative method to facilitate deep breathing and increase vital capacity, hence cough effectiveness, in uncooperative patients. This breathing technique has gained popularity over the years and is used in many hospitals by cardiopulmonary physiotherapists as part of patient care.

4.2.1.3.1. How to perform the technique

The patient should be placed in a comfortable position. A silicon mask with a one-way valve is placed over the patient's face. The valve should be set to allow only inspiration (the expiration branch should be closed) and the patient should be encouraged to perform successive inspiratory efforts over a 20-second period; the result being stacking of breaths on top of each other to increase lung volumes. After the 20-second period the exhalation branch is opened to allow the patient to exhale freely (Dias *et al.*, 2008).

4.2.1.3.2. Contraindications and precautions

No adverse effects have been reported in the literature as a result of the use of breath-stacking.

The effectiveness of breath-stacking compared to incentive spirometry in the physiotherapy management of patients after upper abdominal surgery was investigated by Dias and colleagues. These authors reported the superiority of breath-stacking over incentive spirometry in relation to inspired lung volume in the postoperative period, with more pronounced lung volume reductions in patients who were treated with incentive spirometry (Dias *et al.*, 2008).

4.2.1.4. *Glossopharyngeal breathing*

This is a useful breathing technique for patients following spinal cord injury with paralysis or weakness of the respiratory muscles. The inability to take a deep inspiration is one of the fundamental components of a cough, which is missing in tetraplegic patients. Glossopharyngeal breathing can also be used to maintain or improve lung and chest wall compliance (Pryor *et al.*, 2008).

4.2.1.4.1. How to perform the technique

This technique involves 'gulping' air into the lungs, either voluntarily or with the use of a self-inflating bag with a valve or mask. To perform this technique, the patient is taught to open the mouth and allow air to flow into the oral and pharyngeal cavities. When the mouth is closed, the small volumes of air are propelled into the lower airways through an open glottis (raised during the manoeuvre) using the muscles of the tongue and pharynx. By closing the glottis, the air is trapped inside the lungs while the patient prepares to take the next breath (Maltais, 2011). Glossopharyngeal breathing is therefore a breathing sequence in which the larynx is used as a valve to prevent air escaping from the chest as the mouth is opened for the next 'gulp' or insufflation. The patient should feel their chest filling with air until maximum vital capacity, which may involve taking up to 25 sequential breaths, after which the air is allowed to suddenly escape (similar to FET) (Maltais, 2011). Exsufflation can be enhanced with a manually assisted cough. Glossopharyngeal breathing is taught to patients with spinal cord injury in a reclined position initially (due to postural hypotension) and gradually progressed to the patient breathing in an upright seated position. This technique is not appropriate in the acute phase after traumatic injury or in the presence of an acute chest infection (Pryor *et al.*, 2008), and is only possible in patients with good cognitive function and a normal level of consciousness. This technique can be taught to older children with respiratory muscle paresis or paralysis.

4.2.1.4.2. Contraindications and precautions

- Glossopharyngeal breathing is contraindicated in patients with chronic obstructive pulmonary disease, as the positive pressure could exacerbate air trapping in the lungs (Pryor *et al.*, 2008).
- A fall in blood pressure can occur due to the build-up of intrathoracic pressure and therefore the technique is contraindicated in patients with cardiovascular instability or cardiac dysfunction (Pryor *et al.*, 2008).
- Training sessions should be kept short initially, as learning the technique can be tiring.

4.2.1.5. *Respiratory muscle training*

Respiratory muscle training (RMT) may be useful where there is the potential to strengthen the inspiratory or expiratory respiratory muscles, which might have become weak due to direct or indirect injury and/or prolonged mechanical ventilation. Training of the inspiratory muscles of patients who undergo prolonged mechanical ventilation is effective in reducing the duration of ventilation (Cader *et al.*, 2010). Inspiratory muscle training can be achieved through the adjustment of trigger sensitivity or pressure support settings on the mechanical ventilator or with the use of a spring-loaded resistance device (Caruso *et al.*, 2005; Cader *et al.*, 2010; Martin *et al.*, 2011). A variety of suppliers make inspiratory and expiratory muscle-trainer (IMT/EMT) devices for use in the clinical setting, such as the Threshold® IMT or EMT devices (supplied by Respironics) and POWERbreathe®. These threshold devices are made of plastic, spring-loaded and calibrated (Fig. 4.2). The spring applies resist-

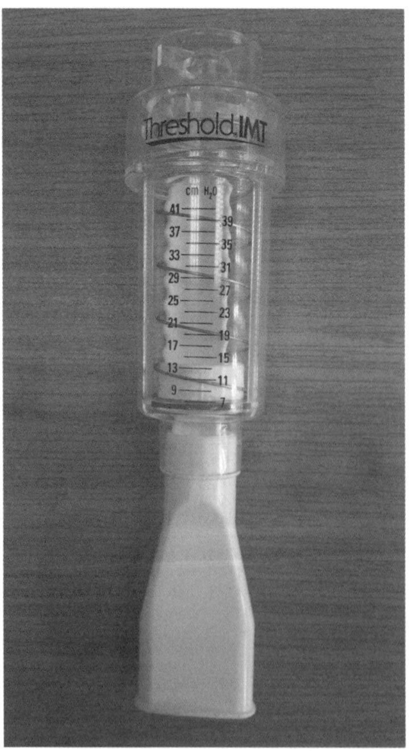

Fig 4.2: Threshold® IMT device.

ance to either inspiratory or expiratory breaths. In some countries electronic respiratory muscle training devices may be available.

4.2.1.5.1. How to perform the technique

4.2.1.5.1.1. *Spring-loaded device.* The patient should be placed in a supported 45° seated position in bed or upright in a chair. To establish baseline inspiratory muscle strength, three measurements of the patient's maximal inspiratory pressure (MIP) should be made using a pressure manometer. The three readings should not vary by more than 20% and the best of the three readings is recorded (ATS/ERS, 2002). The device is attached directly to the endotracheal or tracheostomy tube using a T-piece A-connector. Oxygen therapy can be supplied at the same time through an additional connector attached to the trainer device, if indicated. The patient would need to be able to breathe without support from the ventilator for a few minutes in order to be trained with this device. Spontaneously breathing patients can use this device with a mouthpiece. There are no uniform recommendations in the rehabilitation literature for training with spring-loaded IMT devices. Examples of strategies used by various researchers are summarised in Table 4.5.

Table 4.5: Examples of IMT strategies using spring-loaded devices in patients who are intubated and ventilated*.

Percentage of maximal inspiratory pressure		Highest pressure tolerated
Cader *et al.* (2010)	Condessa *et al.* (2013)	Martin *et al.* (2011)
• Set the spring in the IMT device to 30% of the patient's MIP • The patient breathes through the device for five minutes twice daily • Inspiratory resistance is increased by 10% of baseline MIP daily as tolerated	• Set the resistance in the device to 40% of MIP • The patient performs five sets of 10 breaths, twice daily, for seven days per week	• Set the resistance in the device to the highest pressure level that the patient can tolerate • The patient performs four sets of six to 10 breaths five days per week

*The majority of subjects in all three studies had medical or surgical admission diagnoses.

The optimal dosage of training has not yet been established.

4.2.1.5.1.2. *Adjustment of trigger sensitivity setting on a mechanical ventilator.* This method of IMT was described by Caruso *et al.* (2005). They set the ventilator trigger sensitivity to 20% of baseline MIP and allowed the patients to breathe at this level for five minutes twice daily. The duration of training was increased by five minutes each session until a training duration of 30 minutes was achieved. Resistance was gradually increased by 10% of baseline MIP to a maximum of 40% of baseline MIP. The authors stated that a modest improvement in MIP was observed but duration of weaning from mechanical ventilation was not influenced. A number of their subjects had decreased levels of consciousness. One can argue that if patients are awake and cooperative and able to perform TEE while intubated, during periods of trigger sensitivity adjustment greater improvements in MIP might be observed. Another limitation of this study is that they used the very low resistance of 10–40%. For muscle force to build, resistance levels of 40–60% should be used. Physiotherapists should discuss the temporary adjustment of ventilator settings for respiratory muscle training purposes with the medical or surgical team looking after the patient to ensure the team members understand the purpose of the intervention and support it.

4.2.1.5.1.3. *Adjustment of pressure support setting on a mechanical ventilator.* Another method of IMT used by physiotherapy clinicians is the temporary adjustment of pressure support while the patient performs deep breathing, observing the ventilator screen and attempting to increase the inspiratory tidal volume values with each deep breath (ventilator biofeedback). Pressure support provides inspiratory assistance to the patient during the inspiratory phase of breathing and in so doing unloads the inspiratory muscles. Therefore, the reduction of pressure support imposes resistance to inspiration and greater inspiratory muscle activity. Pressure support may be reduced with 2–3 cm H_2O in a treatment session while the patient performs deep breathing with ventilator biofeedback. The patient should be closely observed for signs of fatigue. Care must be taken to reset the pressure support to the pre-treatment level at the end of each treatment session. Research evidence to support the effectiveness of this type of IMT could not be found. Again, this type of intervention needs to be discussed with the medical or surgical team looking after the patient, as explained above.

4.2.1.5.2. Contraindications and precautions

- A precaution to RMT is that the intubated patient should not be pushed to the point of respiratory muscle exhaustion during training. This delays the process of weaning from mechanical ventilation.
- Patients should always be pre-oxygenated prior to performing each set of IMT repetitions.

A systematic review and meta-analysis of 11 studies of RMT in 212 participants with cervical spine injury concluded that RMT did appear to be effective for increasing respiratory muscle strength and possibly lung volumes for this population group (Berlowitz and Tamplin, 2013). There were insufficient data to report on the effect of RMT on functional outcomes like dyspnoea, cough efficacy, respiratory complications, hospital admissions and health-related QOL.

There are currently no studies of RMT in the paediatric post-surgical, ICU or trauma populations.

4.2.2. *Devices*

4.2.2.1. *Incentive spirometry*

Incentive spirometry is a method used to encourage deep breathing and mimic a sigh, and is used in postoperative patients (Branson, 2013). Incentive spirometry provides visual feedback in terms of volume attained during a deep breath and might therefore be a useful adjunct to deep breathing exercises (Agostini and Singh, 2009). Flow- and volume-oriented spirometers are available, including spirometers designed specifically with children in mind. Volume spirometers require less effort and lead to more laminar airflow, while flow spirometers can be difficult for the older and weaker patients, as greater muscle work is required to lift up the first ball. This also leads to a turbulent flow which does not penetrate as deeply into the airways as laminar flow.

4.2.2.1.1. How to perform the technique

The patient should be in a supported high-sitting position in bed or seated in an upright position in a chair while holding the incentive spirometer parallel with the floor. Shoulder girdle relaxation exercises should be performed prior to initiating incentive spirometry. The physiotherapist should place their hands on the lateral basal aspects of the patient's thoracic cage (Fig. 4.3) and instruct the patient to take in a long, slow breath while attempting to lift the ball or balls in the chamber of the spirometer. During deep inspiration the patient must attempt to breathe into the physiotherapist's hands in order to facilitate expansion of the basal lung segments. The physiotherapist must ensure that the patient achieves expansion in the basal lung regions without elevation of the shoulder girdle (Fig. 4.4). If the patient manages to perform the technique correctly, with adequate basal lung segment expansion, the volume of the incentive spirometer should be adjusted accordingly, starting at the lowest and progressing to the highest volume.

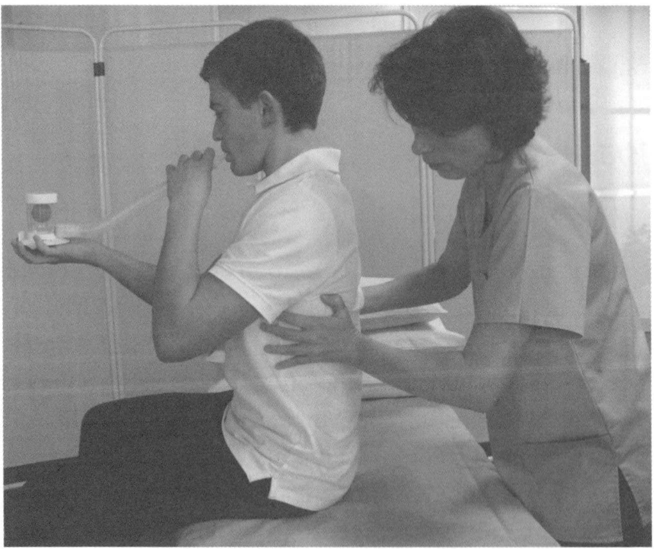

Fig. 4.3: Lateral basal lung segment expansion combined with slow, deep inspiration through the incentive spirometer.

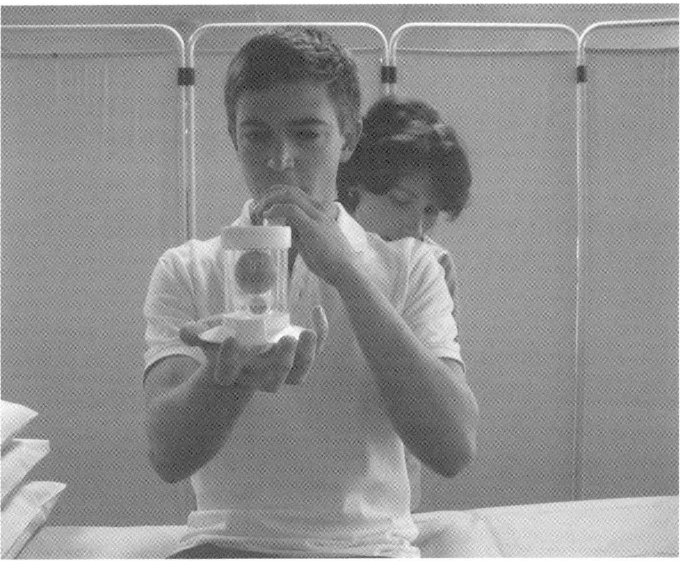

Fig. 4.4: Shoulder girdle relaxation is encouraged while performing deep inspiration with lateral basal lung segment expansion using the incentive spirometer.

As the patient masters the technique under the guidance and supervision of the physiotherapist, they should be encouraged to continue using incentive spirometry on an hourly basis during the day. The physiotherapist should regularly review the patient's technique and changes in their condition in order to provide adequate instruction for the progression of treatment until the desired lung volumes are achieved.

4.2.2.1.2. Contraindications and precautions

- There are no contraindications or precautions to the use of incentive spirometry in awake, cooperative and spontaneously breathing patients with traumatic injury.
- The physiotherapist should stand to the side of or behind the patient during treatment for infection control purposes to prevent the patient from coughing over them.
- Extremely weak trauma patients might become discouraged if they cannot master incentive spirometry due to their weakness. In such cases alternative methods should be considered.

There is currently no high-level evidence for the use of incentive spirometry as stand-alone therapy in patient care (Agostini and Singh, 2009; Branson, 2013). Therefore it is advisable to use incentive spirometry in combination with other physiotherapy treatment modalities.

4.2.2.2. *Intermittent positive pressure breathing*

Intermittent positive pressure breathing (IPPB) refers to the delivery of patient-triggered positive airway pressure throughout inspiration, with airway pressure returning to atmospheric levels during expiration. It is used in the management of spontaneously breathing patients and performed using a positive pressure device such as the Bird Mark 7 or Mark 8 ventilator (Pryor *et al.*, 2008). Patients who suffer from increased work of breathing due to respiratory muscle fatigue or weakness as well as those who breathe at low lung volumes due to postoperative pain find relief of symptoms when using IPPB. By augmenting tidal volume and reducing the work of breathing, IPPB may enhance secretion clearance and re-expand collapsed areas of the lung. Work of breathing is, however, only reduced if the patient relaxes completely and does not 'assist' the machine (Pryor *et al.*, 2008).

4.2.2.2.1. How to perform the technique

The patient is placed in a relaxed supported sitting or side lying position as indicated. A gravity-assisted position may also be used if the patient is not too breathless. The IPPB machine is connected to the oxygen outlet on the wall of the hospital ward or ICU. The breathing circuit is attached to the Bird ventilator and a mouth piece or tight-fitting face mask may be attached to the patient side of the circuit. The IPPB machine delivers dry oxygen to the patient and therefore humidification of the airways is important. Ensure the nebuliser in the circuit is filled with four ml of saline or a mucolytic or bronchodilator drug, if indicated. Auscultate the patient's chest to identify areas of decreased breath sounds.

Some physiotherapists may find using the IPPB machine a daunting task due to all the dials on the machine (Figs 4.5A and B); however, with practice, the use of IPPB becomes second nature.

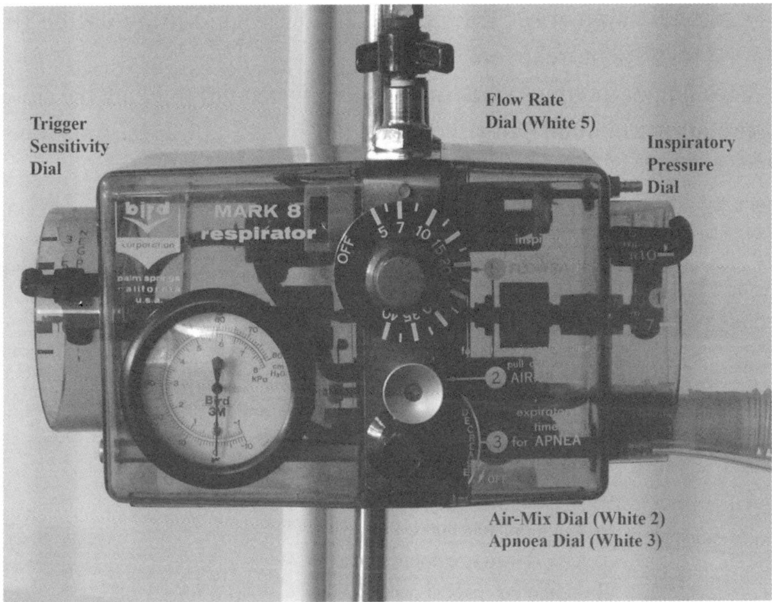

Fig. 4.5A: Front panel display of the Bird Mark 8 IPPB machine.

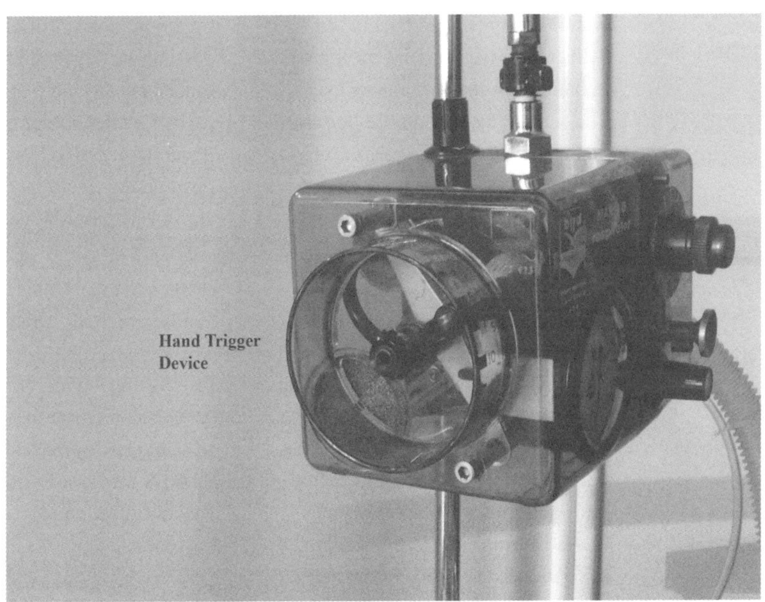

Fig. 4.5B: Hand-triggering device on the side of the Bird Mark 8 IPPB machine.

Table 4.6 summarises the steps to follow when setting up the IPPB machine for patient treatment.

Throughout treatment the patient is instructed not to block the flow of air through the circuit with their tongue, but to allow the machine to

Table 4.6: General steps to follow in setting up an IPPB machine for patient treatment and guidance for progression of management.

Dials on IPPB machine	Initial settings	Progression of settings
Air mix control	The control should be pulled outwards to its fullest length to ensure that a mixture of approximately 45% oxygen is delivered to the patient. If the air mix control is pushed back to its shortest length, it delivers approximately 100% oxygen, which is inappropriate for physiotherapy patient care.	Air mix control remains unchanged at 45% oxygen.
Sensitivity or 'trigger'	The patient needs to generate a negative flow (sucking pressure) with minimal effort through the circuit to trigger the machine to deliver positive pressure during the remainder of the inspiratory cycle. The sensitivity dial should be set to a low value (usually –5 to –7 cmH_2O) and should be adjusted for each individual patient.	If strengthening of the respiratory muscles becomes an aim of treatment, the sensitivity dial can be adjusted to a higher number so that the patient works harder to generate negative flow through the circuit at the start of inspiration.
Flow rate	This dial regulates the rate of flow of inspiratory gas into the patient's airways. The lower the flow rate, the deeper the gas penetrates down the tracheobronchial tree; therefore the patient takes a long slow breath. The breathless patient may initially not manage to breathe at low flow rates and thus a higher flow rate (15–20 L/min) is chosen to match the patient's own respiratory rate.	As the patient settles on the IPPB machine, flow rate can be gradually adjusted to a lower setting (5–7 L/min) to allow for longer inspiration in order to re-expand collapsed airways and assist with the mobilisation of secretions.

(*Continued*)

Table 4.6: *(Continued)*

Dials on IPPB machine	Initial settings	Progression of settings
Inspiratory pressure	The Bird ventilator delivers a range of positive pressure from 0 cmH_2O to 40 cmH_2O. An inspiratory-positive pressure of 10 cmH_2O is initially selected for treatment. The pressure gauge on the front of the IPPB machine indicates whether the desired pressure is being delivered to the patient. After the patient has breathed at this level of pressure for a few minutes, re-auscultate the chest to assess if airflow has increased in areas of the lungs that initially presented with decreased breath sounds.	If the changes in breath sounds are minimal, increase the inspiratory pressure gradually by 2–3 cmH_2O until a level of pressure is reached that results in improved breath sounds.
Hand-triggering device	This device should be used to test that there are no leaks in the circuit before patient treatment is initiated. It is also used to stop the device from cycling at any time during treatment, if indicated.	Not applicable.
Apnoea dial	Must be switched off, as during physiotherapy treatment the IPPB machine is not used as a ventilator.	
Expiratory time dial	Must be switched off, as during physiotherapy treatment the IPPB machine is not used as a ventilator.	

inflate their lungs. On expiration the machine stops cycling to allow the patient to exhale fully. The duration of treatment is dependent on the time taken to deliver the medication in the nebuliser to the patient. Intermittent positive pressure breathing can be combined with expiratory chest wall vibrations and gravity-assisted or modified gravity-assisted positioning to further enhance expiratory flow and improve the clearance of retained secretions.

4.2.2.2.2. Contraindications and precautions

- Undrained pneumo- or haemothorax (Pryor *et al*., 2008).
- Active tuberculosis as it may contaminate the equipment.
- Large bullae in patients with chronic obstructive pulmonary disease, as positive pressure may lead to rupture of the bullae and result in a pneumothorax (Pryor *et al*., 2008).
- Lung abscesses, as positive pressure may lead to an increase in the size of the abscess (Pryor *et al*., 2008).
- Haemoptysis or pulmonary haemorrhage until the bleeding has stopped. Always discuss with the medical team under these conditions.
- Presence of a bronchial tumour in the proximal airways (Pryor *et al*., 2008). On inspiration, air may flow around the tumour into the airways due to the natural expansion of the diameter of the airways by contraction of the elastin and collagen fibres attached to the outside of the airways. Flow of air out of the airways may be prohibited by the tumour during expiration as airway diameter reduces (relaxation of elastin and collagen fibres) and there is risk of the development of a 'ball valve' effect and air trapping.
- Before use in patients who had recent thoracic surgery, discuss the appropriateness of IPPB therapy with the surgical team.
- Reduction in cardiac output may result from IPPB due to the increased intrathoracic pressures and therefore IPPB should be used with care in haemodynamically unstable patients.
- Intermittent positive pressure breathing is not indicated for the treatment of young children due to the potential danger of pneumothorax. There are insufficient safety studies to support using this technique in this vulnerable population. If the physiotherapist deems treatment with IPPB to be necessary, it should only be used in older, cooperative children and maximal inspiratory pressures should be kept lower than or equal to 30 cmH_2O.

There is currently little research evidence for the use of IPPB in patients with traumatic injuries, although it remains a frequently used adjunct to physiotherapy treatment in some clinical settings.

4.2.2.3. *Mechanical insufflation-exsufflation*

Mechanical insufflation-exsufflation is the delivery of positive and negative pressure to a patient's airways through an insufflator-exsufflator machine (CoughAssist In-exsufflator® or Nippy Clearway®) in order to augment a weak or absent cough. Positive pressure is delivered to the airways during inspiration to augment lung volumes and the sudden switch to negative pressure initiates expiration and augments peak cough expiratory flow (Pryor *et al.*, 2008; Morrow *et al.*, 2013).

4.2.2.3.1. How to perform the technique

The patient should be seated in a comfortable position. Non-invasive patient administration of mechanical insufflation-exsufflation can be achieved using a tight-fitting face mask or mouth piece; alternatively, the machine may be attached to an artificial airway such as an endotracheal or tracheostomy tube. The delivery of mechanical insufflation-exsufflation through a face mask or mouth piece involves the patient's active participation to augment their weak, ineffective cough through partially closing the glottis. If glottis control is totally absent in a spontaneously breathing patient, therapy with this device will be ineffective (Toussaint, 2011). The delivery of mechanical insufflation-exsufflation through an artificial airway is effective even in the absence of a patient's spontaneous cough or glottis control (Toussaint, 2011). It should be noted that laboratory data suggests that the inner diameter of the artificial airway reduces peak expiratory flow during mechanical insufflation-exsufflation therapy and therefore cough effectiveness; the narrower the diameter, the lower the peak flow for a given expiratory pressure (Guérin *et al.*, 2011). These findings remain to be verified in *in vivo* studies.

It is recommended that inspiratory positive pressure be set at 15–20 cmH_2O or at a level that is comfortable for the patient during the initial treatment session (Pryor *et al.*, 2008; Bott *et al.*, 2009), and that the negative expiratory pressure should be set at the same value. Treatment progression, if suitable for the individual patient, involves a gradual increase in positive pressure level to achieve a negative pressure level that is 10–20 cmH_2O higher than the positive pressure level (Pryor *et al.*, 2008).

Treatment pressures as high as +40 cm H_2O and −40 to −45 cmH_2O have been reported in all age groups. Some clinicians measure the patient's MIP and then calibrate the inspiratory and expiratory pressure settings as a percentage of MIP instead of using pre-determined set pressures as mentioned above; however, evidence to support this method of calibration could not be sourced.

Ventilator-induced lung injury is a well-known topic of discussion in critical care literature. The use of low inspiratory tidal volumes, maintenance of positive end-expiratory pressure (PEEP) and of wide-pressure swings are recommended to protect the lungs from injury (Carpenter, 2004; Fuller *et al.*, 2013; Park *et al.*, 2013). The high pressures delivered during mechanical insufflation-exsufflation, therefore, raise concern about the long-term effects that this therapy might have on lung mechanics and patient outcomes (Morrow *et al.*, 2013). Lower comfortable pressures may be more beneficial and safer, particularly in the paediatric population.

Patients with spinal cord injury, neuromuscular disease or thoracic cage deformity probably derive the greatest benefits from mechanical insufflation-exsufflation in relation to improved peak cough expiratory flow and maintenance of lung volumes (Morrow *et al.*, 2013). The combination of mechanical exsufflation with manual chest shaking and vibrations and suctioning further enhances secretion clearance (Anderson *et al.*, 2005; Finder, 2010). Patients tend to prefer treatment with mechanical insufflation-exsufflation over airway suction alone, as the device assists with the mobilisation of secretions into the central airways, which are easily and effectively cleared with superficial suction instead of deep airway suction (Schmitt *et al.*, 2007; Toussaint, 2011).

4.2.2.3.2. Contraindications and precautions

- Mechanical insufflation-exsufflation should not be used in the presence of an undrained pneumothorax, haemothorax or pleural effusion, fresh haemoptysis or cardiovascular system instability.
- In addition, the physiotherapist should monitor the patient closely for the development of complications such as abdominal distension, gastro-oesophageal reflux, pneumothorax, cardiac arrhythmia and changes in

mean arterial pressure (MAP). If these complications arise, appropriate assistance should be sought from the other members of the interprofessional team (Morrow *et al.*, 2013).
- Active tuberculosis, due to contamination of the equipment.
- In children, pressures should be carefully increased from an initial low level, with observation and monitoring of clinical response, in order to prevent barotrauma. Pressures should be kept at the lowest level possible that is effective for clearing secretions.
- Do not perform mechanical insufflation-exsufflation therapy within 30 minutes of the patient's last meal.

The effects of mechanical insufflation-exsufflation on outcomes of patients in the ICU have not been studied (Gosselink *et al.*, 2011).

4.2.2.4. *Positive expiratory pressure therapy*

Positive expiratory pressure (PEP) therapy is believed to improve secretion clearance by increasing gaseous pressure behind the secretions using the collateral ventilation channels in the lung periphery or by preventing airway collapse during exhalation (McCool and Rosen, 2006). It is reasonable to assume that PEP therapy improves patient oxygenation, as FRC increases when partially collapsed peripheral airways are recruited through collateral ventilation pathways, with a resultant enlargement of the surface area available for gas exchange. Most studies of PEP therapy have been done in adults and children with chronic lung disease, particularly cystic fibrosis. Apparatus for PEP therapy includes a mask, one-way valve and expiratory resistors (PEP resistors) for continuous PEP; alternatively, bubble PEP (underwater PEP or 'blow bottles') or flutter devices for oscillating PEP. 'Fun' PEP devices and toys (e.g. windmills or bubbles), providing uncontrolled PEP levels, can also be used with children to optimise compliance.

4.2.2.4.1. How to perform the technique

The patient should be placed in a supported high-sitting position in bed or seated in an upright position in a chair when using PEP therapy.

4.2.2.4.1.1. *Continuous PEP therapy.* Expiratory airway pressure remains at a pressure level above atmospheric pressure when continuous PEP therapy is applied. The PEP mask is a popular form of application of continuous PEP. The PEP mask consists of a one-way valve onto which expiratory (outflow) resistors of various diameters (ranges: 1 mm to 5 mm) can be attached. The opposite end of the resistor is attached via tubing to a manometer, through which the generated expiratory pressure is monitored (Figs 4.6A and B).

The PEP mask is a flow resistor device, as the expiratory pressure generated through the mask is determined by expiratory airflow and the diameter of the outflow resistor (Sehlin *et al.*, 2007). The patient is instructed to seal the mask to the face and to perform a sequence of 10 breaths at a time. During each sequence of breaths the PEP mask keeps the alveoli pressurised, which adds benefit compared to methods in which positive pressure is only maintained for a few seconds during expiration (oscillatory PEP). The patient is instructed to perform two to three breathing sequences during one treatment session, with a pause period between each breathing sequence. The desired starting pressure to be generated

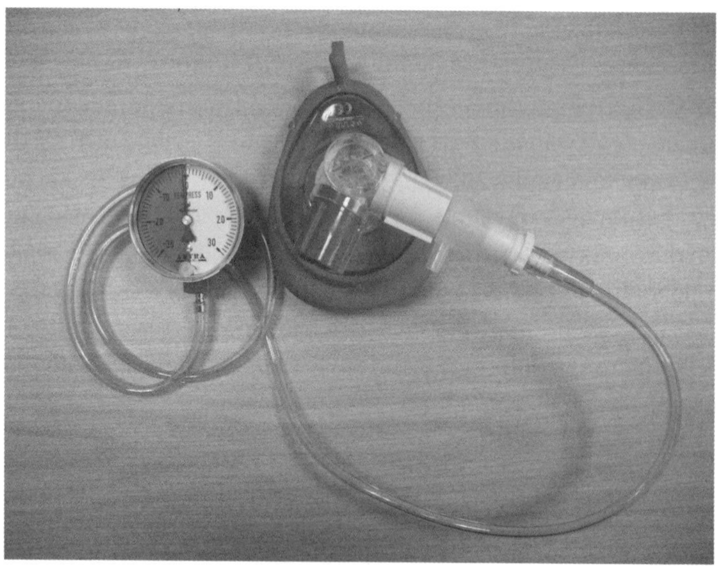

Fig. 4.6A: PEP mask with expiratory flow resistor attached to pressure manometer.

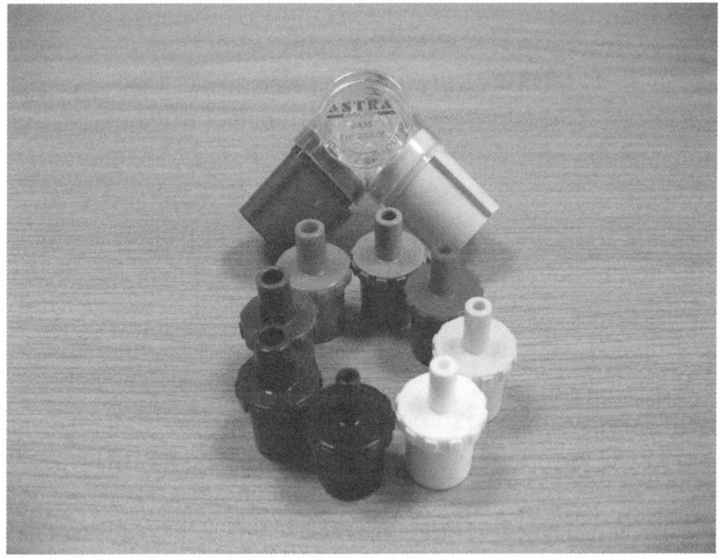

Fig. 4.6B: Flow resistors of various sizes that can be used with PEP mask therapy.

through the mask is 10 cmH_2O (Sehlin *et al.*, 2007), but individual patient assessment is important to establish whether a patient is able to achieve this pressure level during the first session; lower starting pressures may be required, especially if the patient is in pain. Progression to higher levels of PEP should be done in subsequent treatment sessions to achieve the desired patient outcome.

Continuous PEP therapy can also be administered using a spring-loaded device that applies resistance to the expiratory cycle of respiration, such as the Threshold® PEP (supplied by Respironics). The exact level of resistance can be set for each patient. The patient is instructed to perform 10 breaths per breathing cycle (similar to that described for the PEP mask), followed by a rest period before the next breathing cycle. The aim is to perform two to three breathing cycles per treatment session.

4.2.2.4.1.2. *Oscillatory PEP therapy.* At the start of expiration airway pressure is at a level above atmospheric pressure when using oscillatory PEP therapy. Towards the end of expiration, however, airway pressure returns to atmospheric pressure. Oscillatory PEP therapy can be administered using a bubble PEP bottle or a flutter device.

4.2.2.4.1.2.1. Bubble PEP bottle. A bubble PEP bottle can be made by filling a bottle (top open) partially with 10 cm of water and placing the bottom end of a 30 cm length of plastic tubing (1 cm inner diameter) 10 cm below the water surface. The inner diameter of the tube as well as the top of the bottle should be equal to or greater than 8 mm. This is to ensure that the PEP pressure is less than the water column pressure so that the recommended pressure is delivered to the patient (Mestriner *et al.*, 2009). The PEP bottle is a threshold resistor device, as total expiratory pressure is determined not only by expiratory airflow but also by air pressure generated in the airways to overcome the resistance posed by the water column in the bottle (Sehlin *et al.*, 2007). Patients may, therefore, become dyspnoeic when using the PEP bottle and should be monitored closely. The patient is instructed to perform a deep inspiration with or without an inspiratory hold, followed by an active exhalation. This is repeated 10 times and followed by a rest period. Bubbles are created in the water as the patient exhales through the plastic tubing. Exhalation only to the level of FRC is recommended, as exhalation further than FRC may lead to airway collapse as intraluminal pressures are exceeded (Westerdahl *et al.*, 2005). The patient should be instructed to perform bubble PEP breathing every waking hour during the day. Progression to higher levels of PEP may be done in subsequent treatment sessions, if indicated, to achieve the desired patient outcome. Progression is achieved by increasing the water column level in the bottle.

4.2.2.4.1.2.2. Flutter device. The flutter device was developed for the management of people with cystic fibrosis, but is now used in many other clinical scenarios. It is a small plastic pipe containing a steel ball, resting in a circular cone, which creates a valve effect when the patient blows through the device (Figs 4.7A and B). There are flutter devices on the market that have a mouth piece attached that can rotate to allow a patient to perform therapy in side-lying positions.

Exhaling through the flutter creates oscillations in the airway which serve to loosen secretions and increase the resistance to exhalation results

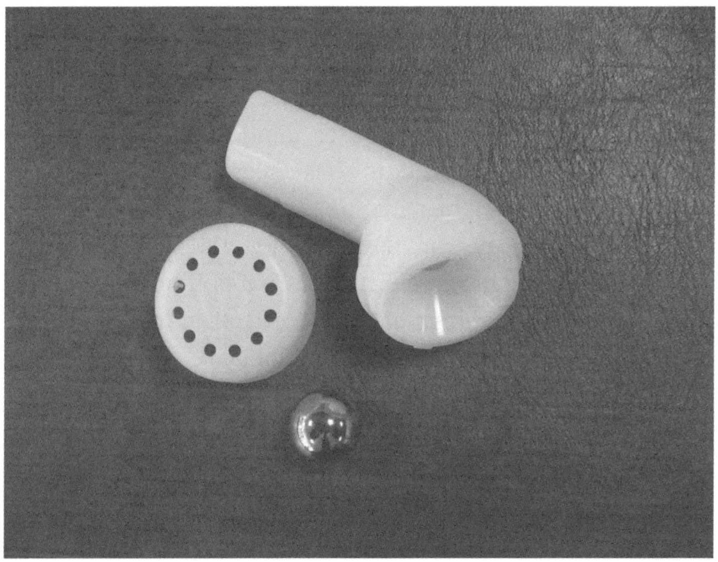

Fig. 4.7A: The flutter device is a plastic pipe-like device with an inner steel ball.

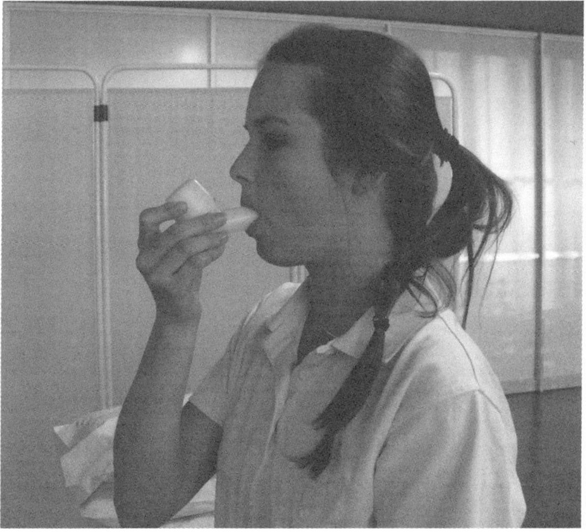

Fig. 4.7B: The flutter device should be kept in a horizontal position to the floor when performing exhalation.

in oscillatory PEP. The patient is instructed to perform four exhalation breaths through the device, starting from a slightly larger than normal inspiratory breath. These four exhalation breaths are followed by a maximal exhalation breath through the flutter, mimicking FET. The aim of the four normal exhalation breaths is to shake secretions loose from the airway walls. The maximal exhalation breath aims to evacuate the loosened secretions from the airways. In young children, the therapist may have to support their cheeks to prevent the cheeks from puffing out and absorbing the vibrations, thereby making treatment ineffective. In a single treatment session, the patient is instructed to repeat the cycle of exhalation breaths until all retained secretions are removed from the airways. The patient should be advised to use the flutter device regularly during the day to mobilise and clear retained secretions.

The Shaker® (supplied by POWERbreathe) and Acapella® (supplied by Smiths Medical) devices also deliver oscillatory PEP.

4.2.2.4.2. Contraindications and precautions

- Positive expiratory pressure therapy should not be used in the presence of an undrained pneumothorax, haemothorax or pleural effusion.
- Use of PEP in the presence of fresh haemoptysis is not advised until the cause of bleeding has been identified and managed.
- Use of PEP in the presence of cardiovascular system instability is not advised, as the added intrathoracic pressure may further impede cardiac function.
- Active tuberculosis is a contraindication for use of the PEP mask due to contamination of equipment.
- When using a bubble PEP bottle, the patient should be instructed not to drink the water from the bottle.

There is limited evidence supporting the use of PEP in acute or post-operative conditions, but it remains popular in the management of patients with chronic respiratory disease (Orman and Westerdahl, 2010). Positive expiratory pressure therapy is often used in conjunction with other breathing exercises and FET.

4.2.2.5. *Percussive ventilation*

Intrapulmonary percussive ventilation (IPV) uses high-frequency oscillatory ventilation to produce percussion-like effects in the lower airways. The percussion-like effects are produced by small bursts of gas delivered to the airways at a frequency of 100–300 bursts per minute (National Institute of Health, 2000). The gas bursts are finely balanced with the patient's passive exhalation. The intrapulmonary wedge pressure, which is created in the airways, reflects the relationship between gas bursts and exhalation. It is believed to be the intrapulmonary wedge pressure that assists with mobilisation and clearance of secretions as the airway pressure oscillates at 5–35 cmH_2O. The airway walls vibrate in synchrony with these oscillations (National Institute of Health, 2000; Vargas *et al*., 2005).

The device associated with the delivery of IPV therapy is the Percussionator®. The Percussionator® has a sliding venturi device, called the Phasitron®, which generates the airway wall oscillations (National Institute of Health, 2000). Medication such as normal or hypertonic saline or bronchodilator therapy may be delivered to a patient with IPV therapy. The effectiveness of drug delivery during IPV is questioned due to the variability of IPV (Kacmarek *et al*., 2013).

Spontaneously breathing patients as well as patients who are intubated and ventilated may benefit from IPV. The manual mode setting of IPV is used for spontaneously breathing patients and the continuous mode setting for those on mechanical ventilation. Intrapulmonary percussive ventilation should only be used in ventilated patients who are on ventilation modes that allow for spontaneous breaths to be taken, such as synchronised intermittent mandatory ventilation, pressure support ventilation or continuous positive airway pressure ventilation (National Institute of Health, 2000). Various patient–machine interfaces can be used in the delivery of IPV, such as mouth piece, mask or an artificial airway. Intrapulmonary percussive ventilation is used to treat active pulmonary disease or to prevent the development of pulmonary disease. Other indications for its use are summarised in Table 4.7 (National Institute of Health, 2000; Kacmarek *et al*., 2013).

Table 4.7: Indications for the use of IPV therapy.

- Atelectasis
- Pneumonia
- Chronic respiratory diseases
- After thoracic or abdominal surgery
- Neuromuscular disorders
- Inability to independently clear airway secretions

4.2.2.5.1. How to perform the technique

Intrapulmonary percussive ventilation is a technique better known to respiratory therapists than physiotherapists and anecdotally does not seem to be used much in the treatment of patients with traumatic injuries. However, it is important that physiotherapists understand how it is used in the event that they come across such a device in their clinical practice. Table 4.8 summarises the steps to follow when using IPV therapy for patient care (National Institute of Health, 2000; Kacmarek *et al.*, 2013). It is important to determine the frequency and dose of IPV treatment with the medical team looking after the patient and to discuss the type of medication to be delivered to the patient during IPV.

Further instructions on how to set up IPV therapy for patient care can be found at https://www.youtube.com/watch?v=ARJLALFf2e0. Potential side-effects of IPV therapy include fatigue, stress, sore ribs and irritation (Kacmarek *et al.*, 2013).

4.2.2.5.2. Contraindications and precautions (National Institute of Health, 2000; Vargas *et al.*, 2005)

- Undrained pneumothorax.
- Haemoptysis.
- Active tuberculosis as it may contaminate the equipment.
- Fractured ribs or unstable chest wall.
- Respiratory arrest or rapid deterioration in neurological status.
- Haemodynamic instability or cardiac arrhythmia.
- Do not use within one hour after a meal. If the patient is on nasogastric tube feed, switch off the feed at least one hour prior to IPV.

Table 4.8: Steps to follow when using IPV therapy.

- Document the patient's pre-treatment clinical presentation, especially chest x-ray status, vital signs and auscultation findings.
- Assemble the IPV circuitry according to manufacturer guidelines and connect the unit pressure hose to a 50 psi outlet.
- Set the driving pressure to 25 psi (children: maximum driving pressure of 30 psi; adults: maximum of 45 psi).
- Set the 'percussive rate' control to 'full easy' to initiate treatment. As the patient grows accustomed to the machine, turn the 'percussive rate' control to the 12h00 position for optimal therapeutic effect.
- Instil the medication, at a total volume of 20 ml, in the aerosol generator.
- Perform a functional check of the IPV machine and circuitry before initiating patient treatment.
- Place the patient in a comfortable seated position.
- Attach the patient to the IPV device using the required interface.
- If the patient is using a mouth piece, instruct them to 'splint' their cheeks.
- Depress the 'remote switch' prior to inspiration and keep it depressed throughout the patient's inspiratory cycle.
- The percussion interval should initially be maintained for 5–10 seconds and then progressed to reach the point at which it is maintained throughout the entire inspiratory cycle.
- During non-percussive intervals the patient should continue to inhale the medication.
- Assessment of the patient's chest excursion and auscultation breath sounds should be done at regular intervals during the treatment session. The driving pressure should be adjusted until it produces visible 'chest shaking'.
- If the patient has a tracheostomy or endotracheal tube, make sure that the cuff is deflated to allow sputum plugs to pass the tube while maintaining a patent airway. If the patient desaturates during treatment, a PEEP valve may be placed on the expiratory side of the IPV circuit.
- Allow the patient time to cough and expectorate secretions or to be suctioned as needed during the IPV treatment session.
- After 20–30 minutes of treatment, or when the medication has finished, the treatment session is terminated and re-assessment of the patient's clinical condition is performed.
- The IPV device should be cleaned, according to manufacturer guidelines, after each treatment session.

- Minimise the risk of aspiration by keeping the patient in a 45° head up seated or upright sitting position.
- Monitor the patient's vital signs closely during the treatment.
- Suction equipment and oxygen therapy should be immediately available for use during treatment.

The combination of increased airway pressure, humidification, oscillation and ventilation and cough stimulation may improve secretion clearance, although this has not been well studied (McCool and Rosen, 2006). One case series documented the utility and feasibility of IPV to treat persistent pulmonary atelectasis associated with hypoxemia after smoke exposure in spontaneously breathing patients with burn injuries. This study used high-frequency IPV with a positive pressure level of 6–12 cmH_2O. There was no control group on which to base a comparison (Reper and Van Looy, 2013).

4.2.3. *Positioning*

Positioning is commonly used in unwell and critically ill patients in order to optimise ventilation and ventilation/perfusion (V/Q) matching (Gosselink *et al.*, 2008), and gravity-assisted positioning (postural drainage) is used to drain pulmonary secretions. Body positioning is therefore an important component of chest physiotherapy management.

4.2.3.1. *Body positioning*

Frequent position changes of the patient with traumatic injury has long been advocated (Kigin, 1981). Different body positions change the orientation of the lungs with respect to gravity, thereby affecting the distribution of ventilation and perfusion (Bryan *et al.*, 1966). Ventilation/perfusion matching is optimal when ventilation and perfusion is as close to 1:1 (matched) as possible in any given lung zone. A defect in ventilation (e.g. consolidation, excessive secretions or atelectasis) results in the shunting of blood away from the affected lung segments towards areas of the lungs that are better ventilated. A defect in perfusion (e.g. embolus) results in dead space, as ventilation is optimal but blood supply around the alveolus is absent; either of these scenarios results in V/Q mismatch and poor oxygenation (Broad *et al.*, 2012).

4.2.3.1.1. How to perform the technique

4.2.3.1.1.1. *Spontaneously breathing adults.* The distribution of ventilation, toward the dependent (lower) lung, in spontaneously breathing adults without pulmonary disease has been well established and described (Riedel *et al.*, 2005). In this population, in the upright standing position, air flows preferentially to the dependent lung zones, as alveoli in the dependent lung zones have greater capacity to expand and take on a larger volume of air than those in the apical and upper lung zones, which are almost stretched to maximum capacity due to the effect of gravity on the airways. Due to the effects of gravity on pulmonary blood flow, perfusion is also optimal in the dependent lung zones. Therefore the upright position optimises V/Q matching and hence oxygenation, as in this position FRC is optimal (Frownfelter and Dean, 2006; Broad *et al.*, 2012).

In spontaneously breathing adults without pulmonary disease, the side-lying position increases airflow to the dependent (bottom) lung, as alveoli in the dependent lung have a greater capacity to expand and take on larger volumes of air than those in the top lung, which are almost stretched to maximum capacity due to the effect of gravity on the airways. Side-lying perfusion is also optimal in the dependent lung due to the effect of gravity on the low-pressure pulmonary circulation; therefore both ventilation and perfusion are better matched in the dependent lung, which results in improved oxygenation (Frownfelter and Dean, 2006). This underscores the use of the 'good lung down' principle in patients with unilateral lung disease in order to improve oxygenation. Take note that FRC is approximately half of the volume in supine than its volume in standing and therefore standing is the most advantageous position for optimising oxygenation (Frownfelter and Dean, 2006).

The effects of body positioning on oxygenation in side lying described above do not apply for patients with moderate to severe obesity, as excessive body weight leads to compression of the dependent lung if this position is maintained for a prolonged time period.

4.2.3.1.1.2. *Ventilated adults.* In ventilated adults, perfusion remains optimal in the dependent lung regions but ventilation is reversed, as air now flows to areas of the lung in which least resistance to air flow is encountered (Broad *et al.*, 2012). The uppermost lung zones are preferentially ventilated and the dependent lung zones are preferentially perfused (due to gravity) (Frownfelter and Dean, 2006; Broad *et al.*, 2012). In unilateral disease or injury, placing the affected lung of a ventilated patient uppermost using side lying leads to improved ventilation in the uppermost lung and improved perfusion in the dependent (unaffected) lung; hence V/Q mismatch and poor oxygenation (Broad *et al.*, 2012) if the position is maintained for a prolonged time period. In ventilated adults, a supported high sitting position (45° head elevation) results in improved ventilation in the upper zones of both lung fields and improved perfusion in the dependent zones of both lungs (Frownfelter and Dean, 2006); hence a ventilated patient always experiences some degree of V/Q mismatch. Improving V/Q matching, therefore, should be considered a dynamic process, as the initial position might increase ventilation to the desired lobe while the secondary position would aim to direct perfusion to that lobe.

4.2.3.1.1.3. *Paediatric patients.* Studies by Davies *et al.* (1985) and Heaf *et al.* (1983) have, until very recently, formed the basis of our understanding of the distribution of ventilation in the paediatric population. These studies were performed over 20 years ago on heterogeneous populations. These authors proposed that ventilation is preferentially distributed to the non-dependent (upper) lung in children; the reversal of that seen in adults. However, recent studies in neonates, infants and children using electrical impedance tomography (EIT), a non-invasive imaging tool, reported contradictory findings with neonates and infants, demonstrating a similar distribution of ventilation to adults (Frerichs *et al.*, 2003; Schibler *et al.*, 2009; Pham *et al.*, 2011; Hough *et al.*, 2012), and great variability occurring in older infants and children (Lupton-Smith *et al.*, 2014). Given the differences found between the recent studies and the older ones, one has to question whether clinical practice in children has been correctly guided. It should now be recommended that optimal positioning in children is determined based on individual assessment of response to positional changes. A 'one size fits all' approach is not appropriate for therapeutic positioning in children.

4.2.3.1.1.4. *Prone positioning in adults and children.* The use of prone positioning for patients who are hypoxic is effective in improving oxygenation in adults and children with acute respiratory distress syndrome (Kornecki *et al.*, 2001; Casado-Flores *et al.*, 2002; Gillies *et al.*,

2012; Gattinoni *et al.*, 2014). No proven effect on paediatric patient outcome has been reported (Curley *et al.*, 2005), but recently prone positioning has been associated with 10–17% absolute survival in adults (Gattinoni *et al.*, 2014). The improvement in oxygenation observed through prone positioning may be due to the recruitment of dorsal lung segments, limited anterior chest wall movement, and reduced effects of abdominal pressure on the thoracic cavity, thereby promoting more uniform ventilation (Gattinoni *et al.*, 2014). In addition, perfusion remains mostly constant (gravity-dependent), thereby improving V/Q matching and reducing intrapulmonary shunt (Marraro, 2003; Gattinoni *et al.*, 2014).

Body positioning is used in combination with other physiotherapy treatment modalities that facilitate secretion clearance and optimise lung volumes to ensure that oxygenation is improved. Body positioning for V/Q matching should be performed at the end of a treatment session to enhance ventilation in areas in which sputum plugs and partial atelectasis were present.

4.2.3.1.2. Contraindications and precautions

- Each patient's response to body position changes should be monitored closely and if adverse reactions are noted, the patient should be positioned back to supine with head elevation.
- Sudden infant death syndrome is associated with sleeping in the prone position; therefore if it is used in infants, they should be placed under continuous cardiorespiratory monitoring (Gillies *et al.*, 2012).

4.2.3.2. *Gravity-assisted positioning (postural drainage)*

This technique involves positioning the patient in a manner in which gravity can act to assist with the clearance or drainage of secretions from peripheral airways (Stiller, 2000). The position chosen depends on the specific lung segments in which secretions are retained.

4.2.3.2.1. How to perform the technique

Standard positions for different lung segments have been advocated (O'Sullivan and Schmitz, 2001; Pryor *et al.*, 2008), with very little scientific evidence to support their use. Table 4.9 provides a description of each specific postural drainage position used to drain secretions from individual lung segments.

Some of these positions require tilting the head downwards into an inverted position; however, studies have shown an increased rate of

Table 4.9: Gravity-assisted body positions to enhance secretion clearance from individual lung segments.

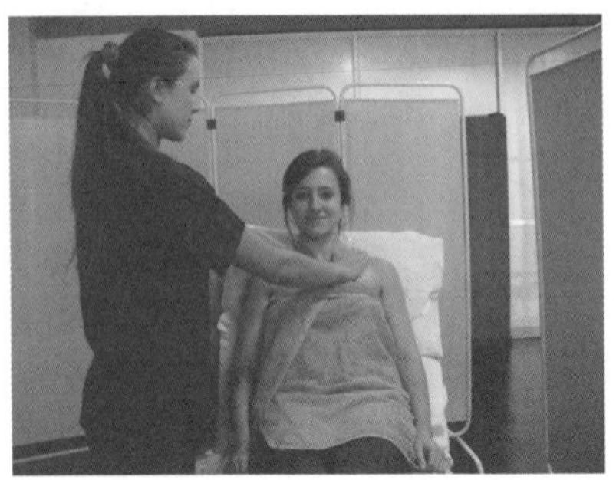	Apical segment of the upper lobe • The patient is placed in a comfortable upright seated position with the back supported.
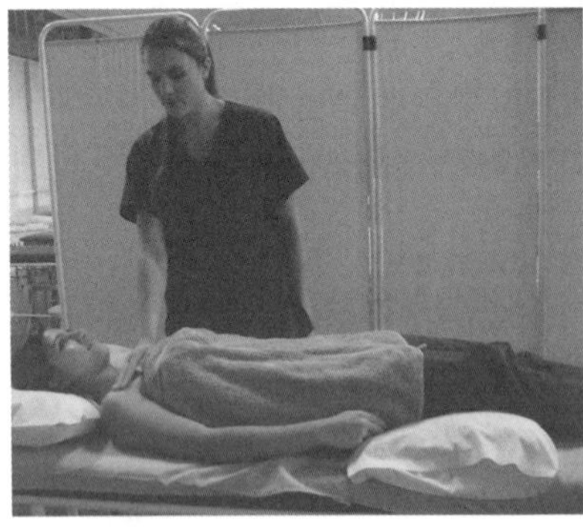	Anterior segment of the upper lobe • The patient lies in a supine position with the knees supported with a pillow.
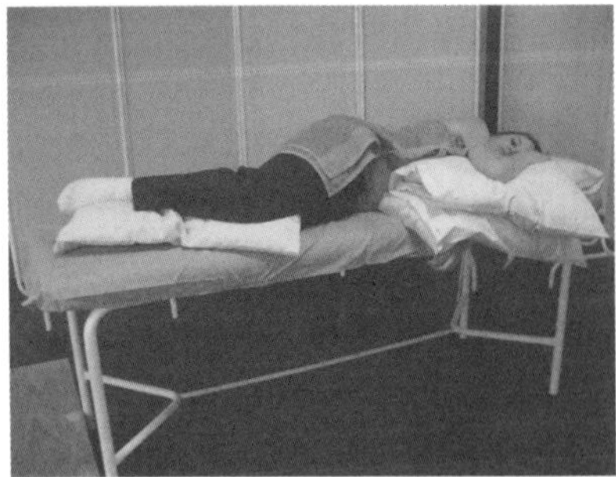	Posterior segment of the right upper lobe • The patient lies in a left–side-lying position with a 45° turn towards prone. • The right shoulder and arm are supported with two pillows.

(*Continued*)

Table 4.9: *(Continued)*

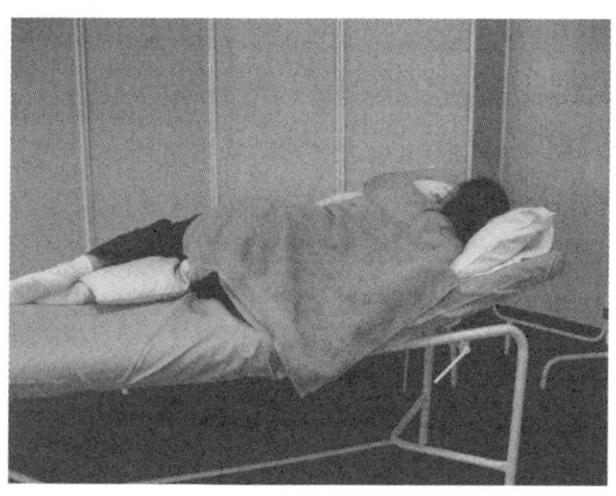	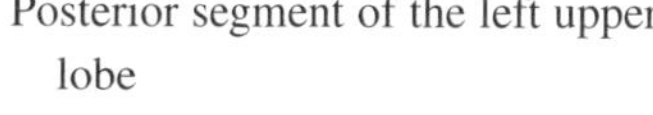 Posterior segment of the left upper lobe • The patient lies in a right–side-lying position with a 45° turn towards prone. • The left shoulder and arm are supported with two pillows. The head of the bed is tilted upwards to elevate the left posterior upper lobe to 30 cm from the horizontal plane.
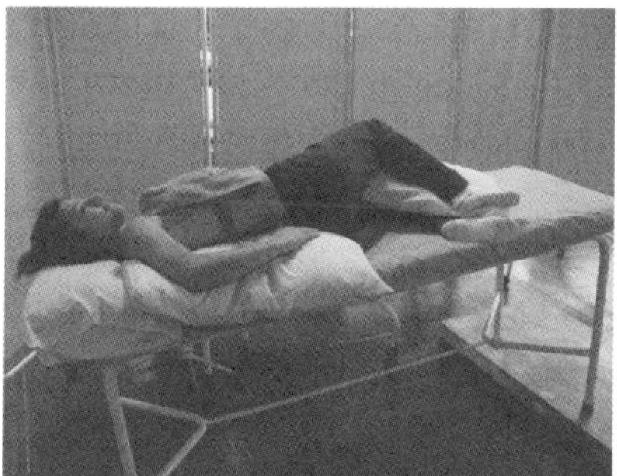	Middle lobe • The bed is elevated onto a platform to produce a chest-down tilt of 15°. • The patient lies in supine and turns the body a quarter turn towards the left side. The right arm and upper torso are supported with a pillow and the head with another pillow. Lingula lobe • The patient assumes the same position but with a quarter turn towards right–side lying.
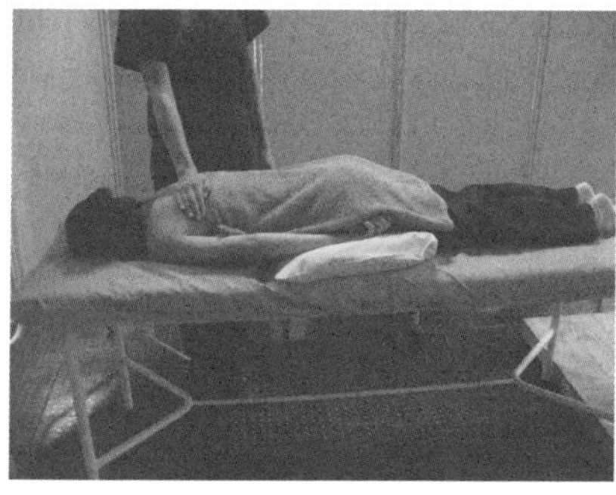	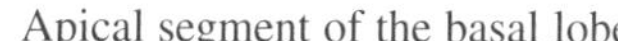 Apical segment of the basal lobe • The bed is positioned horizontally to the floor. • The patient lies in a prone position with one pillow supporting the lower abdominal region and pelvis.

(Continued)

Table 4.9. (*Continued*)

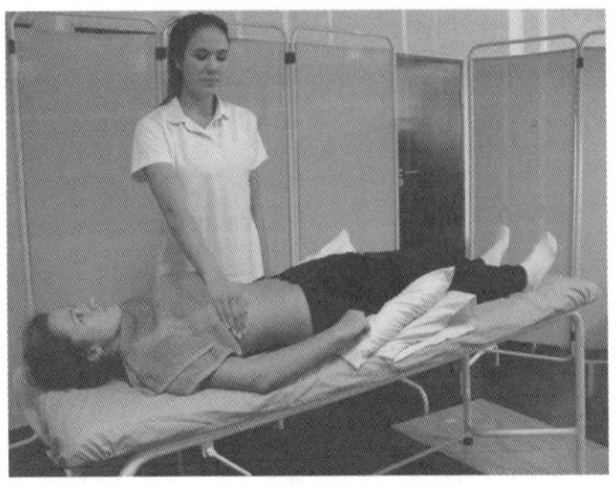	Anterior segment of the basal lobe • The bed is tilted to produce a 20° chest-down tilt. • The patient lies supine.
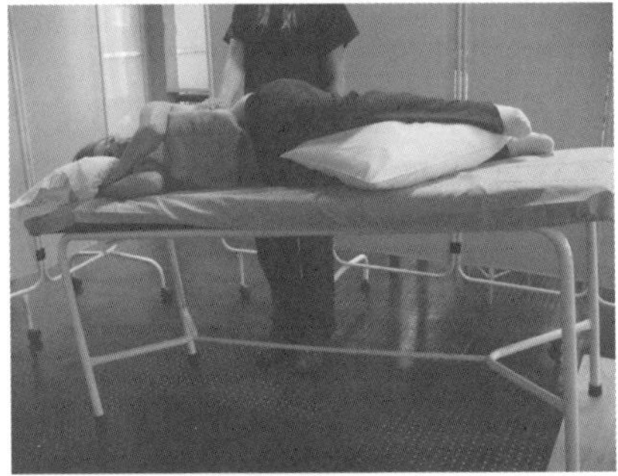	Lateral segment of the basal lobe • The bed is tilted to produce a 20° chest-down tilt. • The patient lies in a comfortable side-lying position. • One pillow is placed under the head and another between the knees for comfort.
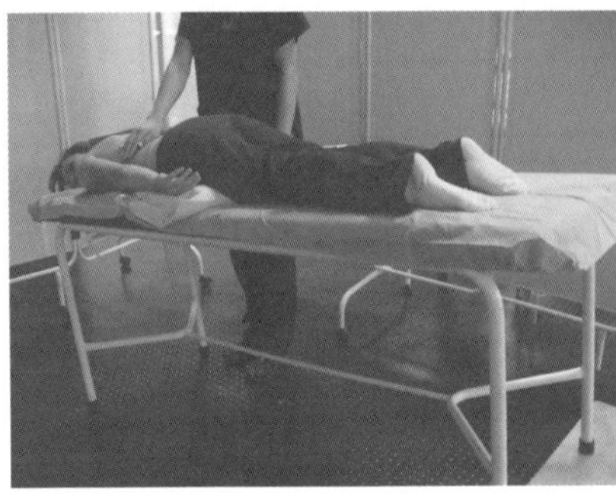	Posterior segment of the basal lobe • The bed is tilted to produce a 20° chest-down tilt. • The patient lies prone with one pillow under the lower abdominal and pelvic regions for comfort.

complications, particularly in the paediatric population, when using the Trendellenberg position. These complications include: gastro-oesophageal reflux (Button *et al.*, 2003); hypoxia; shortness of breath; raised intracranial pressure (Emery and Peabody, 1983); increased load on the diaphragm, predisposing to respiratory failure, particularly in young children (Vivian-Beresford *et al.*, 1987); and the potential for increased vascular return leading to increased work of the heart (Button *et al.*, 2003). By contrast, the use of head-down tilt positions in the adult critical care population for specific affected lobes resulted in increased expiratory flow and sputum clearance, faster resolution of atelectasis and better oxygenation, without the development of haemodynamic instability (Krause *et al.*, 2000; Berney *et al.*, 2004). There is currently very little supporting evidence for the use of the standardised postural drainage (PD) positions, and therefore it is recommended that the drainage position chosen be individualised according to efficacy of secretion production.

4.2.3.2.2. Contraindications and precautions

- Trendellenberg positions are not recommended in:
  - the paediatric population;
  - those with raised (or potentially raised) intracranial pressure or cerebral aneurysms;
  - those with abdominal distension, obesity or a history of gastro-oesophageal reflux;
  - those with severe hypertension, congestive heart failure or aortic aneurysms;
  - those with recent trauma or surgery to the head and neck; and
  - frank haemoptysis.
- Trendellenburg positions should be used with caution in the acutely injured patient.
- When positioning critically ill or injured patients, care must be taken not to dislodge lines, drains, tubes or any invasive devices, and to avoid pressure sores resulting from lying on these attachments.

4.2.4. *Manual chest therapy techniques*

Chest wall percussion, vibration and shaking are the most common manual techniques used in patient bronchopulmonary hygiene. These techniques are often used in conjunction with aerosol administration, body- or gravity-assisted positioning, breathing exercises, manual hyperinflation (MHI) and directed cough (Pryor *et al.*, 2008). The goals of manual chest therapy techniques are to assist in the mobilisation of excessive retained central and peripheral airway secretions, to decrease airflow resistance and to reduce the risk of bronchopulmonary infection (Pryor *et al.*, 2008).

The various forms of percussion, vibrations and shaking are labour intense, time consuming and sometimes challenging to perform effectively. The theory is that these techniques relate to the thixotrophic nature of pulmonary secretions (sputum liquefies on agitation). By applying percussion or vibrations to the chest wall, mechanical energy is transmitted into the airways, where secretions are loosened and can then be moved centrally by positioning, cough or FET (Stiller, 2000). Vibrations have been shown to increase expiratory flow rate through the creation of increased intrapleural pressures in a small sample of healthy adults (McCarren *et al.*, 2006a). It is recommended that percussion, vibration and shaking be interspersed with deep breathing in spontaneously breathing patients to prevent bronchospasm, desaturation and airway closure (Pryor *et al.*, 2008). This recommendation is supported by Guimarães and Zin (2008), who reported decreases in dynamic pulmonary compliance when thoracic percussion was applied for two minutes to the lateral aspects of the chest walls of 12 healthy subjects positioned in left–side lying. Pulmonary compliance normalised when these subjects performed deep breathing immediately after cessation of thoracic percussion (Guimarães and Zin, 2008). The use of percussion or any external vibration method is still considered to be unfounded and unsupported by scientific evidence (Stiller, 2000; Branson, 2007).

Manual chest therapy techniques may be used in the treatment of:

- infants and small children who are unable to voluntarily perform breathing exercises;
- patients with neuromuscular weakness or paralysis;
- intellectually impaired patients;
- patients with suppressed levels of consciousness;
- mechanically ventilated patients who are unable to perform breathing exercises or are required to maintain immobility due to the nature of their injuries; and
- patients with retained secretions, in combination with breathing exercises.

4.2.4.1. *Percussion*

4.2.4.1.1. How to perform the technique

Percussion, also called 'clapping' or 'cupping', is the action of rhythmically striking the chest wall with cupped hands, using flexion and extension movements of the wrists. In infants, two or three fingers are used when performing percussion. It should be applied to the specific area on the thorax that corresponds to the underlying involved lung segment. Percussion can be performed single- or double-handed and the force of percussion should be adapted to suit each individual patient (Pryor *et al.*, 2008). Patients with traumatic brain injury respond better to lower frequency percussion. Percussion should be performed over a layer of towel to avoid skin irritation and should never be uncomfortable or lead to breath-holding. In spontaneously breathing patients, percussion should be combined with three or four TEE to prevent oxygen desaturation and decreases in pulmonary compliance (Guimarães and Zin, 2008; Pryor *et al.*, 2008). In mechanically ventilated patients, percussion should be followed with expansion manoeuvres such as ventilator-assisted breaths with increased tidal volume or manual hyperinflation.

4.2.4.2. *Vibration*

4.2.4.2.1. How to perform the technique

Mechanical or manual vibration involves the application of a fine oscillation (generated through contraction of the physiotherapist's forearm muscles) to the exposed chest wall on expiration along with a slight compression of the chest wall (McCarren *et al.*, 2006a, 2006b; Pryor *et al.*, 2008). In adults, the technique should be performed throughout expiration and ceased when inspiration starts. In children, owing to a faster respiratory rate, it may be necessary to continue vibrating throughout inspiration and expiration, interspersed by a few recovery breaths. Chest vibrations may mobilise loosened secretions towards the central airways by increasing expiratory flow rates (McCarren *et al.*, 2006a).

4.2.4.3. *Shaking*

4.2.4.3.1. How to perform the technique

Chest wall shaking involves the physiotherapist using their hands to apply a coarse oscillatory compression to the exposed chest wall over the involved lung segment during expiration (Fig. 4.8). The technique should be performed rhythmically throughout expiration and ceases at the end of expiration to allow for the next inspiratory breath. It is believed to result in similar enhancements of expiratory flow as mentioned above for chest wall vibrations.

Vibrations and shaking of the chest wall should never be uncomfortable and the intensity of application should be adapted for each individual patient.

4.2.4.4. *Contraindications and precautions for the use of manual chest therapy techniques*

- Frank haemoptysis (Pryor *et al.*, 2008).
- Excessive pain (Pryor *et al.*, 2008).

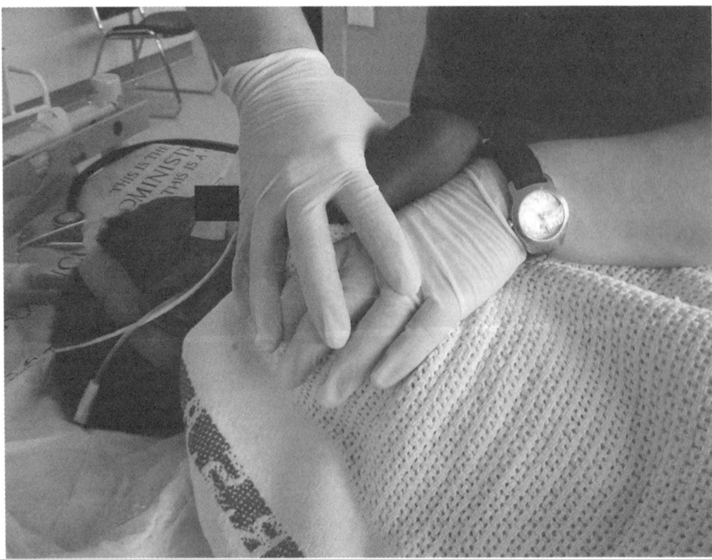

Fig. 4.8: A ventilated child in the paediatric intensive care unit receiving manual vibrations and shaking.

- Acute head injuries with uncontrolled intracranial pressure (Pryor *et al.*, 2008).
- Multiple rib fractures or flail rib segments (Pryor *et al.*, 2008).
- Acute bronchospasm that does not respond to bronchodilator therapy (Pryor *et al.*, 2008).
- Patient with pulmonary embolism not on anti-coagulant therapy (Pryor *et al.*, 2008).
- Severe clotting disorders such as platelet count below 50×10^9\L (50000 cm^3) and international normalised ratio (INR) greater than 1.4 seconds.
- Manual techniques should be used with extreme caution in patients with unstable spinal cord injuries. Techniques performed bilaterally on the chest wall in the supine position potentially cause less harm to the spinal cord than unilaterally performed techniques.
- Loss of skin integrity such as recent burns or open wounds on the chest wall (Pryor *et al.*, 2008).
- Subcutaneous emphysema indicative of an undrained pneumothorax, haemothorax or pleural effusion.
- Severe osteoporosis, as it may result in rib fractures (Pryor *et al.*, 2008).
- Unstable angina or cardiac arrhythmias (Pryor *et al.*, 2008).
- Non-communicating lung abscesses (Pryor *et al.*, 2008).
- Preterm infants.
- Pulmonary oedema or unstable pulmonary hypertension (Pryor *et al.*, 2008).

4.2.5. *Assisted and supported coughing*

Cough effectiveness is often reduced in patients who suffer from respiratory or neuromuscular diseases and may lead to the development of pneumonia or respiratory failure (Cardoso *et al.*, 2012). The measurement of peak expiratory cough flow provides important clinical data to determine changes in respiratory muscle function. Peak expiratory cough flow values for healthy individuals range from 240–500 L/min and must be higher than 160 L/min for an effective cough to be produced (Cardoso *et al.*, 2012). Physiotherapists therefore need to ensure that this minimum peak expiratory cough flow is produced when assisted or supported coughing manoeuvres are used for secretion clearance.

4.2.5.1. *Manually assisted cough*

Outward (paradoxical) movement of the abdomen is observed during coughing in patients with cervical or high thoracic spinal cord injury or neuromuscular weakness. This paradoxical movement is due to a loss of abdominal muscle tone, paralysis or weakness of the expiratory muscles and contributes to poor cough effort (McCool and Rosen, 2006). Assisted cough manoeuvres can improve cough effectiveness by increasing peak expiratory cough flow by 14–100% (McCool and Rosen, 2006), thereby enhancing secretion clearance in such patients.

4.2.5.1.1. How to perform the technique

Assisted cough manoeuvres aim to reduce the abdominal paradox during cough through the application of manual pressure to the upper abdomen and/or the lower thorax (McCool and Rosen, 2006; Gosselink *et al.*, 2011) following inspiration and, ideally, glottic closure; Figs 4.9A and B illustrate the various methods of application.

Manually assisted coughs may be ineffective in patients with stiff chest walls and thoracic deformities (e.g. scoliosis). It is a very useful

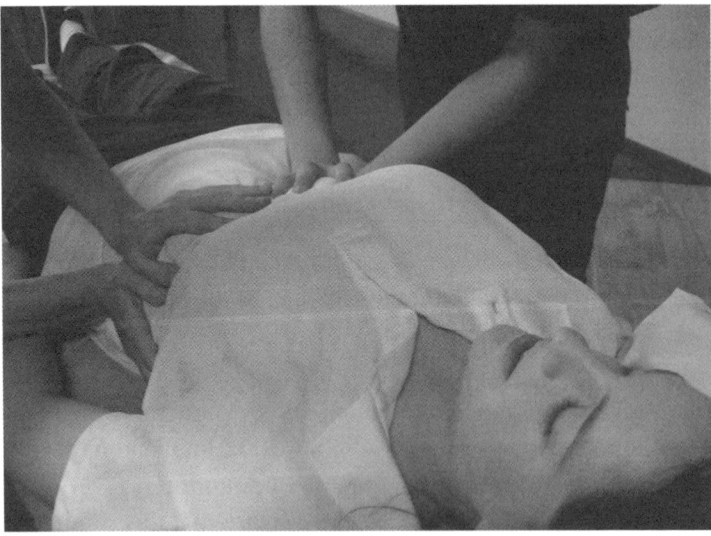

Fig. 4.9A: Manually assisted cough applied by two physiotherapists using bilateral lower chest wall compression.

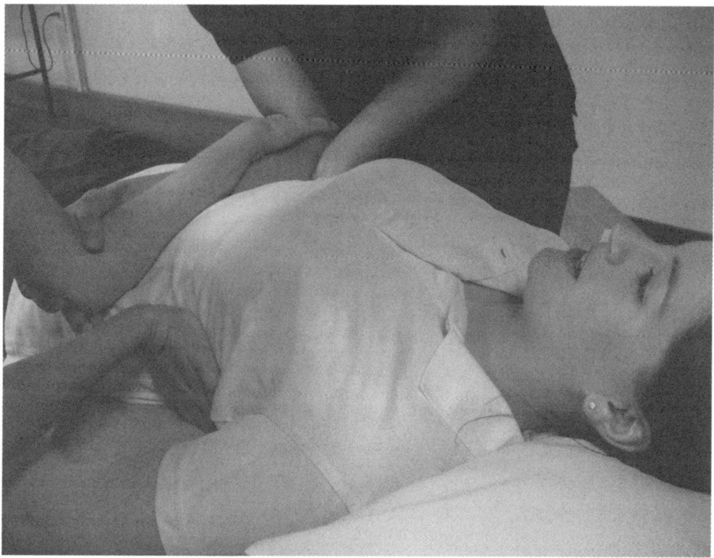

Fig. 4.9B: Manually assisted cough applied by two physiotherapists using a combination of abdominal thrust and lower chest wall compression.

technique in patients with high spinal cord injuries after stabilisation of the spine (McCrory *et al.*, 2001). A low level of scientific evidence supports the use of assisted cough manoeuvres to reduce the incidence of, or treatment of, respiratory complications in patients with expiratory muscle weakness (McCool and Rosen, 2006).

4.2.5.1.2. Contraindications and precautions

- This technique should be avoided or performed with great care in patients following abdominal or thoracic trauma or surgery.
- In young children, abdominal thrusts should be avoided and thoracic compression used as the preferred method of assisted cough.

4.2.5.2. *Supported cough*

After abdominal or thoracic trauma or surgery, patients find it painful to take deep inspiratory breaths and cough effectively. Supporting a surgical incision or unstable chest wall during coughing anecdotally reduces pain experienced by the patient and may make them less anxious that the wound will re-open during coughing.

4.2.5.2.1. How to perform the technique

It is generally recommended that either the physiotherapist or the patient him/herself brace their surgical incision (abdominal or thoracic) or rib cage (in the case of rib fractures) during coughing, either with their hands or with a pillow or towel for extra support (Figs 4.10A and B).

4.2.5.2.2. Contraindications and precautions

- No inwards compression of the chest wall during bracing should be done in the presence of rib fractures.

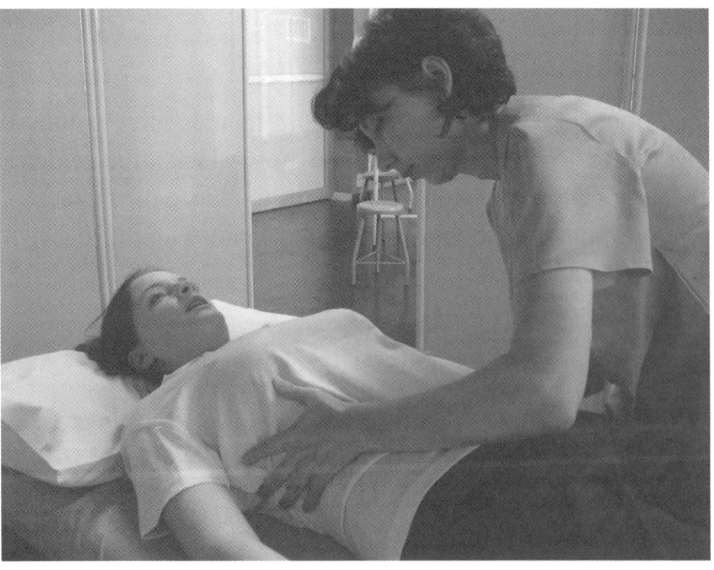

Fig. 4.10A: Supported cough technique applied by a physiotherapist using bilateral chest wall bracing.

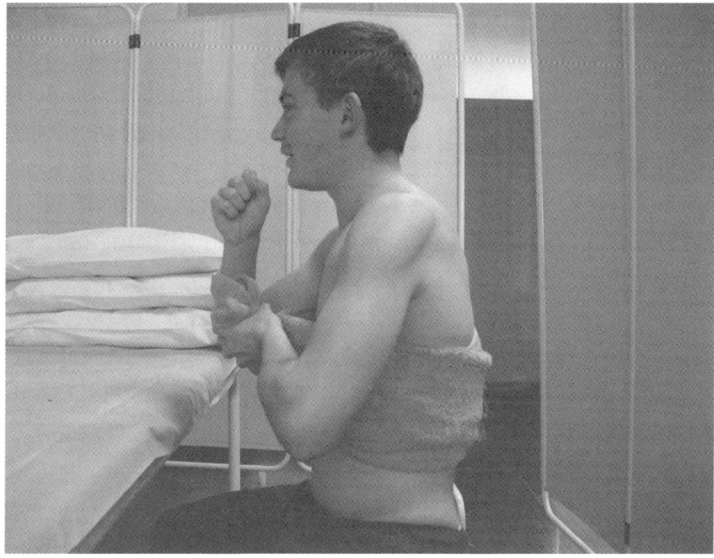

Fig. 4.10B: Supported cough performed independently using a towel positioned around the rib cage.

4.2.6. *Hyperinflation techniques*

4.2.6.1. *Manual hyperinflation*

Manual hyperinflation is commonly used in the ICU and high care settings in conjunction with other physiotherapeutic techniques, with the intention of re-expanding collapsed areas of the lung, mobilising peripheral secretions towards the central airways, improving oxygenation and static and dynamic lung compliance, reducing airway resistance and preventing atelectasis (Choi and Jones, 2005; Maa *et al*., 2005; Gosselink *et al*., 2011; Stiller, 2013).

4.2.6.1.1. How to perform the technique

Manual hyperinflation usually consists of the delivery of larger than tidal volume breaths (using a resuscitation, anaesthetic or self-inflating bag) during slow inspiration, reaching a predetermined set pressure or volume, followed by a brief inspiratory hold to recruit collateral ventilation channels and alveoli, and a rapid release of the bag to enhance expiratory flow, thereby mimicking FET and stimulating a cough (Maa *et al.*, 2005). It is recommended that an in-line pressure manometer be used to monitor the pressure delivered to the airways during the performance of MHI (Maa *et al.*, 2005) (Fig. 4.11). Peak inspiratory pressure (PIP) is only a proxy for tidal volume, and even if PIP is controlled and measured, the tidal volume delivered cannot be directly extrapolated, as this depends on a number of other variables, including compliance of the respiratory system. In adults it is generally recommended that PIP should be less than 40 cmH_2O (Gosselink *et al.*, 2011).

To prevent alveolar derecruitment when the patient is disconnected from the ventilator for MHI, a PEEP valve, set at a similar level to that which the patient receives from the ventilator, should be attached to the MHI circuit (Savian *et al.*, 2005) (Fig. 4.11).

The principles of lung protective ventilator strategies require that delivered tidal volumes be kept low (6–8 ml/kg ideal body weight)

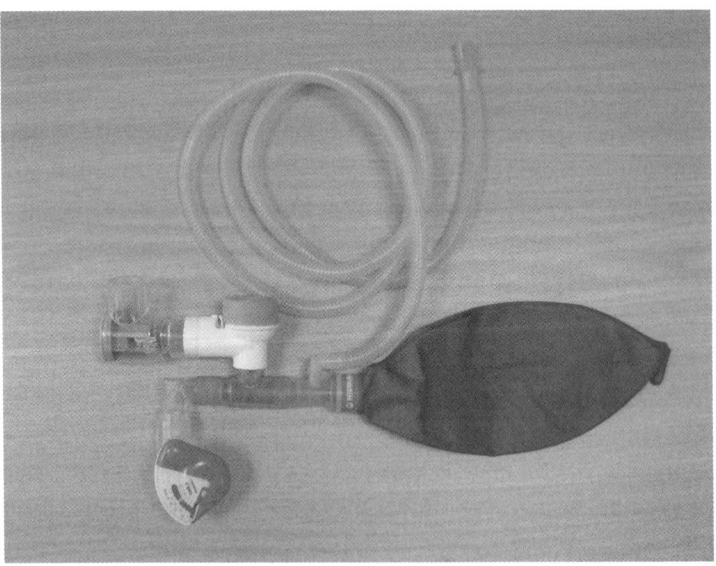

Fig. 4.11: Pressure manometer and PEEP valve connected to a Mapleson-C MHI circuit.

(Carpenter, 2004; Fuller *et al.*, 2013) and that the lung is opened and kept open using adequate PEEP and conservative PIP levels, without the opening and closing of lung units, which can lead to lung injury (Park *et al.*, 2013). If the tidal volume delivered is too large, it may contribute to lung damage, regardless of the pressure applied, particularly with low lung compliance and fragile or immature lungs (O'Donnell *et al.*, 2003). By these mechanisms, repeated application of MHI without a PEEP valve could theoretically lead to lung injury. Savian *et al.* (2005) reported that peak expiratory flow from the airways is enhanced when PEEP less than or equal to 10 cmH_2O is used. They found that PEEP greater than 10 cmH_2O was associated with less secretion clearance, as the positive expiratory pressure posed resistance to the flow of peripheral secretions towards the central airways for clearance. Table 4.10 summarises the steps to follow when performing MHI on an intubated adult patient.

Table 4.11 summarises the steps to follow when performing MHI on a paediatric patient (Elrauf, 2010).

The patient may be positioned in prone, side-lying or supine position during MHI. The position chosen is guided by the lung lobes in which pathology was noted during assessment. If lung volumes are reduced in

Table 4.10: Procedure for the performance of manual hyperinflation for adult patients.

- Before the patient is disconnected from the ventilator:
  - Assemble the MHI circuit and connect it to an oxygen flow meter
  - Set the flow on the flow meter to 15 L/minute
  - Attach a pressure manometer and suitable PEEP valve to the MHI circuit
  - Test that the MHI circuit works correctly before attaching it to the patient's artificial airway
- Monitor the patient's chest wall movements; disconnect the ventilator circuit at the peak of inspiration and immediately connect the patient to the MHI circuit.
- Synchronise the delivered MHI breaths with the patient's own inspiratory efforts.
- If the patient was able to take a few spontaneous breaths while connected to the mechanical ventilator, allow them to do spontaneous breaths between MHI breaths.
- If the patient had no spontaneous respiratory efforts while on mechanical ventilation, the physiotherapist should perform every breath for them using the MHI circuit.
- At the end of the treatment session, the patient should be reconnected to the ventilator.
- The physiotherapist should observe that the patient is stable before leaving the patient's bedside.

Table 4.11: Procedure for the performance of manual hyperinflation for paediatric patients.

- An appropriately sized bag should be used:
  - 0.5L for babies
  - 1L for children
  - 2–3L for children older than 7 years
- An appropriate flow rate through the MHI circuit should be selected:
  - Less than 6L for neonates
  - Less than 10L for babies
  - Less than 15L for older children with stiff lungs
- A pressure manometer and PEEP valve should be used.
- When the patient is attached to the MHI circuit, they should be given two tidal breaths followed by one larger than tidal volume breath, and this sequence should be continued throughout the treatment session.
- The rest of the procedure is similar to that described for adults.

the lower lobe segments of the left lung in adult patients, MHI performed in the supine position may not be successful in re-inflating these lung segments. In a randomised crossover trial, Van Aswegen *et al.* (2013) investigated airflow distribution through the lung fields of critically ill adult patients when MHI was performed with two frequently used MHI circuits. Visualisation of airflow distribution was achieved through the administration of radioactive technetium and gamma camera imaging. They reported that the least amount of technetium deposition was measured in the lower segments of the left lung in the supine position, regardless of the type of MHI circuit used (Van Aswegen *et al.*, 2013).

A cycle of six to seven MHI breaths should be delivered to the patient in between suction passes to allow the patient time to recover from coughing and increase oxygenation before the next suction pass. The duration of MHI in a single treatment session is dependent on the patient's response to MHI and whether the aims of treatment were achieved.

Manual hyperinflation can be used in combination with expiratory rib cage compression. This treatment combination is reported to shorten the duration of mechanical ventilation and ICU length of stay of adult patients (Berti *et al.*, 2012). Physiotherapists who work in the paediatric ICU and paediatric cardiac ICU often use MHI combined with expiratory vibration as chest physiotherapy intervention (McCord *et al.*, 2013).

4.2.6.1.2. Contraindications and precautions (Pryor *et al.*, 2008; Dennis *et al.*, 2012)

- Acute pulmonary oedema.
- Bullae in patients with chronic obstructive pulmonary disease or cystic fibrosis.
- Undrained pneumothorax, haemothorax or large pleural effusion or intercostal drain with an air leak.
- Bronchopleural fistula.
- Obstructing airway tumour or lung tumour.
- Potential bronchospasm, especially in patients with a history of asthma.
- Cardiovascular instability (MAP < 60 mmHg; total inotrope requirement ≥ 15 ml/hour of adrenaline or noradrenaline (dilution 3 mg/50 ml); patients on extracorporeal membrane oxygenation).
- Frank haemoptysis.
- Care should be taken in performing MHI for any patient with PEEP greater than 15 cmH_2O or requiring high levels of ventilator support ($FiO_2 > 0.7$) to maintain oxygenation, as the MHI circuit may not be able to meet the patient's high ventilatory needs.
- High-frequency oscillatory ventilation.

4.2.6.1.3. Safety and efficacy of MHI in adults

Studies in adults have reported varying results with regards to the efficacy of MHI, with earlier studies reporting no improvements in atelectasis, compliance and gas exchange (Stiller, 2000; Barker and Adams, 2002), whilst more recent studies have reported such changes (Choi and Jones, 2005; Maa *et al.*, 2005; Dennis *et al.*, 2012; Stiller, 2013). Earlier studies on MHI in adults reported adverse events such as raised intracranial pressure and cardiovascular complications (Singer *et al.*, 1994; Stiller, 2000), whilst more recent studies reported no adverse events in relation to aspiration, cardiovascular instability, neurological deterioration, oxygen desaturation or pneumothorax when MHI was used (Maa *et al.*, 2005; De Godoy *et al.*, 2011; Berti *et al.*, 2012; Van Aswegen *et al.*, 2013). Paulus *et al.* (2010) investigated the rate of adverse events when MHI was conducted by 57 experienced and trained ICU nurses on

74 stable critically ill patients. They found a low rate of 6% adverse events during the study, which were mostly associated with patient-related anxiety that developed during the procedure. The authors concluded that cardiovascular and respiratory adverse events occurred rarely when MHI was administered by experienced and trained ICU nurses. It would be reasonable to conclude that the same would apply when MHI is performed by experienced and trained ICU physiotherapists.

4.2.6.1.4. Safety and efficacy of MHI in the paediatric population

In infants and children MHI can be particularly hazardous, as this population has an increased risk of both volutrauma and barotrauma. There is minimal scientific evidence supporting MHI in the paediatric population. A recent systematic review (De Godoy *et al.*, 2013) could only include three articles, only one of which was a randomised clinical trial (Main *et al.*, 2004) which was not designed to evaluate the effects of MHI specifically, as patients received a range of non-standardised interventions, some of which included MHI. Gregson *et al.*, (2007, 2012) conducted two observational studies of chest physiotherapy, including MHI, in children. Gregson *et al.* (2012) observed children during chest physiotherapy sessions that consisted of a combination of manual lung inflation (they avoid the term 'hyperinflation'), compression–vibrations, saline delivery and endotracheal suction, with physiotherapists applying treatments according to clinical judgement (therefore not standardised). Despite the limitations of the study, these authors reported that there was a significant increase in peak expiratory flow by an average of 22% during manual inflations compared to baseline; but the increase was much larger, at 76%, when compression–vibrations were added on expiration. It is concerning that the highest inflation volumes and pressures recorded during physiotherapy in Gregson *et al.*'s (2012) study exceeded those believed to cause lung injury (Wolthuis *et al.*, 2008). The authors postulated that lung injury is more likely to occur as a result of prolonged changes in pressure or volume, whereas physiotherapy treatments tend to be brief and intermittent.

Insufficient safety and efficacy data currently exist to support MHI as a standard component of chest physiotherapy in critically ill and injured children. When this intervention is deemed essential, it should only be performed by trained, experienced individuals and the self-inflating bag should be equipped with a pressure manometer and be appropriately sized to limit volutrauma. It is the authors' opinion that 'normo-inflation' may be better than hyperinflation in children, as hyperinflation has a negative impact on lung function, whilst inflation to normal, homogenous volumes offers the potential to recruit collapsed areas and clear secretions without the damage caused by over-inflation.

4.2.6.2. *Ventilator hyperinflation*

Hyperinflation may also be delivered through a mechanical ventilator and is a technique frequently used by Australian physiotherapists (Dennis *et al.*, 2012; De Godoy *et al.*, 2013).

4.2.6.2.1. How to perform the technique

Table 4.12 summarises the steps to follow when performing ventilator hyperinflation (VHI) (Dennis *et al.*, 2012).

Four sets of eight VHI breaths may be delivered during one treatment session, depending on the patient's response to treatment (Dennis *et al.*, 2012).

Table 4.12: Ventilator hyperinflation procedure.

- Use the synchronised intermittent mandatory ventilation mode to deliver VHI breaths
- Adjust the airway pressure alarm to 45 cmH_2O
- Adjust the tidal volume alarm to 250% of the initial tidal volume
- Increase the fraction of inspired oxygen to one for the duration of treatment
- Leave the PEEP setting unchanged
- Adjust inspiratory time on the ventilator to 3–5 seconds
- Adjust respiratory rate on the ventilator to 6–8 breaths per minute
- Adjust the tidal volume setting on the ventilator to deliver hyperinflation breaths that are 15 ml/kg, as calculated using lean body weight
- Incrementally increase tidal volume by 150 ml at a time until the target volume or a peak airway pressure of 40 cmH_2O is reached

4.2.6.2.2. Contraindications and precautions

- The same contraindications and precautions as listed for MHI apply for the use of VHI.
- The use of VHI should be discussed with the medical team looking after the patient prior to implementation.
- Ventilator hyperinflation should only be performed by trained physiotherapists.

Ventilator hyperinflation is reported to be just as safe and effective as MHI in the adult population and produces similar beneficial effects on oxygenation, secretion clearance and lung compliance (Berney and Denehy, 2002; Dennis *et al.*, 2012; Stiller, 2013). No evidence could be found to support the use of VHI in children.

4.2.7. *Airway suctioning*

Most intubated and ventilated patients will need airway suctioning to maintain a patent airway. Compromised mucociliary clearance, lack of glottis closure and sometimes reduced levels of consciousness will all influence cough effectiveness. Closed or open (Fig. 4.12) suction systems may be used, but there have been no proven benefits of either system in terms of the prevention of nosocomial infection or other clinical outcome measures in adult or paediatric patients (Jongerden *et al.*, 2007; Pedersen *et al.*, 2009; Morrow *et al.*, 2012).

Although suctioning is often necessary, it is associated with a number of complications, including hypoxia, cardiac arrhythmia, raised intracranial pressure, mucosal trauma, blood pressure changes, atelectasis and impaired ciliary function (Morrow and Argent, 2008; Gosselink *et al.*, 2011). Suctioning should therefore never be done routinely, but rather only when clinically indicated (Branson, 2007; Pedersen *et al.*, 2009; Gosselink *et al.*, 2011).

Clinical indications for suctioning include the following.

- Audible or visible secretions in the endotracheal or tracheostomy tube.
- Coarse breath sounds on auscultation.
- Coughing with difficulty in clearing secretions from the airways.

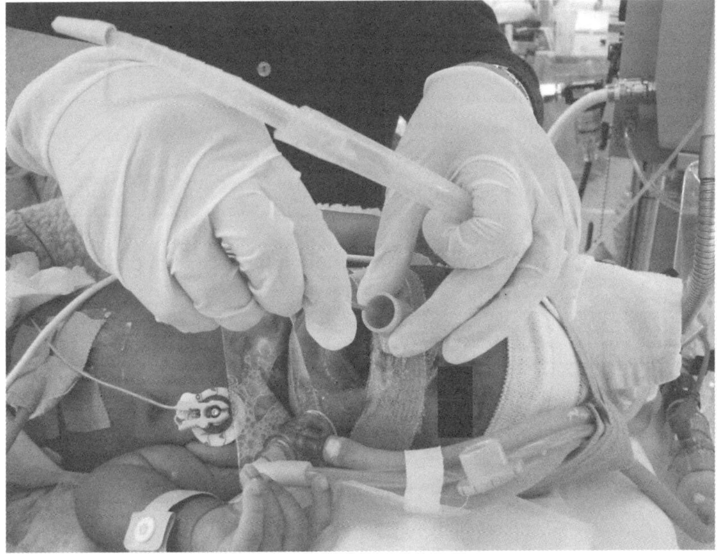

Fig. 4.12: A ventilated infant undergoing open endotracheal suctioning via nasal endotracheal tube.

- Increased work of breathing.
- Desaturation or bradycardia as a result of airway secretions.
- Decreased tidal volume observed during pressure-controlled ventilation.
- 'Saw-tooth' pattern changes in the pressure waveform on the ventilator display panel indicate the presence of secretions in the central airways and will be visible in any mode of mechanical ventilation.

4.2.7.1. *Suction of artificial airways*

4.2.7.1.1. How to perform the technique

Table 4.13 lists the equipment required to perform suctioning of patients with endotracheal or tracheostomy tubes.

It is good practice to prepare your suction equipment prior to patient treatment so that the patient can be suctioned promptly when secretions are mobilised, without developing respiratory distress due to airway occlusion. The patient can be suctioned in any position.

Table 4.13: Equipment required for suction of artificial airways.

- Sterile gloves, mask and eye protection
- Sterile suction catheter of an appropriate size
- Suction unit (wall-mounted or portable) in good working condition
- Sterile gauze and water to clean the catheter with between suction passes during open suction (in a single treatment session) if a closed suction catheter is not available

Table 4.14: Guideline for suction catheter selection for paediatric patients from three months of age*.

Age	ETT size (mm internal diameter)	Catheter size range (French gauge)
Birth to 3 months	2.5–3.5	5–7
3 months	3.5	7
1 year	4.0	7–8
2 years	4.5	7–8
3 years	4.5	7–8
4 years	5	8
6 years	5.5	8
8 years	6	10
10 years	6.5	10–12
12 years	7	10–12

*Taken from Morrow and Argent (2008), with permission.

4.2.7.1.1.1. *Select the correct suction catheter size.* In adults, the size of the catheter used for suctioning should not exceed half the internal diameter of the endotracheal or tracheostomy tube (Pedersen *et al.*, 2009). One example of a formula for calculating catheter size is: suction catheter size (Fr) = [endotracheal tube size (mm) — 1) × 2] (Pedersen *et al.*, 2009). This formula does not apply to the paediatric population. In children, the smallest catheters are often larger than half the internal diameter of the smallest endotracheal tubes (Morrow and Argent, 2008). A guideline for selection of suction catheters (for medium to thick mucus consistency) in children is presented in Table 4.14.

4.2.7.1.1.2. *Pre-oxygenate the patient prior to suctioning.* Pre-oxygenation is recommended in adults and children to prevent hypoxia during suctioning (Oh and Seo, 2003; Pedersen *et al.*, 2009). The patient should receive FiO_2 of one for at least 30 seconds prior to and after the suction procedure (Pedersen *et al.*, 2009).

4.2.7.1.1.3. *Suction pressure.* Suction pressures should be kept low enough so as not to damage mucosa, but sufficiently high to effectively evacuate secretions (Morrow and Argent, 2008). Suction pressure ranges of 80–150 mmHg (10.6–20 kPa) are recommended for adult patients (Pedersen *et al.*, 2009; Moffatt, 2011).

4.2.7.1.1.4. *Instillation of normal saline during suction.* Saline should not be used routinely for suctioning as it has been shown to increase hypoxia in adults and children, with no physiological benefit, as saline and mucus are essentially immiscible (Akgul and Akyolcu, 2002; Ji *et al.*, 2002; Ridling *et al.*, 2003; Pedersen *et al.*, 2009). It is suggested that saline might be indicated in specific circumstances only, for example to dislodge an adherent plug from the airway wall through cough stimulation. In order to ensure pulmonary secretions are manageable, adequate humidification is essential, as well as ensuring systemic hydration (Branson, 2007).

4.2.7.1.1.5. *Depth of catheter insertion.* To minimise the risk of mucosal trauma, the depth of catheter insertion should generally be limited to the length of the endotracheal or tracheostomy tube and 1 cm beyond, at which point a cough is normally stimulated (Morrow and Argent, 2008; Pedersen *et al.*, 2009). The catheter is retracted when a cough is stimulated and suction pressure is applied after the catheter is retracted 1 cm (Pedersen *et al.*, 2009).

4.2.7.1.1.6. *Duration of suction.* The duration of suction application should be kept to a minimum and should not exceed 15 seconds per suction pass (Pedersen *et al.*, 2009). Continuous suction pressure should be applied through the closure of the thumb port on the catheter until the length of the catheter has protruded from the artificial airway. Intermittent suction pressure is not recommended, as the risk of alveolar collapse increases when intermittent suction is applied through a closed suction system (Pedersen *et al.*, 2009). The technique of 'tromboning' (inward and outward sliding of the catheter on withdrawal from the airway) is not appropriate.

In between suction catheter passes, the patient should be reconnected to the mechanical ventilator or MHI circuit to prevent the onset of hypoxaemia. The patient should be allowed to adequately recover from coughing before the next suction pass is performed. It is essential that all patients are continually monitored during endotracheal suctioning to assess for any clinical or physiological changes. The physiotherapist should re-auscultate the patient's chest during and following completion of the suction procedure to establish if the aims of treatment were achieved.

4.2.7.2. *Nasotracheal and orotracheal suctioning*

It may become necessary at times to suction a patient who does not have an artificial airway in place. In this instance, airway suction can be performed by passing the suction catheter down the nasal passages or the oral cavity into the upper respiratory tract. The equipment required for suction, suction procedure and precautions to suction are similar to that described for endotracheal suctioning. Because suctioning is an unpleasant procedure for the patient, the physiotherapist needs to carefully explain to the patient what the procedure entails, including the expected duration of the procedure. The patient should be pre-oxygenated prior to suctioning using a face mask.

4.2.7.2.1. Nasopharyngeal and nasotracheal suction

The tip of the suction catheter is lubricated with water-soluble jelly before it is passed through the nose. The physiotherapist should gently aim the direction of the catheter medially and downwards through the nasal passage to guide it down the pharynx towards the trachea. The suction catheter is passed downwards during inspiration without applying suction pressure. As soon as the patient coughs the catheter should be withdrawn 1 cm, before suction pressure is applied. Some patients have no cough reflex while the catheter passes down the pharynx and therefore it may become necessary to pass the catheter through the vocal cords to stimulate a cough. Position the patient's neck into extension and ask her/him to stick their tongue out while the suction catheter is being inserted to prevent it from going down the oesophagus (Pryor *et al.*, 2008). The patient will cough vigorously as soon as the catheter passes through the vocal cords. Suction pressure should then be applied and the catheter may be removed from the airways.

Some clinicians prefer not to remove the catheter from the trachea once it is inserted past the vocal cords in order to reduce the amount of discomfort experienced by the patient. In these circumstances the catheter remains *in situ* after insertion into the trachea and is connected via oxygen tubing to an oxygen flow meter at the bedside. The thumb port on the top of the catheter is occluded and oxygen is delivered directly into the trachea while the patient recovers from coughing. When the patient is ready for the next suction, the catheter is disconnected from the oxygen and reconnected to the suction tubing. This process continues until all secretions have been removed and only then is the catheter withdrawn from the trachea. Insertion of a nasopharyngeal airway, if available locally, can be used if frequent suction is anticipated. The presence of this airway will also reduce patient discomfort during suction when the catheter is repeatedly passed into the nasal passages.

4.2.7.2.2. Oropharyngeal suction

Suctioning of the mouth can be done with a hard plastic suction device called a Yankauer. Deeper suction into the pharynx, larynx or trachea is performed with a soft suction catheter and an oropharyngeal or Guedel pattern airway. This is a plastic tube that is shaped to fit the patient's curved palate and is available in different sizes (Fig. 4.13).

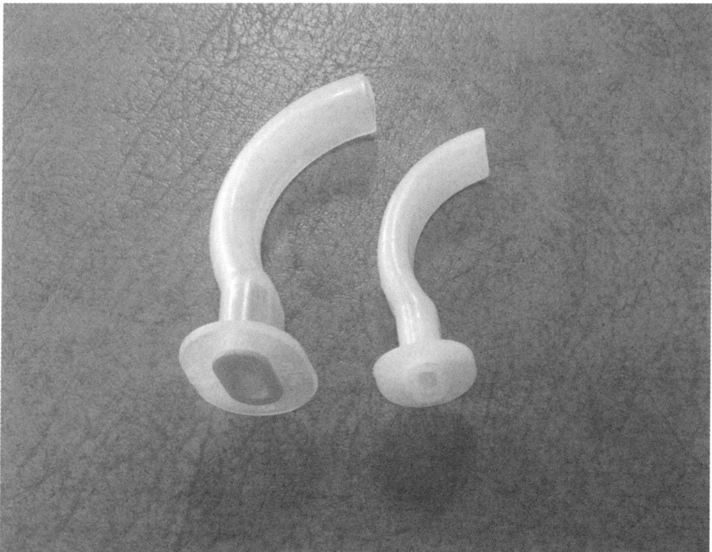

Fig. 4.13: Examples of adult- and paediatric-sized Guedel oral airways.

Choosing the correct size of oral airway is done by measuring the distance between the middle of the patient's mouth and the angle of the mandible. The oropharyngeal airway is too short if its tip ends in the middle of the cheek when measured from the middle of the mouth. If the patient's mouth is dry, the airway should be lubricated with water prior to insertion. Insertion of the oropharyngeal airway should be performed with the airway angled in the position of use, in other words in line with the curvature of the tongue, and gently slid into the mouth. If the patient's tongue poses obstruction to the insertion of the airway, use two or three wooden tongue spatulas held together and push down on the tongue to displace it anteriorly while the oropharyngeal airway is inserted.

The suction catheter is inserted through the opening on the front of the oral airway and passed down the pharynx or through the vocal cords, as necessary. The rest of the suction procedure is similar to that described for nasopharyngeal and nasotracheal suction. Oropharyngeal suction is chosen over nasopharyngeal suction in patients with fractures to the base of skull or with occluded nasal passages.

4.2.7.3. *Contraindications and precautions for suction*

Considering that all intubated patients are likely to require suctioning to maintain a patent airway and non-intubated patients may be unable to clear their airway with resultant detrimental consequences, there can be no absolute contraindications to the procedure. Special care should be taken when the following is present (Morrow and Argent, 2008; Moffatt, 2011).

- Haemoptysis or pulmonary haemorrhage.
- Suction should be considered with caution in patients with clotting derangements.
- Pulmonary oedema.
- Severe bronchospasm.
- Cardiovascular instability.
- Raised intracranial pressure.
- Pulmonary hypertension.
- Nasopharyngeal, nasotracheal and oropharyngeal suction should not be used in patients with recent oesophageal or tracheal anastomoses or tracheo-oesophageal fistula.

4.2.7.4. *Complications associated with suction* (*Moffatt, 2011*)

- Vagal nerve stimulation and resultant bradycardia and hypotension. The patient's heart rate and blood pressure should be monitored closely during the suction procedure. If these complications arise the procedure should be stopped to allow the patient to recover. Immediate assistance should be sought from the nursing or medical staff if the patient's condition continues to deteriorate.
- Hypoxaemia. The patient should be placed on oxygen therapy in between each suction pass.
- Vomiting. The patient should immediately be turned on their side to avoid vomitus from being aspirated into the lungs. The physiotherapist should suction all vomitus from the oral cavity and thereafter suspend the suction procedure until the patient stabilises.
- Bronchospasm. Immediate access to bronchodilator therapy is essential.
- Misdirection into the oesophagus. The catheter should be withdrawn and carefully re-inserted into the trachea if deep suction is required.

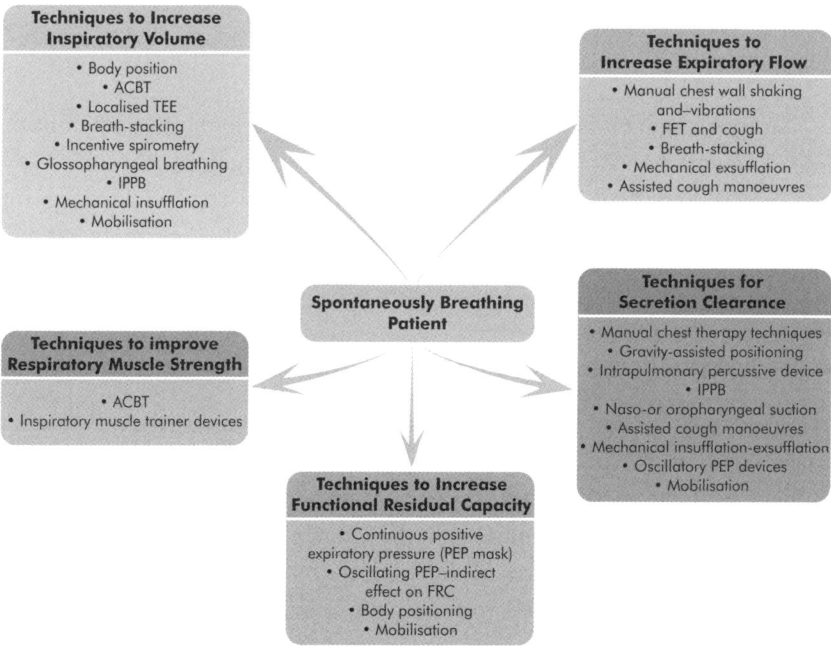

Fig. 4.14: Cardiopulmonary physiotherapy techniques and their effects on the pulmonary system when used in spontaneously breathing patients.

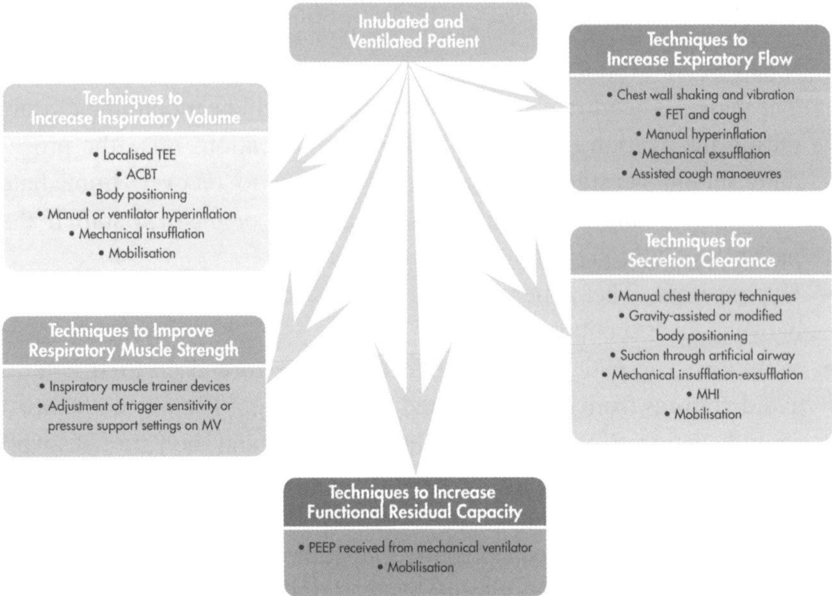

Fig. 4.15: Cardiopulmonary physiotherapy techniques and their effects on the pulmonary system when used in intubated and ventilated patients.

In conclusion of this section and as quick reference for physiotherapists, Figs 4.14 and 4.15 summarise the various cardiopulmonary physiotherapy techniques and their effects on the pulmonary system when used for patients who are spontaneously breathing or those who are intubated and ventilated.

4.3. Markers and Outcome Measures

An important component of physiotherapy patient management is regular assessment of the patient's response to treatment intervention. Various subjective and objective markers can be used to assess adult and paediatric patients' responses to treatment on a daily basis. These are appropriate for use in the trauma population. Varieties of outcome measures are available to assess patients' responses to treatment interventions over longer time periods, and these are also appropriate for use in patients who have suffered traumatic injury. Tables 4.15 and 4.16 list a selection of subjective and objective markers that can be used for patient management, both in

Table 4.15: Examples of subjective markers to assess the effectiveness of physiotherapy interventions.

Marker	Adults	Paediatrics
Patient feedback	• Verbal	• Verbal
Breathlessness	• Borg breathlessness scale (CR10) • Medical Research Council (MRC) breathlessness scale	• Visual analogue scale (VAS) for dyspnoea
Pain	• Visual Analogue Scale (10 cm) • Wong–Baker faces pain rating scale • McGill pain questionnaire (MPQ) • Numeric pain rating scale (NPRS) • Behavioural pain scale for sedated critically ill patients • Critical care pain observation tool	• Wong–Baker faces pain rating scale • CRIES scale for infants • Neonatal infants pain scale • Faces pain scale (FPS) • Riley infant pain scale
Clearance of excessive secretions	• Auscultation • Consistency, colour and volume of secretions	• Auscultation • Consistency, colour and volume of secretions
Reversal of partial or complete segmental or lobar collapse	• Auscultation	• Auscultation

Table 4.16: Examples of objective markers to assess the effectiveness of physiotherapy interventions.

Marker	Adults	Paediatrics
Changes in neurological status	• Glasgow coma scale (GCS) • Intracranial pressure value • Cerebral perfusion pressure value	• GCS • Intracranial pressure value • Cerebral perfusion pressure value
Cognitive and behavioural recovery	• Rancho Los Amigos level of cognitive function scale • Awareness questionnaire • Coma recovery scale	• Child behaviour checklist (CBCL)

(Continued)

Table 4.16. (*Continued*)

Marker	Adults	Paediatrics
Level of cooperation	• S5Q test (see Table 4.17) • GCS	• S5Q in older children • Ability to follow simple instruction (age appropriate)
Oedema of the extremities	• Tape measure	• Tape measure
Range of motion	• Goniometry	• Goniometry
Muscle length	• Thomas test (hip flexors) • Ober test (iliotibial band) • Passive straight leg raise (hamstring)	• Thomas test • Passive straight leg raise
Muscle strength (awake and cooperative patient)	• MRC scale • Manual muscle test (MMT) • Hand-held dynamometry* • PFIT	• MRC scale • Hand-held dynamometry* • MMT
Spasticity	• Ashworth and modified Ashworth scales	• Ashworth and modified Ashworth scales
Breathing pattern	• Observation	• Observation
Breathing rate, heart rate and blood pressure	• Observation of values on bedside monitor • Measurement (in absence of bedside monitor)	• Observation • Bedside monitor • Measurement
Clearance of excessive secretions	• Amount of secretions cleared during treatment	• Amount of secretions cleared during treatment
Reversal of partial or complete segmental or lobar collapse	• Thoracic expansion • Chest x-ray • Thoracic ultrasound	• Thoracic expansion • Chest x-ray • Thoracic ultrasound
Oxygenation (see Appendix II for equations)	• Peripheral oxygen saturation (SpO_2) • PaO_2/FiO_2 • $P(A–a)O_2$ • Oxygenation index	• SpO_2 • PaO_2/FiO_2 • $P(A–a)O_2$ • Oxygenation index

(*Continued*)

Table 4.16. (*Continued*)

Marker	Adults	Paediatrics
Respiratory mechanics (patient on mechanical ventilation)	• Pulmonary compliance • Tidal volumes • Airway resistance • Peak inspiratory pressure	• Pulmonary compliance • Tidal volumes • Airway resistance • Peak inspiratory pressure
Alveolar ventilation	• Capnography (end-tidal CO_2 monitoring)	• Capnography
Respiratory muscle strength	• Maximal inspiratory pressure • Maximal expiratory pressure • Peak cough flow (Measured using a pressure manometer or the mechanical ventilator)	• Maximal inspiratory pressure • Maximal expiratory pressure • Peak cough flow in older children
Exercise endurance	• PFIT • Six-step exercise test combining perceived effort with the modified Borg scale (Roos *et al.*, 2002, 2004) • Six-minute walk test • Ten-meter walk test • Three-minute step test • Treadmill test (modified Bruce protocol) • Six-minute arm test • Timed up and go test (TUG)	• Two-minute walk test • TUG • Energy expenditure index (EEI)

*It is important to note that accuracy of dynamometry measurements might be influenced by the patient's level of consciousness and ability to cooperate.

clinical practice and research (Cole *et al.*, 1995; Practice Committee, 2005; Pollack *et al.*, 2009; Rehabilitation Measures Database, 2014).

A useful method of assessing cooperation in a critically ill patient is the S5Q test. This test was described by Gosselink *et al.* (2011) and is summarised in Table 4.17.

Table 4.18 lists examples of outcome measures that may be used in clinical practice and research (Cole *et al.*, 1995; Practice Committee, 2005; Pollack *et al.*, 2009; Rehabilitation Measures Database, 2014).

Table 4.17: S5Q to evaluate cooperation in an ICU patient*.

Score	Question
1	Open and close your eyes
2	Look at me
3	Open your mouth and stick out your tongue
4	Shake yes and no (nod your head)
5	I will count to five, frown your eyebrows afterwards

*Interpretation of the S5Q score:
- S5Q = 0/5: no cooperation
- S5Q < 3/5: no to low cooperation
- S5Q = 3/5: moderate cooperation
- S5Q = 4/5: close to full cooperation
- S5Q = 5/5: full cooperation

Table 4.18: Examples of outcome measurement tools.

Outcome	Adults	Paediatrics
Functional ability in the ICU and in the ward	• Chelsea critical care physical assessment (CPAx) tool • Berg balance scale • Functional ambulation score • Functional independence measure (FIM) • Quadriplegia index of function and spinal cord independence measure • Glasgow outcomes score-extended • Clinical outcome variable scale (COVS) • Barthel index • Functional independence measure • American Spinal Injury Association (ASIA) charting	• Functional status scale (see Table 4.19) • Functional outcomes assessment grid • Bailey scales of infant development (psychomotor scale) • Alberta infant motor scale (AIMS) • Test of motor and neurological functions (TMNF) • Functional independence measure for children (WeeFIM) • King's outcome score for head injury • Gross motor function measure (GMFM) • Gross motor performance measure (GMPM) • Paediatric evaluation of disability inventory (PEDI) • Peabody gross motor scale and Peabody scales of infant development
Physical morbidity	• CPAx tool	• Functional status scale (Table 4.19) • Paediatric musculoskeletal functional health questionnaire (POSNA)

(*Continued*)

Table 4.18: (*Continued*)

Outcome	Adults	Paediatrics
Anxiety	• Burn specific anxiety scale • Hospital anxiety and depression scale (HADS)	• VAS • Hamilton anxiety rating scale (HAM-A) • Modified short state-trait anxiety inventory (STAI)
Quality of life	• Medical outcomes study short form 36 (SF-36) • Medical outcomes study short form 12 (SF-12) • EuroQol-5D (EQ-5D) • Quality of well-being • Sickness impact profile • Nottingham health profile • Community integration questionnaire • Satisfaction with life scale • Life satisfaction questionnaire • World Health Organisation QOL-BREF scale • Perceived QOL questionnaire • Global QOL questionnaire	• EQ-5DY • The paediatric quality of life inventory (PedsQL) • KIDSCREEN-27 • Childhood health assessment questionnaire (CHAQ) • Child health questionnaire (CHQ) • Health utilities index, mark 3 (HUI-3)

More information about the paediatric functional status scale is provided in Table 4.19.

4.4. Conclusion

The physiotherapy management of patients with traumatic injury in the acute care setting should be aimed at early mobilisation, prevention of respiratory complications and other complications associated with immobility and the return of the patient to optimal functional ability as they recover from injury. A variety of cardiopulmonary physiotherapy interventions were discussed and the choice of which to use should be determined by each individual patient's needs and response to treatment. This

Table 4.19: Paediatric functional status scale*.

	Normal score = 1	Mild dysfunction score = 2	Moderate dysfunction score = 3	Severe dysfunction score = 4	Very severe dysfunction score = 5
Mental status	Normal sleep/wake cycles, appropriate responsiveness	Sleepy but rousable to noise/touch/ movement and/or periods of social non-responsiveness	Lethargic and/or irritable	Minimal arousal to stimuli (stupor)	Unresponsive, coma and/or vegetative state
Sensory functioning	Intact hearing and vision and responsive to touch	Suspected hearing or vision loss	Not reactive to auditory or visual stimuli	Not reactive to auditory or visual stimuli	Abnormal responses to pain or touch
Communication	Appropriate non-crying vocalisations, interactive facial expressions or gestures	Diminished vocalisation, facial expression and/or social responsiveness	Absence of attention-getting behaviour	No demonstration of discomfort	Absence of communication

Motor functioning	Coordinated body movements, normal muscle control, awareness of action and reason	One limb functionally impaired	Two or more limbs functionally impaired	Poor head control	Diffuse spasticity, paralysis or decerebrate/ decorticate posturing
Feeding	All food taken by mouth with age-appropriate help	Nothing by mouth or need for age-inappropriate help with feeding	Oral and tube feedings	Parenteral nutrition with oral or tube feedings	All parenteral nutrition
Respiratory status	Room air and no artificial support or aids	Oxygen treatment and/or suctioning	Tracheostomy	Continuous positive airway pressure (CPAP) for all or part of the day and/ or mechanical ventilation for part of the day	Mechanical ventilatory support for the whole day and night

*Adapted from Pollack *et al*. (2009).

chapter also provided strategies for the use of exercise therapy in the acute care setting as well as markers and outcome measures to assess each patient's response to treatment. This information should equip physiotherapists with adequate knowledge to successfully manage patients with traumatic injury in the acute care setting.

Bibliography

Agostini, P., and Singh, S. (2009). Incentive spirometry following thoracic surgery: what should we be doing? *Physiotherapy,* **95**, 76–82.

Akgul, S., and Akyolcu, N. (2002). Effects of normal saline on endotracheal suctioning, *J. Clin. Nurs.,* **11**, 826–830.

American College of Sports Medicine (ACSM). (2009). Special communications: progression models in resistance training for healthy adults, *Med. Sci. Sports Exerc.,* **41**, 687–708.

American College of Sports Medicine (ACSM). (2014). *ACSM's Guidelines for Exercise Testing and Prescription*, 9th edn., Wolters Kluwer/Lippincott Williams & Wilkins, Philadelphia, PA.

American Thoracic Society/European Respiratory Society (ATS/ERS). (2002). ATS/ERS statement on respiratory muscle testing, *Am. J. Resp. Crit. Care Med,* **166**, 518–624.

Anderson, J.L., Hasney, K.M., and Beaumont, N.E. (2005). Systematic review of techniques to enhance peak cough flow and maintain vital capacity in neuromuscular disease: the case for mechanical insufflation-exsufflation, *Phys. Ther. Rev.,* **10**, 25–33.

Bailey, P., Thomson, G.E., Spuhler, V.J., *et al.* (2007). Early activity is feasible and safe in respiratory failure patients, *Crit. Care Med.,* **35**, 139–145.

Barker, M., and Adams, S. (2002). An evaluation of a single chest physiotherapy treatment on mechanically ventilated patients with acute lung injury, *Physiother. Res. Int.,* **7**, 157–169.

Berlowitz, D.J., and Tamplin, J. (2013). Respiratory muscle training for cervical spinal cord injury. *Cochrane Database Syst. Rev.,* **23**, 7: CD008507.

Berney, S., and Denehy, L. (2002). A comparison of the effects of manual and ventilator hyperinflation on static lung compliance and sputum production in intubated and ventilated intensive care patients, *Physiother. Res. Int.,* **7**, 100–108.

Berney, S., Denehy, L., and Pretto, J. (2004). Head-down tilt and manual hyperinflation enhance sputum clearance in patients who are intubated and ventilated, *Aust. J. Physiother.,* **50**, 9–14.

Berney, S., Haines, K., Skinner, E.H., *et al.* (2012). Safety and feasibility of an exercise prescription approach to rehabilitation across the continuum of care for survivors of critical illness, *Phys. Ther.,* **92,** 1524–1535.

Berti, J.S.W., Tonon, E., Ronchi, C.F., *et al.* (2012). Manual hyperinflation combined with expiratory rib cage compression for reduction of length of ICU stay in critically ill patients on mechanical ventilation, *J. Bras. Pneumol.,* **38**, 477–486.

Bott, J., Blumenthal, S., Buxton, M., *et al.* (2009). Guidelines for the physiotherapy management of the adult, medical, spontaneously breathing patient, *Thorax,* **64**, i1–i51.

Branson, R.D. (2007). Secretion management in the mechanically ventilated patient, *Respir. Care,* 52, 1328–1342.

Branson, R.D. (2013). The scientific basis for postoperative respiratory care, *Respir. Care,* **58**, 1974–1984.

Broad, M.A., Quint, M., Thomas, S., *et al.* (2012). *Cardiorespiratory Assessment of the Adult Patient: A Clinician's Guide, The Physiotherapist's Toolbox Series*, Churchill Livingstone Elsevier, London.

Bryan, A.C., Milic-Emili, J., and Pengelly, D. (1966). Effect of gravity on the distribution of pulmonary ventilation. *J. Appl. Physiol.,* **21**, 778–784.

Button, B.M., Heine, R.G., Catto-Smith, A.G., *et al.* (2003). Chest physiotherapy in infants with cystic fibrosis: to tip or not? A five-year study, *Pediatr. Pulmonol.,* **35**, 208–213.

Cader, S.A., Vale, R.G., Castro, J.C., *et al.* (2010). Inspiratory muscle training improves maximal inspiratory pressure and may assist weaning in older intubated patients: a randomised trial, *J. Physiother.,* **56**, 171–177.

Cardoso, F.E.F., De Abreu, L.C., Raimundo, R.D., *et al.* (2012). Evaluation of peak cough flow in Brazilian healthy adults, *Int. Arch. Med.,* **5**, 25. [Online] Available at: http://www.intarchmed.com/content/5/1/25 [Accessed 13 November 2014].

Carpenter, T. (2004). Novel approaches in conventional mechanical ventilation for paediatric acute lung injury, *Paediatr. Respir. Rev.,* **5**, 231–237.

Caruso, P., Denari, S.D.C., Al Ruiz, S., *et al.* (2005). Inspiratory muscle training is ineffective in mechanically ventilated critically ill patients, *Clinics (Sao Paulo),* **60**, 479–484.

Casado-Flores, J., Martinez de Azagra, A., Ruiz-Lopez, M.J., *et al.* (2002). Pediatric ARDS: effect of supine-prone postural changes on oxygenation, *Intensive Care Med.,* **28**, 1792–1796.

Choi, J.S., and Jones, A.Y. (2005). Effects of manual hyperinflation and suctioning in respiratory mechanics in mechanically ventilated patients with ventilator associated pneumonia, *Aust. J. Physiother.,* **51**, 25–30.

Cole, B., Finch, E., Gowland, C., *et al.* (1995). *Physical Rehabilitation Outcome Measures*, Williams & Wilkins, Baltimore, MD.

Condessa, R.L., Brauner, J.S., Saul, A.L., *et al.* (2013). Inspiratory muscle training did not accelerate weaning from mechanical ventilation but did improve tidal volume and maximal respiratory pressures: a randomised trial, *J. Physiother.*, **59**, 101–107.

Conroy, B., and Earle, R.W. (2000). 'Bone, muscle and connective tissue adaptations to physical activity', in Baechle, T.R., and Earle, R.W. (eds), *Essentials of Strength Training and Conditioning: National Strength and Conditioning Association*, 2nd edn., Human Kinetics, Champaign, IL, pp. 57–72.

Curley, M.A., Hibberd, P.L., Fineman, L.D., *et al.* (2005). Effect of prone positioning on clinical outcomes in children with acute lung injury: a randomized controlled trial, *JAMA,* **294**, 229–237.

Dammeyer, J., Dickinson, S., Packard, D., *et al.* (2013). Building a protocol to guide mobility in the ICU, *Crit. Care Nurse,* **36**, 37–49.

Davies, H., Kitchman, R., Gordon, I., *et al.* (1985). Regional ventilation in infancy, *N. Engl. J. Med.,* **313**, 1626–1628.

De Godoy, A.C., Yokota, C. de O., Araújo, I.I., *et al.* (2011). Can manual hyperinflation manoeuvres cause aspiration of oropharyngeal secretions in patients under mechanical ventilation? *Rev. Bras. Anestesiol.,* **61**, 556–560.

De Godoy, V.C.W.P., Zanetti, N.M., and Johnston, C. (2013). Manual hyperinflation in airway clearance in pediatric patients: a systematic review, *Rev. Bras. Ter. Intensiva.,* **25**, 258–262.

Dennis, D., Jacob, W., and Budgeon, C. (2012). Ventilator versus manual hyperinflation in clearing sputum in ventilated intensive care unit patients, *Anaesth. Intensive Care,* **40**, 142–149.

Dias, C.M., Plácido, T.R., Ferreira, M.F.B., *et al.* (2008). Incentive spirometry and breath stacking: effects on the inspiratory capacity of individuals submitted to abdominal surgery, *Braz. J. Physiother.,* **12**, 94–99.

Elrauf, A.A. (2010). *Physiotherapy Guidelines for Manual Hyperinflation.* NHS Lothian University Hospitals Division Children's services. [Online] Available at: www.scribd.com/doc/97908818/Physiotherapy-Guidelines-for-Manual-Hyperinflation [Accessed 22 July 2014].

Emery, J.R., and Peabody, J.L. (1983). Head position affects intracranial pressure in newborn infants, *J. Pediatr.,* **103**, 950–953.

Fan, E. (2012). Critical illness neuromyopathy and the role of physical therapy and rehabilitation in critically ill patients, *Respir. Care,* **57**, 933–946.

Finder, J.D. (2010). Airway clearance modalities in neuromuscular disease, *Paediatr. Resp. Rev.,* **11**, 31–34.

Frerichs, I., Schiffmann, H., Oehler, R., *et al.* (2003). Distribution of lung ventilation in spontaneously breathing neonates lying in different body positions, *Intensive Care Med.,* **29**, 787–794.

Frownfelter, D., and Dean, E. (2006). *Cardiovascular and Pulmonary Physical Therapy: Evidence and Practice*, 4th edn., Mosby Elsevier, Philadelphia, PA.

Fuller, B.M., Mohr, N.M., Drewry, A.M., *et al.* (2013) Lower tidal volume at initiation of mechanical ventilation may reduce progression to acute respiratory distress syndrome: a systematic review, *Crit. Care,* **17**, R11. [Online] Available at: http://ccforum.com/content/17/1/R11 [Accessed 22 July 2014].

Gattinoni, L., Taccone, P., Carlesso, E., *et al.* (2014). Prone position in acute respiratory distress syndrome: rationale, indications and limits, *Am. J. Respir. Crit. Care Med.,* **188**, 1286–1293.

Gillies, D., Wells, D., and Bhandari, A.P. (2012). Positioning for acute respiratory distress in hospitalised infants and children, *Cochrane Database Syst. Rev.,* **7**, CD003645.

Gosselink, R., Bott, J., Johnson, M., *et al.* (2008). Physiotherapy for adult patients with critical illness: recommendations of the European respiratory society and European society of intensive care medicine task force on physiotherapy for critically ill patients, *Intensive Care Med.,* **34**, 1188–1199.

Gosselink, R., Clerckx, B., Robbeets, C., *et al.* (2011). Review: physiotherapy in the intensive care unit, *Neth. J. Crit. Care,* **15,** 66–75.

Gregson, R.K., Stocks, J., Petley, G.W., *et al.* (2007). Simultaneous measures of force and respiratory profiles during chest physiotherapy in ventilated children, *Physiol. Meas.,* **28**, 1017–1028.

Gregson, R.K., Shannon, H., Stocks, J., *et al.* (2012). The unique contribution of manual chest compression-vibrations to airflow during physiotherapy in sedated, fully ventilated children, *Pediatr. Crit. Care Med.,* **13**, e97–e102.

Guérin, C., Bourdin, G., Leray, V., *et al.* (2011). Performance of the CoughAssist insufflation-exsufflation device in the presence of an endotracheal tube or tracheostomy tube: a bench study, *Respir. Care,* **56,** 1108–1114.

Guimarães, F.S., and Zin, W.A. (2008). Thoracic percussion yields reversible mechanical changes in healthy subjects. *Eur. Appl. Physiol.,* **104**, 601–607.

Hanekom, S.D., Gosselink, R., Dean, E., *et al.* (2011). The development of a clinical management algorithm for early physical activity and mobilisation of critically ill patients: synthesis of evidence and expert opinion and its translation into clinical practice, *Clin. Rehabil.,* **25**, 771–787.

Harman, E. (2000). 'The biomechanics of resistance exercise', in Baechle, T.R., and Earle, R.W. (eds), *Essentials of Strength Training and Conditioning: National Strength and Conditioning Association*, 2nd edn., Human Kinetics, Champaign, IL, pp. 25–56.

Heaf, D., Helms, P., Gordon, I., *et al.* (1983). Postural effects on gas exchange in infants, *N. Engl. J. Med.,* **308**, 1505–1508.

Hough, J.L., Johnston, L., Brauer, S.G., *et al.* (2012). Effect of body position on ventilation distribution in preterm infants on continuous positive airway pressure, *Pediatr. Crit. Care Med.,* **13**, 446–451.

Ji, Y.R., Kim, H.S., and Park, J.H. (2002). Instillation of normal saline before suctioning in patients with pneumonia, *Yonsei Med. J.,* **43**, 607–612.

Jongerden, I.P., Rovers, M.M., Grypdonck, M.H., *et al.* (2007). Open and closed endotracheal systems in mechanically ventilated intensive care patients — a meta-analysis, *Crit. Care Med.,* **35**, 260–270.

Kacmarek, R.M., Stoller, J.K., and Heuer, A.J. (2013). *Egan's Fundamentals of Respiratory Care*, 10th edn, Elsevier, St. Louis, MO.

Kayambu, G., Boots, R., and Paratz, J. (2013). Physical therapy for the critically ill in ICU: a systematic review and meta-analysis, *Crit. Care Med.,* **41**, 1543–1554.

Kigin, C.M. (1981). Chest physical therapy for the postoperative or traumatic injury patient, *Phys. Ther.,* **61**, 1724–1736.

Kirstensen, J., and Franklyn-Miller, A. (2012). Resistance training in musculoskeletal rehabilitation: a systematic review, *Br. J. Sports Med.,* **46**, 719–726.

Kocan, M.J., and Lietz, H. (2013). Special considerations for mobilising patients in the neurointensive care unit, *Crit. Care Nurs.,* **36**, 50–55.

Kornecki, A., Frndova, H., Coates, A.L., *et al.* (2001). A randomized trial of prolonged prone positioning in children with acute respiratory failure, *Chest,* **119**, 211–218.

Knight, J., Nigam, Y., and Jones, A. (2009a). *Effects of Bed Rest 1: Cardiovascular, Respiratory and Haematological Systems.* Nursing Times. [Online] Available at: http://www.nursingtimes.net/nursing-practice/clinical-zones/cardiology/effects-of-bedrest-1-cardiovascular-respiratory-and-haematological-systems/5002005.article [Accessed 15 March 2014].

Knight, J., Nigam, Y., and Jones, A. (2009b). *Effects of Bed Rest 2: Gastrointestinal, Endocrine, Renal, Reproductive and Nervous Systems.* Nursing Times. [Online] Available at: http://www.nursingtimes.net/nursing-practice/clinical-zones/gastroenterology/effects-of-bedrest-2-gastrointestinal-endocrine-renal-reproductive-and-nervous-systems/5002434.article [Accessed 15 March 2014].

Knight, J., Nigam, Y., and Jones, A. (2009c). *Effects of Bed Rest 3: Musculoskeletal and Immune Systems, Skin and Self-Perception.* Nursing Times. [Online] Available at: http://www.nursingtimes.net/effects-of-bedrest-3-musculoskeletal-and-immune-systems-skin-and-self-perception/5003298.article [Accessed 15 March 2014].

Krause, M.W., Van Aswegen, H., and De Wet, E.H. (2000). Postural drainage in intubated patients with acute lobar atelectasis: a pilot study, *S. Afr. J. Physiother.,* **56**, 29–32.

Lewis, L.K., Williams, M.T., and Olds, T.S. (2012). The active cycle of breathing technique: a systematic review and meta- analysis, *Respir. Med.,* **106**, 155–172.

Lupton-Smith, A., Argent, A.C., Rimensberger, P., *et al.* (2014). Challenging a paradigm: positional changes in ventilation distribution are highly variable in healthy infants and children. *Pediatr. Pulmonol.,* **49**, 764–771.

Maa, S.H., Hung, T.J., Hsu, K.H., *et al.* (2005). Manual hyperinflation improves alveolar recruitment in difficult-to-wean patients, *Chest,* **128**, 2714–2721.

MacMahon, C. (1915). Breathing and physical exercises for use in cases of wounds in the pleura, lung and diaphragm, *Lancet,* **2**, 769–770.

Main, E., Castle, R., Newham, D., *et al.* (2004). Respiratory physiotherapy vs. suction: the effects on respiratory function in ventilated infants and children, *Intensive Care Med.,* **30**, 1144–1151.

Maltais, F. (2011). Glossopharyngeal breathing, *Am. J. Respir. Crit. Care Med.,* **184**, 381.

Marini, J.J., Rodriguez, R.M. and Lamb, V.J. (1986). Involuntary breath-stacking. An alternative method for vital capacity estimation in poorly cooperative subjects, *Am Rev Respir Dis.,* **134**, 694–698.

Marraro, G.A. (2003). Innovative practices of ventilatory support with pediatric patients, *Pediatr. Crit. Care Med.,* **4**, 8–20.

Martin, A.D., Smith, B.K., Davenport, P., *et al.* (2011). Inspiratory muscle strength training improves weaning outcome in failure to wean patients: a randomized trial, *Crit. Care,* **15**, R84. [Online] Available at: http://ccforum.com/content/15/2/R84 [Accessed 15 November 2014].

McCarren, B., Alison, J.A., and Herbert, R.D. (2006a). Manual vibration increases expiratory flow rate via increases intrapleural pressure in healthy adults: an experimental study, *Aust. J. Physiother.,* **52**, 267–271.

McCarren. B., Alison, J.A., and Herbert, R.D. (2006b). Vibration and its effect on the respiratory system, *Aust. J. Physiother.,* **52**, 39–43.

McCool, F.D., and Rosen, M.J. (2006). Nonpharmacologic airway clearance therapies: ACCP evidence-based clinical practice guidelines, *Chest,* **129** [Suppl], S250–S259.

McCord, J., Krull, N., Kraiker, J., *et al.* (2013). Cardiopulmonary physiotherapy practice in the paediatric intensive care unit, *Physiother. Can.,* **65**, 374–377.

McCrory, D.C., Samsa, G.P., Hamilton, B.B., *et al.* (2001). *Treatment of Pulmonary Disease following Cervical Spinal Cord Injury: Evidence Report/*

Technology Assessment no. 27. Publication no 01-E014. Agency for Healthcare Research and Quality, Washington, DC.

Mestriner, R.G., Fernandes, R.O., Steffen, L.C., *et al.* (2009). Optimum design parameters for a therapist-constructed positive-expiratory-pressure therapy bottle device, *Respir. Care,* **54**, 504–508.

Moffatt, F. (2011). *Guideline for Adult Nasal and Oropharyngeal Suction.* Nottingham University Hospitals NHS Trust. [Online] Available at: https://www.nuh.nhs.uk/handlers/downloads.ashx?id=50628 [Accessed 23 July 2014].

Morris, P.E., Goad, A., Thompson, C., *et al.* (2008). Early intensive care unit mobility therapy in the treatment of acute respiratory failure, *Crit. Care Med.,* **36**, 2238–2243.

Morrow, B., and Argent, A. (2008). A comprehensive review of pediatric endotracheal suctioning: effects, indications and clinical practice, *Pediatr. Crit. Care Med.,* **9**, 465–477.

Morrow, B.M., Mowzer, R., Pitcher, R., *et al.* (2012). Investigation into the effect of closed-system suctioning on the frequency of pediatric ventilator-associated pneumonia in a developing country, *Pediatr. Crit. Care Med.,* **13**, e25–e32.

Morrow, B., Zampoli, M., Van Aswegen, H., *et al.* (2013). Mechanical insufflation-exsufflation for people with neuromuscular disorders, *Cochrane Database Syst. Rev.,* **12**, CD010044.

National Institute of Health, Critical Care Therapy and Respiratory Care Section. (2000). *Intrapulmonary Percussive Ventilation.* Critical Care Medicine Department. [Online] Available at: http://clinicalcenter.nih.gov/ccmd/cctrcs/pdf_docs/Bronchial%20Hygiene/03-Intrapul.Percussive.pdf [Accessed 23 April 2014].

O'Donnell, C.P., Davis, P.G., and Morley, C.J. (2003). Resuscitation of premature infants: what are we doing wrong and can we do better? *Biol. Neonate,* **84**, 76–82.

O'Sullivan, S.B., and Schmitz, T.J. (2001). *Physical Rehabilitation. Assessment and Treatment*, 4th edn., F.A. Davis Company, Philadelphia, PA.

Oh, H., and Seo, W. (2003). A meta-analysis of the effects of various interventions in preventing endotracheal suction- induced hypoxaemia, *J. Clin. Nurs.,* **12**, 912–924.

Orman, J., and Westerdahl, E. (2010). Chest physiotherapy with positive expiratory pressure breathing after abdominal and thoracic surgery: a systematic review, *Acta Anaesthesiol. Scand.,* **54**, 261–267.

Park, H.Y., Ha, S.Y., Lee, S.H., *et al.* (2013). Repeated derecruitments accentuate lung injury during mechanical ventilation, *Crit. Care Med.,* **41**, e423–e30.

Paulus, F., Binnekade, J.M., Vermeulen, M., *et al.* (2010). Manual hyperinflation is associated with a low rate of adverse events when performed by experienced and trained nurses in stable critically ill patients — a prospective observational study, *Minerva Anestesiol.,* **76,** 1036–1042.

Pedersen, C.M., Rosendahl-Nielsen, M., Hjermind, J., *et al.* (2009). Review: endotracheal suctioning of the adult intubated patient — what is the evidence? *Int. Crit. Care Nurs.,* **25**, 21–30.

Pham, T., Yuill, M., Dakin, C., *et al.* (2011). Regional ventilation distribution in the first 6 months of life, *Eur. Respir. J.,* **37**, 919–924.

Pollack, M.M., Holubkov, R., Glass, P., *et al.* (2009). Functional status scale: new pediatric outcome measure, *Pediatrics,* **124**, e18–e28.

Practice Committee. (2005). *List of Assessment Tools Used in Pediatric Physical Therapy*. Section on Pediatrics. [Online] Available at: http://otpt13.wikispaces.com/file/view/AssessScreenTools_used+by+pedi+PT_r05.pdf [Accessed 18 March 2014].

Pryor, J.A., Prasad, S.A., Bethune, D., *et al.* (2008). 'Physiotherapy techniques', in Pryor, J.A., and Prasad, S.A. (eds), *Physiotherapy for Respiratory and Cardiac Problems: Adults and Paediatrics*, 4th edn., Churchill Livingstone Elsevier, Edinburgh, pp. 134–206.

Rehabilitation Measures Database. (2014). *The Rehabilitation Clinician's Place to Find the Best Instruments to Screen Patients and Monitor their Progress.* Rehabilitation Measures Database. [Online] Available at: http://www.rehabmeasures.org/ [Accessed 18 March 2014].

Reper, P., and Van Looy, K. (2013). Letter to the editor: chest physiotherapy using intrapulmonary percussive ventilation to treat persistent atelectasis in hypoxic patients after smoke inhalation, *Burns,* **39**, 192–193.

Ridley, S.C., and Heinl-Green, A. (2002). 'Surgery for adults', in Pryor, J.A., and Prasad, A. (eds), *Physiotherapy for Respiratory and Cardiac Problems: Adults and Paediatrics*, 3rd edn., Churchill Livingstone Elsevier, Edinburgh, pp. 377–420.

Ridling, D.A., Martin, L.D., and Bratton, S.L. (2003). Endotracheal suctioning with or without instillation of isotonic sodium chloride solution in critically ill children, *Am. J. Crit. Care,* **12**, 212–219.

Riedel, T., Richards, T., and Schibler, A. (2005). The value of electrical impedance tomography in assessing the effect of body position and positive airway pressures on regional lung ventilation in spontaneously breathing subjects, *Intensive Care Med.,* **31,** 1522–1528.

Roos, R., Van Aswegen, H., and Eales, C.J. (2002). Perceived effort of functional activities after a period of mechanical ventilation, *S. Afr. J. Physiother.,* **58**, 33–36.

Roos, R., Van Aswegen, H., Eales, C.J., *et al.* (2004). Exercise testing of patients after a period of prolonged mechanical ventilation. *S. Afr. J. Physiother.,* **60**, 27–35.

Savian, C., Chan, P., and Paratz, J. (2005). The effect of positive end-expiratory pressure level on peak expiratory flow during manual hyperinflation, *Anesth. Analg.,* **100**, 1112–1116.

Schibler, A., Yuill, M., Parsley, C., *et al.* (2009). Regional ventilation distribution in non-sedated spontaneously breathing newborns and adults is not different, *Pediatr. Pulmonol.,* **44**, 851–858.

Schmitt, J.K., Stiens, S., Trincher, R., *et al.* (2007). Survey of use of the insufflator-exsufflator in patients with spinal cord injury, *J. Spinal Cord Med.,* **30**, 127–130.

Schweickert, W.D., Pohlman, M.C., Pohlman, A.S., *et al.* (2009). Early physical and occupational therapy in mechanically ventilated, critically ill patients: a randomised controlled trial, *Lancet,* **373**, 1874–1882.

Sehlin, M., Öhberg, F., Johansson, G., *et al.* (2007). Physiological responses to positive expiratory pressure breathing: a comparison of the PEP bottle and the PEP mask, *Respir. Care,* **52**, 1000–1005.

Singer, M., Vermaat, J., Hall, G., *et al.* (1994). Hemodynamic effects of manual hyperinflation in critically mechanically ventilated patients, *Chest,* **106,** 1182–1187.

Stiller, K. (2000). Physiotherapy in intensive care: towards an evidence-based practice, *Chest,* **118**, 1801–1813.

Stiller, K. (2013). Physiotherapy in intensive care: an updated systematic review, *Chest,* **144**, 825–847.

Ströhle, A. (2009). Physical activity, exercise, depression and anxiety disorders, *J. Neural. Transm.,* **116**, 777–784.

Toussaint, M. (2011). The use of mechanical insufflation-exsufflation via artificial airways, *Respir. Care,* **56**, 1217–1219.

Truong, A.D., Fan, E., Brower, R.G., *et al.* (2009). Bench-to-bedside review: mobilizing patients in the intensive care unit — from pathophysiology to clinical trials, *Crit Care,* **13**, 216. [Online] Available at: http://ccforum.com/content/13/4/216 [Accessed 15 November 2014].

Van Aswegen, H., Van Aswegen, A., Du Raan, H., *et al.* (2013). Airflow distribution with manual hyperinflation as assessed through gamma camera imaging: a crossover randomised trial, *Physiotherapy,* **99**, 107–112.

Vargas, F., Bui, H.N., Boyer, A., *et al.* (2005). Intrapulmonary percussive ventilation in acute exacerbations of COPD patients with mild respiratory acidosis: a randomized controlled trial, *Crit. Care,* **9**, R382–R389.

Vigen, R., Ayers, C., Willis, B., *et al.* (2012). Association of cardiorespiratory fitness with total, cardiovascular and non-cardiovascular mortality across 3 decades of follow-up in men and women, *Circ. Cardiovasc. Qual. Outcomes,* **5,** 358–364.

Vivian-Beresford, A., King, C., and MacCauley, H. (1987). Neonatal post-extubation complications: the preventative role of physiotherapy, *Physiother. Can.*, **39**, 184–190.

Warburton, D.E.R., Nicol, C.W., and Bredin, S.S.D. (2006). Prescribing exercise as preventive therapy, *Can. Med. Assoc. J.*, **174,** 961–975.

Westerdahl, E., Lindmark, B., Eriksson, T., *et al.* (2005). Deep breathing exercises reduce atelectasis and improve pulmonary function after coronary artery bypass surgery, *Chest,* **128**, 3482–3488.

Wolthuis, E.K., Choi, G., Dessing, M.C., *et al.* (2008). Mechanical ventilation with lower tidal volumes and positive end-expiratory pressure prevents pulmonary inflammation in patients without preexisting lung injury, *Anesthesiology,* **108**, 46–54.

Woodward, F.H., and Jones, M. (2002). 'Intensive care for the critically ill adult', in Pryor, J.A., and Prasad, A. (eds), *Physiotherapy for Respiratory and Cardiac Problems: Adults and Paediatrics*, 3rd edn., Churchill Livingstone Elsevier, Edinburgh, pp. 347–373.

Zafiropoulos, B., Alison, J.A., and McCarren, B. (2004). Physiological responses to the early mobilisation of the intubated, ventilated abdominal surgery patient, *Aust. J. Physiother.,* **50**, 95–100.

Chapter 5

Blunt and Penetrating Injuries

*Written by H. van Aswegen,
B.M. Morrow and E. van Aswegen*

Trauma in the form of motor vehicle and pedestrian vehicle crashes, falls from a height, gunshot or stab wounds or physical abuse often result in blunt (non-penetrating) or penetrating injuries to the thoracic cage and/or abdominal organs.

In this chapter information is shared about:

- The causes and mechanisms of blunt or penetrating abdominal or thoracic injuries.
- The complications associated with abdominal or thoracic injuries.
- The medical and surgical management of patients with blunt or penetrating abdominal or thoracic injuries.
- The physiotherapy aims for the management of patients with such injuries in the intensive care unit and surgical or trauma ward.
- The contraindications and precautions related to the physiotherapy management of patients with blunt or penetrating abdominal or thoracic injuries.
- The physiotherapy interventions for patients who have suffered blunt or penetrating trauma.
- Adult and paediatric clinical case scenarios.

5.1. Causes and Mechanisms of Injury

Injuries may be classified according to the site(s) and mechanism(s) of injury. Abdominal and thoracic trauma can be classified according to site as skeletal, pulmonary, heart and great vessels, visceral or diaphragmatic injury; and the mechanisms may be blunt or penetrating injury types. Blunt injuries result from forces distributed over a relatively large area and include deceleration or compression injuries. With penetrating injuries, forces are generally distributed over a small area and the organs injured are usually those that lie along the path of the penetrating object.

Abdominal or thoracic injuries, in the form of blunt or penetrating trauma, are often caused by falls from a height, motor vehicle and motor cycle crashes, pedestrian vehicle crashes, violence or attempted suicide. The epidemiology of thoracic and abdominal trauma varies according to social, economic, cultural and geographical characteristics (Herrera and Langer, 2008). A positive blood alcohol level and the use of drugs remain the highest risk factors for motor cycle, motor vehicle and pedestrian vehicle crashes, as well as for intentional injury caused to others or one-self (Carrasco *et al.*, 2012; Brady and Li, 2013). Children are particularly vulnerable to trauma due to their physical size (smaller bodies result in a greater distribution of force), improper restraining in motor vehicles and issues of neglect or overt violence or abuse (Van As, 2010).

5.1.1. *Penetrating injuries*

Damage caused to the trunk by a penetrating object depends on the shape, size and velocity of the object, as well as the distance between the object and the person. The severity of a bullet injury is directly proportional to the amount of kinetic energy that is delivered to the tissues. The mortality associated with gunshot wounds is eight times higher than that of stab wounds (De Groot and Van Oppell, 2003).

5.1.1.1. *Low-velocity injuries*

Low-velocity penetrating injuries from civilian gunshot wounds or stab wounds damage only those tissues with which they come into direct contact. Axe or machete wounds cause extensive superficial damage without a great deal of internal injury (De Groot and Van Oppell, 2003). Disintegrating bullets are designed to break into small pieces upon contact with a surface harder than the bullet itself. Non-disintegrating bullets do not deliver significant kinetic energy to the tissues and cause less damage than disintegrating bullets. The path that handgun bullets follow through the body is unpredictable due to their low velocity and deflection may occur through bone or parenchymal organs such as the liver (Clarke, 2003; Livingstone and Hauser, 2004).

5.1.1.2. *High-velocity injuries*

High-velocity wounds can be caused by fragments of explosive devices such as grenades, bombs or high-velocity bullets from machine guns or rifles. High-velocity bullets cause damage to tissues in the path of the bullet, but also to remote organs. Shock waves radiate from the missile tract through the tissues, forcing them to accelerate violently forwards and outwards. A large cavity is formed that is larger than the diameter of the missile (Maiden, 2009; Hauer *et al*., 2011). This creates a vacuum that sucks debris, air and bacteria from the external environment into the primary missile tract and the cavity collapses over a period of a few milliseconds. Blood vessel and nerve damage, as well as shattering of bones, may result without these structures being directly hit by the bullet (Feliciano, 2004; Maiden, 2009; Hauer *et al*., 2011).

Penetrating abdominal and thoracic trauma is much less common than blunt trauma in the paediatric age group (Kadish, 2006; Saladina and Lund, 2006). However, the incidence of gunshot and stab injuries in children and adolescents is increasing at alarming rates in the US and South Africa (Prinsloo *et al*., 2012; Schecter *et al*., 2012), with unchanged rates of injury reported from the United Kingdom (Melling *et al*., 2012).

5.1.2. *Abdominal injury*

5.1.2.1. *Abdominal injury in adults*

Blunt abdominal trauma can result from direct injury, such as the rim of a steering wheel forced into the abdomen during a head-on motor vehicle collision or a tightly drawn seatbelt. These mechanisms can result in a crushing injury, in which the bowel is forced against the vertebral column, or a bursting injury, in which there is a sudden increase in pressure in the bowel. Indirect blunt injury to the abdomen can result from abrupt deceleration injury (fall from a height), with shearing forces causing injury next to sites of fixation of the bowel or solid viscera (Thomson, 2003).

The size of an abdominal organ and its contact with the anterior abdominal wall determine the frequency with which the organ is wounded. The most commonly injured organs are the abdomen, liver, small bowel (most commonly) and the colon (Feliciano, 2003; Thomson, 2003). Abdominal vascular injuries are common following penetrating trunk trauma. Abdominal injuries may accompany chest wounds or vice versa (Feliciano, 2003; Thomson, 2003).

Penetrating abdominal injuries are not immediately life threatening unless a major blood vessel is damaged. Stab wounds to the abdomen are easier to manage than those to the chest and involve injury to the major abdominal vasculature only 10% of the time (Feliciano, 2003). Stab wounds to the back are often accompanied by abdominal injuries. A gunshot wound that penetrates a major artery or vein and the colon is potentially lethal, initially due to haemorrhage and subsequently due to sepsis through the possible contamination of either the vascular wound repair site or the peritoneum (Feliciano, 2004).

5.1.2.2. *Abdominal injury in paediatrics*

Abdominal injuries affect 10–15% of injured children, with the spleen being the most affected organ (Gaines, 2009). Abdominal injuries are a marker of severe trauma in children (Coppola and Gilbert, 2011).

Children are at greater risk of abdominal injury following blunt trauma than adults because of their immature musculoskeletal system (Saladina and Lund, 2006). Children have less soft tissue to absorb the energy transmitted by a traumatic impact; incomplete ossification of the bony skeleton provides less protection to underlying viscera; and the pelvis is small and immature (Gaines, 2009). Another predisposing factor to severe paediatric abdominal injury is the smaller size of children, which results in abdominal organs being closely packed together. A force applied to the abdomen is distributed over a small surface area overlying a number of organs, increasing the risk of injury to multiple structures (Saladina and Lund, 2006; Zamakhshary and Wales, 2008). The spleen and liver are the most commonly injured abdominal organs in children, as they are more anterior and less protected by musculature than in adults, as well as the kidneys, which are more mobile and therefore less protected (Saladina and Lund, 2006; Klein, 2011). The presence of a seat belt sign (bruising of the abdominal wall by the lap belt) correlates with bowel injury in children following motor vehicle accidents, but its absence does not exclude abdominal injury (Chidester *et al.*, 2009; Klein, 2011).

5.1.3. *Thoracic injury*

5.1.3.1. *Thoracic injury in adults*

The severity of injury resulting from thoracic trauma relates to the fundamental importance of the organs and physiological systems situated within the thoracic cavity.

Blunt thoracic trauma involves injuries such as fractured ribs, haemothorax, pneumothorax and pulmonary contusion. High-speed deceleration trauma may lead to cardiac, aortic, diaphragmatic and bronchial injuries. Myocardial contusion may accompany up to 76% of blunt thoracic injuries and, if diagnosed quickly, has a low mortality rate (Bansal *et al.*, 2005). Diaphragmatic rupture occurs in less than 10% of victims of motor vehicle accidents. The left hemi-diaphragm ruptures more frequently than the right hemi-diaphragm, which is protected by the liver (Chughtai *et al.*, 2009).

Penetrating injuries of the chest are the most lethal of injuries. The site and size of the wound to the chest wall determines the condition of the patient. The patient's capacity to ventilate depends on the subsequent ability to sustain a negative intrapleural pressure (due to air leak from the lung into the pleural space), the extent of the parenchymal injury and oxygen delivery to the tissues (ventilation/perfusion (V/Q) ratio) (De Groot and Van Oppell, 2003). Pneumothoraces, lung collapse, diaphragmatic rupture and cardiovascular injury may all contribute to severe respiratory distress, which can be life threatening if left unattended (Livingstone and Hauser, 2004).

5.1.3.2. *Thoracic injury in paediatrics*

Paediatric thoracic trauma differs from adult thoracic trauma in terms of the mechanism and type of injury and the frequency of other organ system involvement (Kadish, 2006). Blunt trauma accounts for the vast majority (about 80%) of thoracic injuries in children (Herrera and Langer, 2008), although, unfortunately, penetrating trauma also occurs (Figs 5.1 and 5.2). The most common thoracic injuries in children are pulmonary contusions, pneumothorax (Fig. 5.3) or haemothorax and fractures. Lacerations of the heart, great vessels and lungs are relatively uncommon (Kadish, 2006). *Commotio cordis* is a rare occurence unique to paediatric thoracic trauma, in which sudden death follows discrete blunt chest trauma. It is postulated that an abrupt strike to the chest will, in some children, results in dysrhythmia followed by rapid cardiovascular collapse (heart- and vessel-related factors that lead to sudden reduction in effective blood flow) (Bliss and Silen, 2002).

Although the pliable cartilaginous rib cage in children makes rib fractures less common than in adults, it also results in the thorax being more vulnerable to serious injury (Kadish, 2006; Klein, 2011). The anterior ribs can actually be compressed to meet the posterior ribs on impact, resulting in severe pulmonary contusions, even without any rib fractures or other

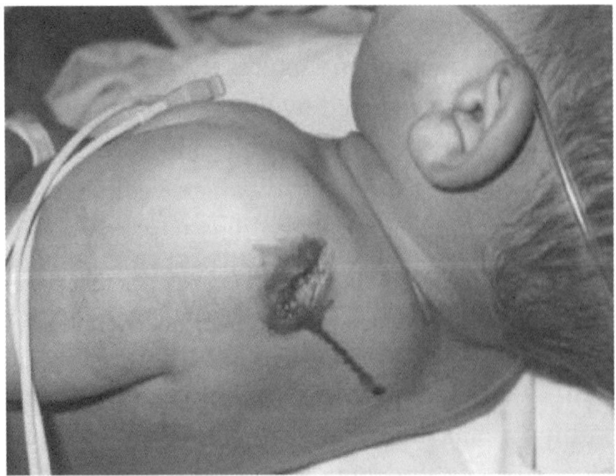

Fig. 5.1: One-year-old child hit by a stray bullet to the chest, whilst asleep at home. Photo courtesy of Prof. A.B. van As, with permission.

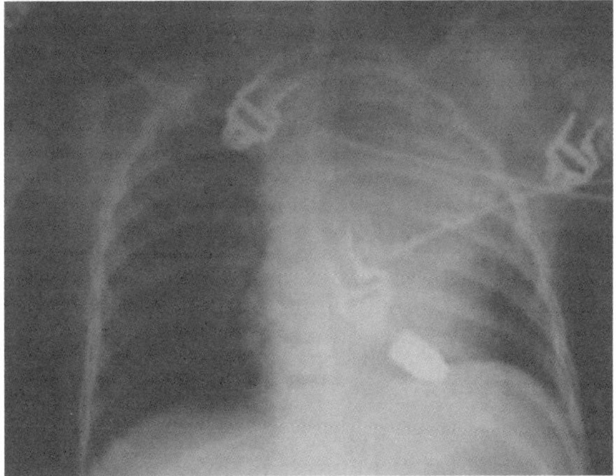

Fig. 5.2: Chest x-ray showing a bullet close to the heart of a young child. Courtesy of Prof. A.B. van As, with permission.

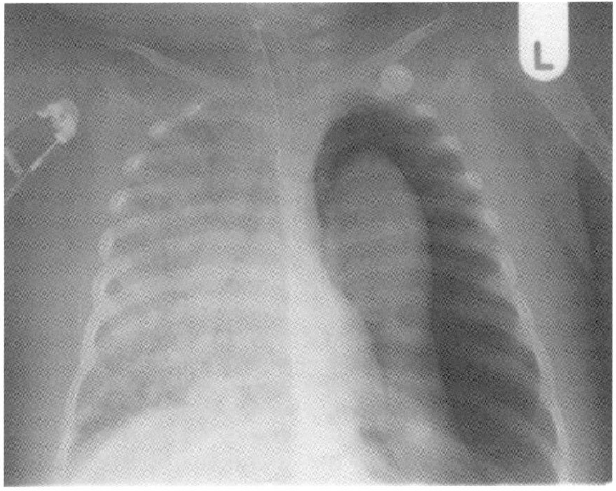

Fig. 5.3: Chest x-ray of a child with a traumatic left-sided tension pneumothorax.

external evidence of trauma such as bruising (Bliss and Silen, 2002; Kadish, 2006; Tovar, 2008). Air and/or fluid in the pleural space more easily displaces the mobile mediastinum in children than adults, predisposing to tension situations with compromised venous return and cardiac output (Kadish, 2006). In children, thoracic trauma is frequently associated with abdominal trauma because of the close proximity of the chest and abdominal cavities (Kadish, 2006). Up to 12% of children will have abdominal injuries following blunt trauma (Zamakhshary and Wales, 2008).

5.2. Causes of Fatality after Abdominal or Thoracic Injuries

On-scene fatality due to traumatic injuries is high in the adult population. Death at the scene is greater with high-energy injuries (motor cycle, motor vehicle or pedestrian vehicle accidents; falls from a height; gunshot or stab injuries) than low-energy injuries (falls from low height), and mostly occurs due to traumatic brain injuries, high-level spinal cord injuries or severe blood loss from injury to the great vessels. In-hospital deaths in adults after trauma-related injuries are usually as a result of hypotension, respiratory distress or low admission Glasgow coma score (GCS) (less than eight) (Søreide *et al.*, 2007; Evans *et al.*, 2010).

In-hospital complications of thoracic and abdominal injuries may arise from impairment of cardiac output or gaseous exchange. Impaired cardiac output occurs due to blood loss, increased intrapleural pressures, blood in the pericardial sac, myocardial valve damage or vascular disruption. Impaired gaseous exchange develops due to atelectasis, contused lung tissue or disruption of the respiratory tract. Thoracic trauma contributes to mortality in a quarter of trauma-related deaths (Zargar *et al.*, 2007; Oikonomou and Prassopoulos, 2011). The mortality rate increases in proportion to the time between injury and surgery (Adesanya *et al.*, 2000). Multiple organ failure is a common cause of late-hospital fatality (Søreide *et al.*, 2007; Evans *et al.*, 2010).

In children, most fatalities at the scene result from lacerations of the heart, lung, blood vessels and bronchi, whilst in-hospital fatalities are mostly caused by cardiac tamponade, injuries to the great vessels and tension haemo- or pneumothoraces (Kadish, 2006). Prompt recognition of these conditions is therefore essential to reduce mortality. Although abdominal injuries are more common than thoracic injuries, they are 40% less fatal in children (Zamakhshary and Wales, 2008). Thoracic injury accounts for up to 12% of traumatic injuries and carries 5% mortality

(Bliss and Silen, 2002). In multi-injured children, thoracic trauma increases mortality 20 times (Herrera and Langer, 2008).

5.3. Medical and Surgical Management of Survivors of Abdominal or Thoracic Trauma

The medical and surgical management of any patient with traumatic injury is divided into:

- primary survey and resuscitation of vital functions;
- detailed secondary survey as adjunct to the primary survey; and
- definitive care.

The specific management of patients with abdominal or thoracic injuries is outlined below in relation to the abovementioned three phases of care.

5.3.1. *Primary survey and resuscitation of vital functions*

On admission to the emergency department, initial assessment and management of the adult and paediatric patient focuses on identifying and reversing hypoxia, which is the most serious problem. Assessment for injuries that are life threatening is also done during the primary survey. Internationally, the 'airways, breathing, circulation, disability, exposure' (ABCDE) approach to basic life support is used for all adult and paediatric patients with trauma-related injuries admitted to casualty (Thim *et al.*, 2012).

During the primary survey, ABCDE are all assessed, regardless of the organ system damaged. The ABCDE approach consists of assessment for (Thim *et al.*, 2012) the following.

- *Airway* patency (with protection of the cervical spine), including the presence of oropharyngeal foreign body obstruction.
- Presence or absence of *breathing*. Respiratory movements and the quality of respirations are assessed using the 'look (observe), feel (palpate) and listen (auscultate)' approach. Shallow respirations are an early

indicator of distress, whilst cyanosis is a late indicator. Pulse oximetry forms part of this assessment.

- *Circulation* by feeling the pulse for quality, rate and regularity. The skin is observed and palpated for colour, temperature and capillary refill. The neck veins are observed to assess whether they are flat or distended. Any active bleeding is stopped with compression over the wound. Penetrating objects are left *in situ* (Herrera and Langer, 2008). Electrocardiography (ECG) monitoring is done and blood pressure is measured.
- *Disability* by determining level of consciousness. This is done through assessing whether the patient is alert, voice responsive, pain responsive or unresponsive (AVPU approach). Pupil shape, size and reactivity to light are assessed as well as quality of limb movements. Blood glucose testing usually forms part of this assessment.
- Injuries by *exposing* the patient through the removal of clothes in order to visualise the skin and identify injuries. The patient's clothes are removed but the patient is kept warm in order to prevent the onset of hypothermia.

Children with thoracic or abdominal injuries may present in respiratory or circulatory failure, but respiratory failure is more common with signs of tachypnoea, chest wall recessions or retractions and agitation secondary to hypoxia (Kadish, 2006).

Radiological investigations such as ultrasound technology, chest x-rays and computed tomography (CT) scans form part of the primary survey in order to identify life-threatening injuries that are not visible. Particularly in paediatric populations, ultrasound is extensively used in the diagnosis of thoracic and abdominal dysfunction and has the advantages of non-invasiveness and lack of radiation (Gaines, 2009). Diagnostic peritoneal lavage (DPL) may also be performed, if indicated, to diagnose intra-peritoneal haemorrhage.

Care provided to the patient in the emergency department during the primary survey includes oxygen therapy, placement of an endotracheal tube (ETT) if indicated, nasogastric tube placement to decompress the stomach if necessary, placement of peripheral intravenous (IV) lines for medication administration and fluid replacement therapy and, lastly, insertion of a urinary catheter. Analgesia is provided for pain relief.

5.3.1.1. *The lethal six injuries as a result of thoracic trauma*

Figure 5.4 illustrates injuries that may result from thoracic trauma which constitute immediate life threats and are often termed 'the lethal six'. Identification of 'the lethal six' injuries forms an important component of the primary survey. These injuries require immediate attention and can often be treated quickly and simply with a tube or needle (Tai and Boffard, 2003; Yamamoto *et al.*, 2005). In the presence of *commotio cordis* in children, defibrillation may be life-saving (Herrera and Langer, 2008).

A description of each of these injuries follows below.

5.3.1.1.1. Airway obstruction

This is managed by positioning the patient's head and neck to open the airway (with protection of the cervical spine) and suctioning to remove obstructions such as blood or vomit. Foreign bodies causing obstruction

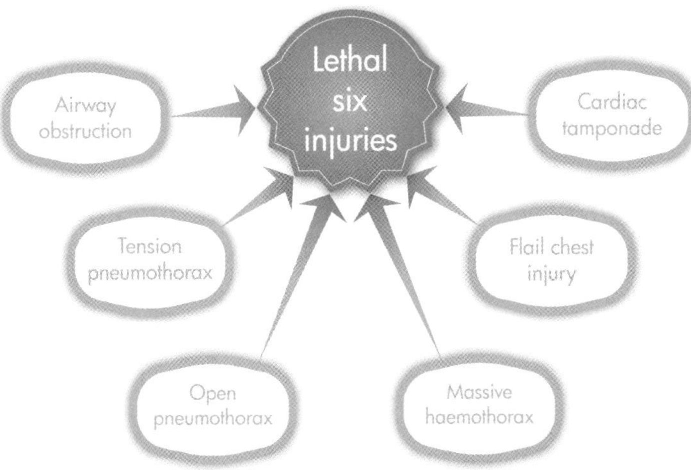

Fig. 5.4: Lethal six injuries associated with thoracic trauma.

should be removed if possible. The insertion of an artificial airway may be indicated for an unconscious patient (Thim *et al.*, 2012).

5.3.1.1.2. Tension pneumothorax

Tension pneumothoraces occur following an injury to the lung, which results in an air leak with a one-way valve effect. This leads to the accumulation of air in the pleural space with a progressive build-up of pressure resulting in mediastinal shift and lung compression (Fig. 5.3). If not resolved it can lead to reduced venous return, decreased cardiac output, diaphragmatic inversion, subcutaneous emphysema and ultimately cardiorespiratory arrest. The presence of a simple pneumothorax can be assessed through the use of ultrasound technology such as extended focussed assessment with sonography for trauma (FAST). This non-invasive assessment tool is also useful in identifying the presence of blood in the pericardium (Rippey and Royse, 2009). In the absence of ultrasound technology, chest x-ray or CT scan can be used for confirmation of diagnosis. Emergency treatment is needle decompression via the second intercostal space in the mid-clavicular line, followed by insertion of an intercostal drain (ICD).

5.3.1.1.3. Open pneumothorax ('sucking chest wound')

Normal ventilation requires a negative intra-thoracic pressure. A large open chest wall defect leads to the equilibration of intra-thoracic and atmospheric pressures, and if the hole is more than two-thirds of the tracheal diameter, the air preferentially flows through the chest defect, leading to severe hypoxia. Emergency treatment requires the defect to be sealed and secured with a dressing on three sides (total occlusion may lead to tension pneumothorax) and placement of an ICD at a site remote from the open chest wound, followed by definitive surgical repair (Smith, 2013; Trauma.Org, 2013b).

5.3.1.1.4. Massive haemothorax

This refers to a rapid accumulation of a large volume of blood in the chest cavity, leading to hypovolaemia and hypoxaemia. On examination the neck veins may be either flat from hypovolaemia or, on rare occasions, distended as a result of the intrathoracic blood. Breath sounds are absent and the thorax is dull to percussion. Extended FAST can be used for diagnosis of a haemothorax (Rippey and Royse, 2009). But again, in the absence of ultrasound technology, chest x-ray or CT scan can be used for confirmation of diagnosis. Emergency management is the insertion of a large-bore (adult 32–36 French gauge (FG); child 16–24 FG; infant 12–16 FG; newborn 8–12 FG) tube to drain the blood, followed by either closed drainage or open thoracotomy.

5.3.1.1.5. Flail chest

Flail chest is usually a result of direct impact to the chest wall. Two or more adjacent ribs are fractured in two or more places, producing a 'free-floating' segment of chest wall which moves paradoxically (opposite to normal chest wall motion) with respiration (Fig. 5.5). This leads to pain

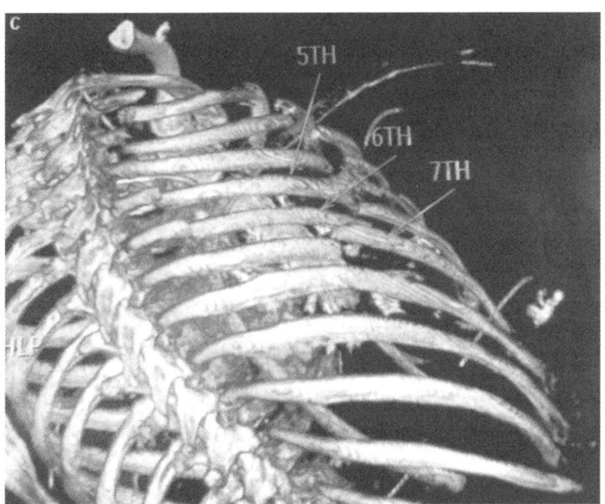

Fig. 5.5: Flail rib fractures.

and restricted chest wall movement, and the underlying pulmonary contusion results in reduced lung compliance and atelectasis. Chest x-ray or CT are used for confirmation of diagnosis. Emergency management involves ensuring adequate ventilation, providing humidified oxygen, fluid resuscitation, pain management and stabilising of the chest. Flail rib segments are rare in children due to the marked pliability of the chest wall, but if present are likely to lead to severe respiratory decompensation (Bliss and Silen, 2002; Kadish, 2006).

5.3.1.1.6. Cardiac tamponade

Blood in the pericardial sac, usually resulting from penetrating injuries, prevents cardiac activity. The patient may present with 'Beck's triad' which constitutes:

- elevated venous pressure;
- decreased arterial pressure; and
- muffled heart sounds.

Furthermore, there may be 'pulsus paradoxus': a decrease of 10 millimetres of mercury (mmHg) or greater in systolic blood pressure (BP) during inspiration. A systolic to diastolic gradient of greater than 30 mmHg is also suggestive of cardiac tamponade. Diagnosis is confirmed through the use of extended FAST (Rippey and Royse, 2009). Emergency treatment is the removal of a small amount of blood from the pericardial sac.

5.3.1.2. *Abdominal trauma*

In the case of abdominal injury, a thorough clinical examination is done to identify signs of internal bleeding, such as stomach distension, rectal bleeding and blood in gastric aspirate or in the urine. Radiological examination includes chest and pelvis x-rays for patients with multiple injuries due to blunt trauma. Those who have penetrating trauma to the abdomen and who are haemodynamically stable also undergo abdominal x-ray (American College of Surgeons Committee on Trauma, 2008). FAST has been shown to be as specific in the diagnosis of the presence of blood in the peritoneum as DPL and abdominal CT scan (American College of Surgeons Committee on Trauma, 2008; Rippey and Royse, 2009; Quinn and Sinert, 2011). Diagnostic peritoneal lavage may be performed in patients with blunt trauma to the abdomen in the presence of haemodynamic instability to identify haemorrhage if FAST is negative or if a CT scan is not available. It is an invasive procedure but is deemed to be 98% accurate in the diagnosis of intraperitoneal bleeding (American College of Surgeons Committee on Trauma, 2008; Quinn and Sinert, 2011).

5.3.2. *Secondary survey as adjunct to primary survey*

The secondary survey also takes place in the emergency department. It begins after the completion of the primary survey, when resuscitation has been carried out and vital functions normalised. The secondary survey is a 'head-to-toe' evaluation of the patient, which involves taking a detailed history of the patient as well as a complete neurological and physical examination.

Care provided to the patient during the primary survey continues in the secondary survey. If the patient's condition is stable, placement of arterial and central venous pressure (CVP) lines are performed. If the patient's condition is unstable, placement of these lines is done in theatre or in the intensive care unit (ICU) as part of definitive care.

The secondary survey is guided by suspicion for injuries missed during the primary survey, especially in patients who are unconscious or unstable. The presence of possible abdominal injury should be confirmed, as serious complications can occur in both adults and children if diagnosis is delayed.

- Computed tomography is used to rule out any undiagnosed injuries to the heart and major thoracic vasculature, injuries to the diaphragm, intra-abdominal haemorrhage and intestinal perforation, as well as injuries to other parts of the body, especially in the case of multiple blunt trauma (American College of Surgeons Committee on Trauma, 2008; Chidester *et al.*, 2009; Van Vugt *et al.*, 2011).
- Computed tomography with contrast may be needed to identify isolated injuries to the duodenum, ascending or descending colon, rectum,

biliary tract and pancreas which were not identified through DPL (American College of Surgeons Committee on Trauma, 2008).

- Multi-detector CT scan may be used, if available in the trauma centre, to identify internal bleeding in haemodynamically stable patients with blunt abdominal organ injury (Van der Vlies *et al.*, 2011).
- Diagnostic laparoscopy may be needed if uncertainty remains following non-invasive diagnostic measures (Gaines, 2009).

5.3.2.1. *The hidden six injuries that result from thoracic trauma*

Figure 5.6 illustrates thoracic injuries that are considered to be potential life threats and are often referred to as 'the hidden six' (Tai and Boffard, 2003; Yamamoto *et al.*, 2005; Nayak, 2008). Suspicion of these injuries guides the secondary survey.

The 'hidden six' injuries follow below.

5.3.2.1.1. Pulmonary contusion

Pulmonary contusion refers to injury of the lung parenchyma without laceration. It is a potentially life-threatening condition with an insidious

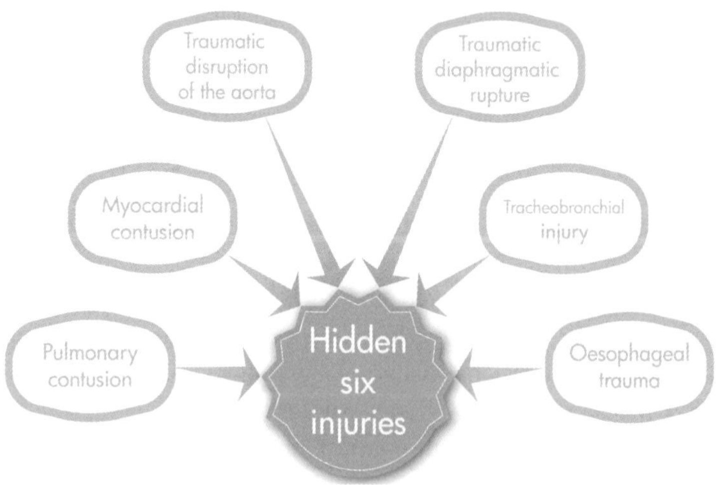

Fig. 5.6: The hidden six injuries associated with thoracic trauma.

onset, and is particularly common in children (Kadish, 2006). Interstitial haemorrhage and oedema fluid that result from the contusion leak into the alveoli and cause reduced pulmonary compliance, atelectasis (exacerbated by decreased surfactant production by injured alveolar cells) and hypoventilation. Bronchospasm may result from bleeding into lung segments that were not affected at the time of injury and this leads to further pulmonary dysfunction. Pulmonary dysfunction may also be compromised by increased mucus production and decreased clearance of mucus (Cohn and DuBose, 2010). More than 50% of adults and 20% of children will develop pneumonia, even with treatment (Bliss and Silen, 2002; Tovar, 2008).

The risk of pulmonary oedema must be considered when managing such patients. In children, it may be difficult to differentiate aspiration from contusion. Aspiration may occur at the time of injury, during intubation or following vomiting whilst in the supine position (Bliss and Silen, 2002). Usually, the right lower lobe is affected due to the structure of the tracheobronchial tree, but diffuse infiltrates may be seen on a chest x-ray. Pulmonary contusion usually resolves by day seven after injury (Cohn and DuBose, 2010). See Fig. 5.7 for a chest x-ray example of pulmonary contusion.

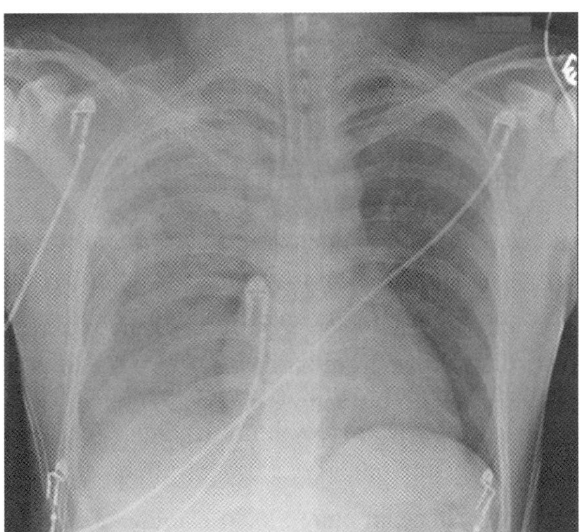

Fig. 5.7: Blunt chest trauma resulting in rib and clavicle fractures, haemothorax and pulmonary contusion on the right.

5.3.2.1.2. Myocardial contusion

Myocardial or cardiac contusions occur as a result of blunt precordial chest trauma and are often difficult to diagnose. There is a risk of dysrhythmias, tamponade, pericarditis and sudden death. Myocardial contusion is diagnosed by ECG and elevated cardiac-specific enzyme levels. Blunt cardiac injury is rare in children, occurring in less than 5% of paediatric trauma patients (Taio *et al.*, 2000; Kadish, 2006).

5.3.2.1.3. Traumatic disruption of the aorta

This type of injury is associated with rapid deceleration-type accidents. It is associated with high mortality at the accident scene, and for those who survive to hospital, mortality increases significantly with each undiagnosed day. Disruption occurs at the ligamentum arteriosum (ductus arteriosus) and results in a contained haematoma of 500–1000 ml of blood. Specific radiographic signs include a widened mediastinum, tracheal and oesophageal deviation to the right, and first and second rib fractures. Definitive surgical repair is required (O'Connor *et al.*, 2009).

Great vessel and cardiac injuries are much less common in children than in adults (Bliss and Silen, 2002; Kadish, 2006). However, more than 80% of children who sustain an aortic tear will also have significant injuries to the lung, heart, abdominal viscera and nervous system, and there is a high associated mortality (Bliss and Silen, 2002; Kadish, 2006).

5.3.2.1.4. Traumatic diaphragmatic rupture

Diaphragmatic tears lead to immediate or delayed visceral herniation and lung compression. Left-sided hemi-diaphragm rupture is more common than right-sided hemi-diaphragm rupture in adults due to the protection provided by the liver (Chughtai *et al.*, 2009; Vilallonga *et al.*, 2011).

In children, diaphragmatic rupture occurs in up to 5% of cases following major chest trauma, particularly blunt trauma. The site of rupture is usually posterolateral (Chughtai *et al.*, 2009; Moore *et al.*, 2009). Surgical repair is the definitive treatment.

5.3.2.1.5. Tracheobronchial injury

Tracheobronchial injury refers to injury involving the larynx, trachea or bronchus. Injury to the larynx is rare. Suspicion is raised if the patient presents with hoarseness of the voice or subcutaneous emphysema and intubation proves to be difficult. Tracheal injury may be accompanied by oesophageal injury. Bronchial injury, usually due to blunt trauma, is rare and may be lethal. Injuries to the tracheobronchial tree are rare in children, but may occur following both penetrating and blunt trauma and are associated with up to 30% mortality (Bliss and Silen, 2002; Tovar, 2008). Up to 80% of all paediatric airway injuries occur in the distal trachea or bronchi. Most injuries show mediastinal air, although more distal injuries may present with pneumothoraces (Bliss and Silen, 2002; Kadish, 2006).

5.3.2.1.6. Oesophageal trauma

This is commonly caused by penetrating injury and may be lethal if not recognised. A high suspicion of oesophageal trauma is raised if the patient has a left pneumothorax and haemothorax without rib fractures. Another cause for concern is the presence of shock out of proportion to apparent blunt chest trauma, and there may be particulate matter in the ICD tube (Bliss and Silen, 2002). Oesophageal injuries are rare in children and are difficult to diagnose. Oesophageal perforation in children is mostly caused by iatrogenic injury followed by penetrating trauma and may have devastating consequences, such as mediastinal sepsis and death (Kadish, 2006).

5.3.3. *Definitive care*

Definitive care is initiated after completion of the primary and secondary surveys. At this point the patient is transferred out of the emergency department either to theatre for surgical intervention or to the ICU for close monitoring and care.

The types of definitive care provided for patients who have suffered blunt or penetrating injuries to the abdomen or thorax are discussed below.

5.3.3.1. *Abdominal injury*

Several adult patients with blunt abdominal organ injury who are haemodynamically stable are successfully managed non-operatively (Van der Vlies *et al.*, 2011). In children, most injuries to the abdominal organs are managed non-operatively with very high success rates (Zamakhshary and Wales, 2008; Gaines, 2009). These patients are admitted to the ICU for monitoring and therapy.

An adult or paediatric patient with blunt abdominal trauma who presents with shock due to intra-abdominal bleeding is immediately taken to theatre for surgical intervention in the form of an exploratory laparotomy. A laparotomy is also performed if a patient with penetrating trauma presents with multiple organ injuries, haemodynamic instability, prolonged hypoxia, significant intra-abdominal blood loss or evidence of hollow visceral injury (Adesanya *et al.*, 2000; Thomson, 2003; Gaines, 2009). The vertical abdominal incision gives the surgeon sufficient exposure to the intra-abdominal organs to identify injuries, control bleeding and contain contamination. Where possible all dead and contaminated tissue is excised to leave healthy tissue behind (Vikram, 2011).

After surgery the patient is transferred to the ICU for further care and monitoring. Special attention is paid to the detection of the development of abdominal compartment syndrome (increased pressure in the abdomen). Abdominal compartment syndrome develops due to increased pressure in the intra-abdominal compartment from large-volume fluid resuscitation after major abdominal surgery and also tight abdominal wall closure after emergency laparotomy procedures. This increase in intra-abdominal pressure leads to symptomatic organ dysfunction such as acute renal failure (Subramanian *et al.*, 2008). Like adults, children can develop abdominal compartment syndrome, with a high associated mortality if not treated timely (Gaines, 2009).

5.3.3.1.1. Damage control surgery

Damage control is a concept that is being used more frequently internationally (Kirkpatrick *et al.*, 2006). Damage control involves a staged approach to the repair of damaged abdominal organs. Initially the surgeon repairs only major organ tears to stop internal bleeding and control contamination. The visceral cavity is packed with dressings to control capillary oozing, the abdominal wall is left open and the patient is taken to the ICU to be stabilised (Fig. 5.8). Repair to smaller organ tears is done in theatre once the patient is in a more stable condition (24–48 hours after initial operation). Definitive repair is completed with closure of the abdominal wall, provided that intra-abdominal swelling had subsided (Cirocchi *et al.*, 2010, 2013).

The administration of large volumes of IV fluid during surgery may result in excessive swelling of the intestines and mesentery and retroperitoneal tissues in patients with severe abdominal trauma. The abdominal walls become less compliant due to oedema and closure of the abdominal fascia may lead to increased intraperitoneal pressure. This may result in decreased blood flow to the hepatic, renal and intestinal organs due to intra-abdominal hypertension or compartment syndrome, as discussed above (Subramanian *et al.*, 2008).

Unplanned relook laparotomy becomes necessary in the presence of intra-abdominal sepsis, intra-abdominal bleeding, missed injuries, small

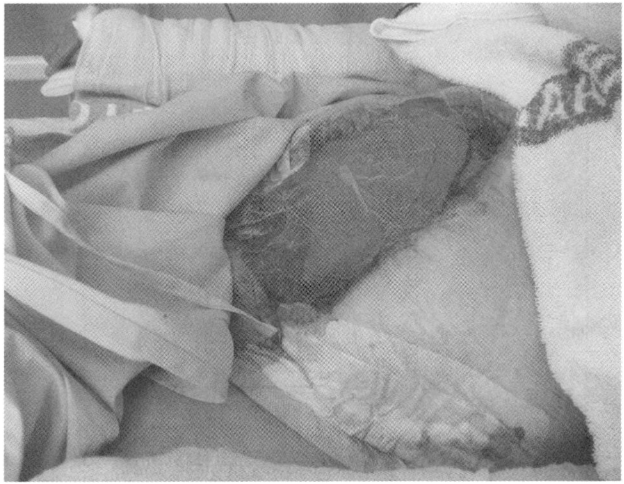

Fig. 5.8: Damage control surgery. Open abdominal wound packed with sterile sponge material and covered with transparent adhesive film.

bowel obstruction and fluid leaks at anastomosis sites. Between surgical interventions, patients are monitored and managed in the ICU until they have stabilised. Patients who undergo unplanned relook laparotomy have a higher mortality rate than those patients who do not. Negative pressure wound therapy may be used as part of wound care for such patients (Figs 5.9A and B) (Roberts *et al.*, 2012). This involves the delivery of negative pressure to the wound site through the placement of patented sponge material inside the wound, together with a drainage tube that is attached to a suction machine at the bedside. This negative pressure assists in removing infectious material from the wound site, promotes the formation of granulation tissue and helps to draw the wound edges closer together (Roberts *et al.*, 2012). The abdominal wound is closed surgically when sepsis is resolved.

5.3.3.2. *Thoracic injury*

The definitive management of blunt and penetrating chest injuries is very similar.

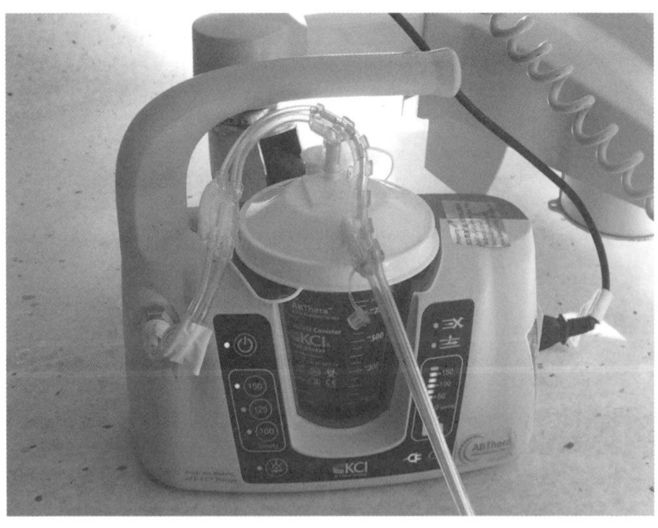

(A)

Fig. 5.9: Negative pressure wound therapy. (A) KCI vacuum device; (B) Wound drainage tube exiting inferior to the sponge material.

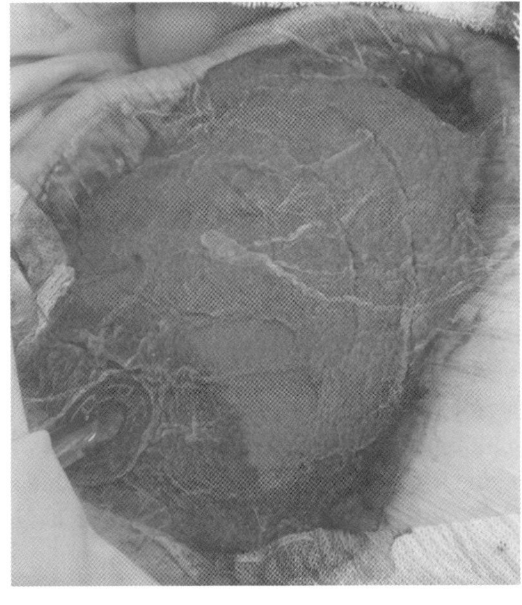

(B)

Fig. 5.9: (*Continued*)

5.3.3.2.1. Pneumothorax or haemothorax

Pneumo- or haemothoraces are managed with the placement of an ICD, as mentioned previously, to release pressure from the pleural space, as part of standard care. Low-pressure, high-volume suction may be necessary to encourage re-expansion of collapsed lung regions (Paramasivan and Bodenham, 2007). Prompt drainage of blood from the pleural space is essential in adults and children with haemothoraces because as the haematoma organises, it may be replaced by fibrous scar tissue, causing lung entrapment, which predisposes the patient to chronic atelectasis, V/Q mismatch, pneumonia or empyema (Bliss and Silen, 2002). Drainage also provides a method to measure and monitor the volume and rate of blood loss. A thoracotomy may be indicated for direct closure of the wound if low-pressure, high-volume suction is unsuccessful (Keilin *et al.*, 2003; Paramasivan and Bodenham, 2007).

5.3.3.2.2. Posttraumatic empyema

Posttraumatic empyema may result from either blunt or penetrating chest injuries in 10–27% of adult cases and contributes to morbidity and mortality (Hoth *et al.*, 2002; DuBose *et al.*, 2012). A retained haemothorax is primarily associated with the development of posttraumatic empyema and is often caused by rib fractures. Blood trapped in the pleural space impairs its own absorption and forms an ideal environment for bacterial growth. The placement of an ICD may lead to contamination of a retained haemothorax and the development of empyema.

The diagnosis of posttraumatic empyema is made through chest CT and the presence of clinical findings such as increased leukocyte count, fever and worsening respiratory function.

The management of posttraumatic empyema includes thoracotomy for decortication and re-expansion of the involved lung, less invasive video-assisted thoracoscopy or intrapleural administration of fibrinolytic agents such as streptokinase or urokinase (Hoth *et al.*, 2002; Paramasivan and Bodenham, 2007; DuBose *et al.*, 2012).

5.3.3.2.3. Cardiac, airway or great vessel injuries

These injuries may be managed conservatively initially with close patient monitoring. The unstable hypotensive patient is managed surgically with a median sternotomy incision or high antero-lateral thoracotomy incision to gain access to the great vessels, trachea or bronchi, oesophagus and the heart to repair damage. Repair of the thoracic aorta requires single lung ventilation and a thoracotomy incision at the fourth intercostal space on the left side of the chest wall (Keilin *et al.*, 2003; O'Connor *et al.*, 2009).

5.3.3.2.3.1. *Myocardial contusion.* Electrocardiography tracing is instituted in patients with myocardial contusion to monitor for cardiac arrhythmias. Echocardiography is undertaken to directly assess the presence of right or left ventricular contusion. The concentration of cardiac enzymes (especially creatinine phosphokinase-myocardial band (CPK-MB)) is monitored to identify the extent of cellular injury of cardiac and skeletal muscles (Bansal *et al.*, 2005).

5.3.3.2.4. Soft tissue injuries of the chest wall

Entrance and exit wounds of gunshot injuries are debrided thoroughly. Necrotic tissue and debris create an ideal focus area for infection. Gas gangrene may develop in neglected wounds or those that have undergone inadequate debridement. Reconstructive surgery may be indicated for wounds with large loss of chest wall integrity (Clarke, 2003; De Groot and Van Oppell, 2003; Mauffrey, 2005).

5.3.3.2.5. Pulmonary contusion

Control of pain originating from the chest wall, accurate fluid management and aggressive bronchial hygiene are important components of the treatment of all patients with pulmonary contusion. Patients with severe pulmonary contusion should be monitored closely to ensure adequate oxygenation and organ perfusion. Intermittent positioning in prone can be used to optimise oxygenation (Cohn and DuBose, 2010).

The use of epidural analgesia has been shown to decrease the duration of mechanical ventilation (MV) and the rate of development of nosocomial pneumonia more so than the use of IV opioids in patients with multiple rib fractures and pulmonary contusion. Regional analgesia is also recommended for pain control in patients with rib fractures and pulmonary contusion (Cohn and DuBose, 2010). The survival rate of adults with pulmonary contusion and rib fractures is reported to change from 60–93.5% when pain is adequately controlled, allowing for early chest physiotherapy intervention and mobilisation (Cohn and DuBose, 2010).

Neutrophil-induced lung injury may be restricted with the early administration of hypertonic saline (Bastos *et al.*, 2008; Cohn and DuBose, 2010), but large clinical trials are needed to confirm this finding. Restricted crystalloid IV fluids are given to prevent the development of pulmonary oedema. Intravenous red packed cells and plasma are given to restore blood volume. Diuretics may be used to treat pulmonary oedema (Bastos *et al.*, 2008). Steroid use for patients with pulmonary contusion is not recommended as it may increase the risk for the development of pneumonia (Cohn and DuBose, 2010).

The use of non-invasive positive pressure ventilation may prevent the need for intubation and MV (Cohn and DuBose, 2010). Patients with pre-existing conditions, such as emphysema or renal failure, may need early intubation. In patients with pulmonary contusion who require MV, the use of alveolar recruitment manoeuvres or high-frequency oscillatory ventilation have been reported to improve oxygenation. It is important that any MV strategy that is decided upon should minimise the risk of induced barotraumas (Cohn and DuBose, 2010).

Between 20 and 35% of children with pulmonary contusion will require MV, fewer than in adults (Bliss and Silen, 2002; Norton *et al.*, 2008). Ancillary measures in paediatrics include fluid restriction, supplemental oxygen, pulmonary toilet and pain control.

5.3.3.2.6. Diaphragmatic injury

Diaphragmatic ruptures are managed through surgical intervention, with laparotomy incision being the golden standard. In some instances thoracotomy is performed for a right-sided hemi-diaphragm rupture (Chughtai *et al.*, 2009; Vilallonga *et al.*, 2011).

5.3.3.2.7. Skeletal injuries of the chest wall

5.3.3.2.7.1. *Rib fractures.* A bone scan performed a few days after the initial injury can assist in identifying rib fractures not seen on a chest x-ray. If the first, second or third ribs are involved, or scapula and sternal fractures are present, there should be concern for injury to the head, neck, spinal cord, lungs, and great vessels. If the tenth, eleventh or twelfth ribs are fractured, there should be a high level of suspicion for associated liver or spleen injuries (Bliss and Silen, 2002; Kadish, 2006). Rib fractures are uncommon in young children, but occur more frequently in adolescents. The presence of rib fractures in children often signifies severe associated thoracic injury, as a very large force is needed to break pliable ribs (Bliss and Silen, 2002; Tovar, 2008; Moore *et al.*, 2009).

Unless rib fractures are causing instability, the main aim of management is pain reduction and prevention of pulmonary complications such as atelectasis and infection. This can be achieved by using the following methods.

- Thoracic paravertebral block. Using a continuous epidural infusion of analgesia on the side of multiple unilateral rib fractures has been reported to improve pain at rest and during coughing and improves oxygenation (Shukla *et al.*, 2008).
- Non-invasive positive pressure ventilation (NIPPV) through a fitted face mask together with adequate analgesic support. This is used to improve chest wall stabilisation for patients with multiple rib fractures or flail chest injuries. Oxygen therapy should be humidified so as not to compromise the function of the mucociliary escalator. Mechanical ventilation through an artificial airway is avoided for as long as possible due to its associated risk of complications (Bastos *et al.*, 2008). Gunduz *et al.* (2005) reported that patients with flail chest injuries who were managed with NIPPV had lower mortality and incidence of nosocomial infection than those with flail chest injuries who were intubated and mechanically ventilated.

Operative stabilisation of flail rib fractures can be performed if a patient continues to suffer with poor oxygenation despite optimal MV support (Fitzpatrick *et al.*, 2010).

Circumferential strapping of the chest wall in the presence of rib fractures is contraindicated for pain relief, as it leads to the development of respiratory complications by restricting chest wall expansion (Clarke, 2003; Trauma.Org, 2013a).

5.3.3.2.7.2. *Clavicle fracture.* The clavicle is the most commonly fractured bone and an isolated fracture of the clavicle is seldom a significant injury. Treatment is usually accomplished with a sling-and-swathe or a figure-of-eight sling that immobilises the affected shoulder and arm. Clavicular fractures usually heal well within four to six weeks; in some cases internal fixation is performed for mid-shaft clavicle fractures (Pujalte and Housner, 2008).

5.3.3.2.7.3. *Scapula fracture.* Scapular fractures are less common in children than in adults because of the marked chest wall compliance. A scapula fracture is managed with analgesia and the arm on the side of the fracture is immobilised in a sling (Kadish, 2006; Dandy and Edwards, 2009).

5.3.3.2.7.4. *Sternal fracture.* Sternal fractures occur more commonly in adults than children due to reasons previously mentioned. Sternal fractures are managed with analgesia and oxygen therapy. Open reduction and internal fixation is indicated for overlapping sternal fractures (Kadish, 2006; Panté *et al.*, 2010).

5.3.4. *Prolonged intensive care unit stay*

The severity of injury following blunt or penetrating trauma and increasing patient morbidity due to the development of infection or sepsis can lead to prolonged duration of MV, resulting in longer ICU stay. Under these circumstances the inter-professional team may consider replacing the patient's endotracheal tube with a tracheostomy tube to make the process of weaning from MV easier for the patient. The care of the patient's tracheostomy should be a priority for each member of the interdisciplinary ICU team, as poor standards of care directly influence the patient's mortality (Mitchell *et al.*, 2013).

5.3.4.1. *Tracheostomy care*

5.3.4.1.1. Indications for tracheostomy

A tracheostomy involves the creation of an opening (stoma) on the neck, through which a tracheostomy tube is inserted into the trachea. The main components of adult and paediatric tracheostomy tubes are displayed in Figs 5.10A and B.

Permanent tracheostomy may be used for patients with cancer of the upper airways (adults) or other forms of upper airway obstruction (e.g. Pierre Robin sequence, laryngeal webs etc.) to assist with the maintenance of an intact airway. This is beyond the scope of this text and will not be discussed further. Temporary tracheostomy can be used in a variety of patients, but is performed in the trauma population under the following circumstances.

- To protect the airways from swelling and compression after traumatic injury or surgical procedures performed to the head or neck.

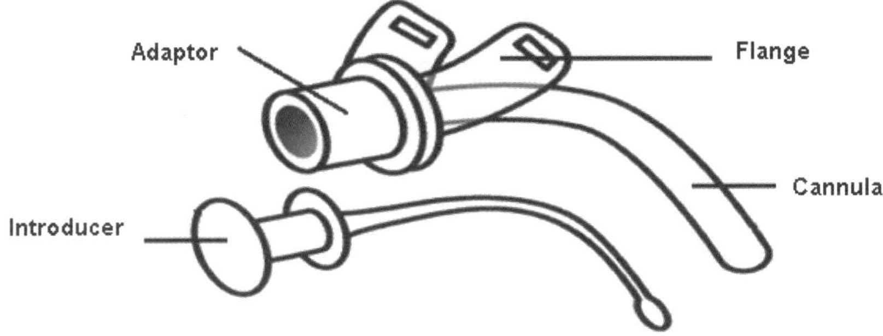

Fig. 5.10A: Paediatric uncuffed tracheostomy tube and introducer (obturator).

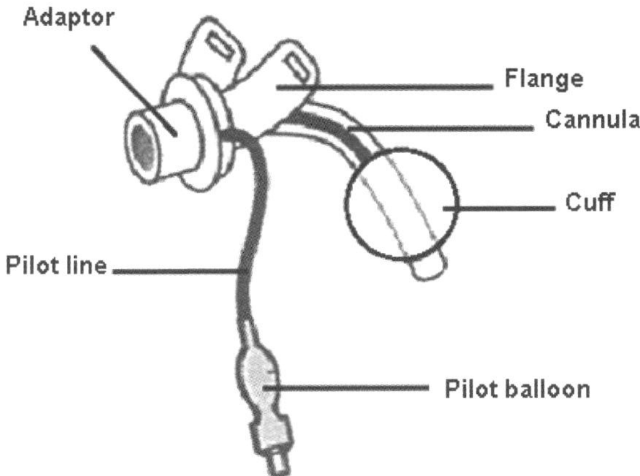

Fig. 5.10B: Adult cuffed tracheostomy tube.

- Prolonged duration of MV (> 10 days in adults; variable in young children) (Fig. 5.11).
- To facilitate weaning from MV, as tracheostomy reduces the need for sedation and reduces dead space and the resistance to airflow created by the ventilator circuit.

A tracheostomy is performed either through a traditional surgical approach or percutaneous dilatational techniques (Mitchell *et al.*, 2013). The reader is referred to Section 5.8 for additional sources that discuss the

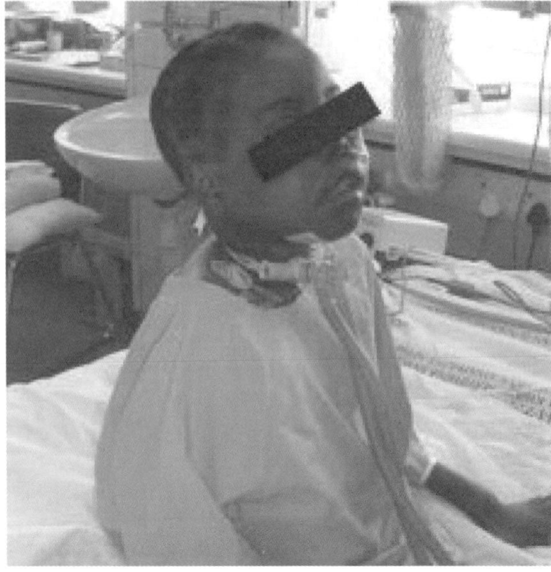

Fig. 5.11: Ten-year-old girl with tracheostomy for long-term ventilation.

types of tracheostomy tubes, sizes of tracheostomy tubes and the emergency equipment that should be kept by the patient's bedside in the case of unforeseen circumstances.

5.3.4.1.2. Positioning of the tracheostomy tube

On chest x-ray assessment the tracheostomy tube tip should extend more than half the distance between the stoma and the carina. The tracheostomy should be positioned parallel to the long axis of the trachea and should be two-thirds the diameter of the trachea in size (Kacmarek *et al.*, 2013).

The tracheostomy tube should be securely fastened to the patient's neck with tracheostomy tape. Tracheal injury and accidental decannulation (removal) can occur if the ventilator tubing pulls excessively on the tracheostomy tube. Good clinical practice involves reducing the leverage of the ventilator tubing on the tracheostomy by securing the tubing to drip stands above or next to the patient's bedside.

5.3.4.1.3. Tracheostomy chart

Care of the patient with a tracheostomy can be enhanced by placing a clearly visible tracheostomy chart above the patient's bed in the ICU or on the ward. Information that should be communicated through this chart includes the following:

- the type of procedure used for insertion of the tracheostomy (surgical or percutaneous);
- the date on which the tracheostomy was performed;
- the tracheostomy tube size; and
- people to contact in case of an emergency, e.g. anaesthesia department, ICU, ear-nose-throat specialist, maxilla-facial surgeon or the hospital emergency department.

5.3.4.1.4. Red flags

The physiotherapist should immediately alert the other members of the interdisciplinary team if they observe any of the following red flag indicators of tracheostomy problems in the patient under their care:

- an inability to pass the suction catheter down the tracheostomy;
- patient able to vocalise: in adults in the presence of an inflated tracheostomy cuff, and in children in the absence of a speaking valve;
- patient exhibiting signs of increasing respiratory distress; and
- desaturation or bradycardia.

5.3.4.1.5. Interdisciplinary team responsibilities in tracheostomy care

Table 5.1 outlines the roles of various interdisciplinary team members in the daily management of a patient with a tracheostomy.

The involvement of physiotherapists in tracheostomy care procedures may vary according to an individual country's scope of practice for physiotherapists. More information is provided below for the tracheostomy care procedures that physiotherapists are directly involved with. The reader is

Table 5.1: Interdisciplinary team responsibilities regarding tracheostomy care.

Responsibilities related to tracheostomy care	Team members
Humidification of tracheostomy	Nurses and physiotherapists
Communication, methods	Speech and language therapist
Communication with patient	All team members
Cuff management, using cuff manometer	Nurses and physiotherapists
Cleaning of the tracheostomy tube (including the inner tube if double lumen tracheostomy is used)	Nurses and physiotherapists
Oral hygiene	Nurses
Secretion clearance	Nurses and physiotherapists
Care of the stoma and application of appropriate dressings and tape	Nurses
Changing a tracheostomy tube	Only staff that have advanced airway skills training or those who have immediate access to someone with those skills. Such a person should be notified beforehand that a tube change will be done and they must avail themselves to immediately assist if an emergency arises
Weaning	Nurses, physiotherapists and speech and language therapists
Decannulation	Nurses and physiotherapists

referred to Section 5.8 for additional sources of information about the rest of the procedures related to tracheostomy care.

5.3.4.1.5.1. *Humidification.* Various forms of humidification can be used for a patient with a tracheostomy (Table 5.2).

5.3.4.1.5.2. *Secretion removal.* Deep suctioning of the tracheostomy tube should not be a routine procedure but should rather be done when there is an indication for suction. If the patient is able to independently cough secretions into the top of the tube, the secretions should be removed using a tissue or a Yankauer suction device. If deep suction is indicated, an

Table 5.2: Methods of humidification for a patient with tracheostomy*.

Tracheostomy and mechanical ventilation	Self-ventilating patient with tracheostomy on supplemental oxygen therapy	Self-ventilating patient with tracheostomy without oxygen therapy
• If the patient has loose secretions or no secretions, a heat moisture exchanger device should be used. • If the patient presents with thick secretions, 4–6 hourly saline nebulisation should be added. • If the secretions become difficult to clear or the patient has consolidative changes on chest x-ray, the heat moisture exchanger should be replaced with a heated water humidifier. • If the secretions remain difficult to clear, additional mucolytic therapy should be added.	• If the patient has no secretions or loose secretions, cold water venturi humidification should be used. • If the patient's secretions become thick, add 4–6 hourly saline nebulisation. • If the patient's condition worsens, follow the steps as outlined for the mechanically ventilated patient in relation to heated water humidification and additional mucolytic therapy.	• If the patient has loose or no secretions, an adequately sized heat moisture exchanger should be placed over the tracheostomy. • The patient should be encouraged to regularly drink fluids during the day to improve systemic hydration. • If the patient's condition worsens, the steps outlined for the self-ventilating patient on oxygen therapy should be followed.

*Adapted from St George's Healthcare NHS Trust Tracheostomy Guidelines (see Section 5.8).

appropriately sized suction catheter should be used. The therapist should begin to withdraw the catheter from the tracheostomy and apply suction pressure as soon as a cough reflex is stimulated with the catheter. The reader is referred to Chapter 4 (Section 4.2.7.1.) for additional information about the suctioning of an artificial airway.

5.3.4.1.5.3. *Communication.* Non-verbal and verbal communication methods (Table 5.3) should be used to make communication between the patient and the interdisciplinary team members more effective. A speech-and-language therapist should be consulted for guidance on the selection of the most appropriate communication method to use for individual patients.

Table 5.3: Communication methods for patients with tracheostomy*.

Non-verbal communication	Verbal communication
• Lip reading • Coded eye blink • Coded hand gestures • Alphabet board • Picture board • Phrase book	• Cuff deflation (adults) • Fenestrated tracheostomy • Intermittent finger occlusion • One-way speaking valve

*Adapted from the St George's Healthcare NHS Trust Tracheostomy Guidelines (see Section 5.8).

5.3.4.1.5.4. *Weaning of tracheostomy.* Weaning a patient from a tracheostomy tube should be an interdisciplinary team approach, as each professional has valuable information to share regarding the patient's ability to cope with the different stages of the weaning process. Weaning a patient from tracheostomy is successful if the patient meets most of the criteria listed in Table 5.4.

The stages of weaning a tracheostomy include the following.

- Cuff deflation (adults): initially for short time periods to re-accustom the patient to managing their own saliva and to swallow. The cuff deflation time is gradually prolonged until the patient is able to tolerate deflation for longer than 24 hours (including overnight).
- Gloved finger occlusion: this test is performed to establish the adequacy of airflow through the patient's upper respiratory tract. The patient should be able to breathe comfortably through the upper respiratory tract while the tube opening is occluded.
- One-way speaking valve: weaning is progressed to this step when the finger occlusion test is successful. The time spent on the speaking valve is determined by each individual patient's work of breathing.
- Decannulation cap: when the patient tolerates cuff deflation for longer than 24 hours and at least four hours at a time on the speaking valve, the tracheostomy is temporarily closed with the decannulation cap. If the patient manages to breathe for four hours or longer using the cap, without any signs of breathlessness or distress, decannulation may be considered.

Table 5.4: Indications for weaning of a tracheostomy*.

- Original indication for tracheostomy is resolved
- Spontaneous breathing with a regular respiratory pattern and respiratory rate < 30 breaths/minute
- Fraction of inspired oxygen (FiO_2) < 35% with adequate oxygenation
- Strong cough and able to clear secretions to the top of the tracheostomy tube
- No signs of excessive secretions or a new or deteriorating chest infection
- Adequate nutrition
- Swallow assessment done by speech-and-language therapist and patient able to cope with own saliva

*Adapted from St George's Healthcare NHS Trust Tracheostomy Guidelines (see Section 5.8).

5.3.4.1.5.5. *Decannulation.* Decannulation is removal of the tracheostomy tube. Determinants of successful decannulation are the patient's level of consciousness, presence of a strong cough and minimal secretions (Stelfox *et al.*, 2008).

5.4. Physiotherapy Aims of Management

Early during any patient's stay in the ICU, a short clinical assessment should be performed to identify the patient's risk of developing physical (e.g. muscle weakness, joint stiffness, poor endurance) and non-physical (e.g. anxiety, panic attacks, delusions) morbidity. Those patients who are identified as 'at risk' should undergo a comprehensive clinical assessment. Short-term and medium-term rehabilitation goals should be set based on clinical assessment findings for those who are 'at risk'. The patient, as well as their family members, should be involved with goal setting. The use of SMART goals is recommended: specific, measureable, attainable, realistic, time-based. Rehabilitation for 'at risk' patients in the ICU should start as soon as clinically possible (National Institute for Health and Clinical Excellence, 2009).

The interdisciplinary team approach to patient rehabilitation in the ICU should include prevention of avoidable physical and non-physical morbidity, regular review of previous and current medication that the patient is receiving, nutritional support and an individualised, structured rehabilitation programme with regular follow up reviews and clear documentation in the patient's clinical records (National Institute for Health and Clinical Excellence, 2009).

For the purposes of this textbook, physiotherapy-specific aims of intervention for patients with abdominal or thoracic trauma are included in this section.

Patients who undergo surgery and, in particular, those who have surgery for injuries sustained due to blunt or penetrating trauma to the abdomen or thorax are at risk of developing postoperative pulmonary complications (PPC) such as atelectasis or pneumonia. The aims of physiotherapy intervention for such patients in the ICU and the ward should therefore include the prevention of the development of PPC as far as possible. The aims of physiotherapy intervention provided here are based on expert opinion as well as the review published by Gosselink *et al.*, (2008) on the research evidence available for the management of the adult patient in the ICU setting. The effects of trauma, anaesthesia and immobility are the same in infants and children as in adults; however, the potential for respiratory complications may be greater because of anatomical and physiological differences between these populations.

Important aims of management of patients with abdominal or thoracic injury, which need to be considered by the physiotherapist based on individual patient assessment findings in the ICU environment, are listed in Table 5.5.

Before discharge from the ICU, patients who started rehabilitation should be re-assessed for physical, sensory and communication problems, pre-existing psychological distress or symptoms such as anxiety, delusions and panic attacks, which may have developed since admission to the ICU. Ward-based care should include a rehabilitation approach that incorporates the assessment findings of the 'prior to ICU discharge' assessment and is individualised and structured (National Institute for Health and Clinical Excellence, 2009).

Important aims for progression of management that need to be considered by the physiotherapist in the surgical or trauma ward environment, based on each individual patient's 'prior to ICU discharge' assessment findings, are listed in Table 5.6.

Table 5.5: Aims of physiotherapy management for patients with abdominal or thoracic traumatic injury in the ICU.

- Enhance mucociliary escalator function through adequate humidification of the airways
- Mobilise and remove excessive retained secretions from the airways of patients who are intubated in order to prevent the development of secondary chest infections
- Enhance the patient's cough effort in order to assist with secretion clearance
- Increase posterior and basal lung volumes of patients who are intubated and sedated (often nursed in a supine position in bed) in order to prevent the development of atelectasis
- Increase the patient's lung compliance in order to optimise and restore lung function
- Improve the patient's oxygenation
- Improve respiratory muscle strength as soon as the patient becomes conscious and cooperative, in order to assist with weaning from MV where the patient has been on prolonged MV
- Maintain or restore passive range of motion (ROM) of all limbs in order to prevent or reduce joint stiffness in patients who are intubated and sedated
- Restore muscle power of the limbs when the patient regains consciousness and is cooperative
- As the patient regains consciousness and their condition stabilises, aim to restore functionality in order for them to gain independence in activities of daily living (ADL)

Table 5.6: Aims for progression of management for patients with abdominal or thoracic traumatic injury in the surgical or trauma ward setting.

- Continue with humidification of the airways for as long as the patient receives oxygen therapy
- Enhance the patient's self-dependence by teaching them to mobilise and remove excessive retained secretions independently
- Maintain optimal lung volumes during the patient's stay in the ward
- Maintain optimal lung compliance during the patient's stay in the ward
- Improve the patient's self-reliance through encouragement of active and active-resisted ROM exercises of the limbs and ensure that end-of-range motion is achieved
- Continue with restoration of muscle power in all peripheries
- Continue with restoration of independent function on the ward
- Improve and restore cardiorespiratory exercise endurance in order to obtain the health benefits of exercise

5.4.1. *Paediatric considerations*

The aims of physiotherapy intervention are similar in both adults and children, but the premorbid functional and developmental level of the child must be taken into account when devising short-term and long-term aims of treatment.

5.4.2. *Functional assessment prior to discharge*

Prior to discharge the adult or paediatric patient should undergo a functional assessment as per recommendations made by National Institute for Health and Clinical Excellence (NICE) (Table 5.7).

The impact of the functional assessment outcomes on the patient's ability to perform ADL should be assessed. Based on these findings, the rehabilitation goals for post-discharge care should be discussed with the patient and their family and agreed upon (National Institute for Health and Clinical Excellence, 2009). Guidelines for exercise rehabilitation for patients after hospital discharge can be found in Chapter 10 (Section 10.6).

5.5. Precautions and Contraindications related to Physiotherapy Management

Recommendations provided in this section are mostly based on expert opinion derived from clinical practice due to paucity in the literature.

5.5.1. *General precautions to physiotherapy in intensive care*

- The patient should be haemodynamically stable (no major fluctuations in vital sign parameters or cardiac rhythm) for the 24 hours before physiotherapy treatment is initiated.
- The patient's response (vital signs and facial expressions) to treatment should be monitored and the physiotherapist should be aware of any adverse responses to treatment that the patient may develop during the session.
- If the patient is attached to a bedside heart rate monitor, the beat volume (QRS trace volume) on the monitor should be increased so that the physiotherapist can hear any sudden changes in heart beat rhythm during

Table 5.7: NICE recommendations for functional assessment of patients after critical care prior to discharge from hospital*.

Physical dimensions

- Physical problems
- Sensory problems
- Communication problems
- Social care or equipment needs

Non-physical dimensions

- Anxiety
- Depression
- Post-traumatic stress-related symptoms
- Behavioural and cognitive problems
- Psychosocial problems

*Adapted from National Institute for Health and Clinical Excellence (2009, Clinical Guideline number 83).

the treatment session, especially if they stand in a position that obscures their direct view of the monitor display.

- If the patient is being fed through a nasogastric tube, the tube feed should be switched off prior to treatment for the duration of the treatment. This helps to prevent any aspiration of feed into the airways during the use of body position changes such as postural drainage or modified postural drainage positions. The tube feed can be resumed at the end of the physiotherapy treatment session.
- Physiotherapists should adhere to the infection control protocols of the ICU that they work in to prevent cross-infection between patients, as well as for personal safety.
- Physiotherapists are reminded to pre-oxygenate a patient prior to airway suction procedures to prevent episodes of hypoxaemia. At completion of the suction procedure the physiotherapist should remember to return the amount of oxygen therapy delivered to the pre-treatment level (AARC, 2010).
- The duration of each suction event should be less than 15 seconds (AARC, 2010).
- Sterility should be maintained during airway suctioning to minimise the risk of nosocomial infections.

- If the use of manual hyperinflation (MHI) is necessary, the patient should be screened for the presence of contraindications or precautions associated with this treatment modality (see Section 4.2.6.1.2.).
- A pressure manometer should be attached to the manual hyperinflation circuit to ensure that inspiratory airway pressures do not exceed the recommended level of 40 cm H_2O (Gosselink *et al.*, 2008). In most cases adequate visual chest expansion can be achieved with inspiratory airway pressures of 25 cm H_2O (Van Aswegen *et al.*, 2013).
- At the end of the physiotherapy treatment session the intubated patient should be positioned in a 30–45° head-up supported sitting position to prevent the risk of aspiration of feed with resultant development of ventilator-associated pneumonia (Minei *et al.*, 2006).
- If a bubble PEP bottle is indicated for use in a spontaneously breathing patient, it is important to change the water in the bottle on a daily basis. The patient should also be advised not to drink the water from the bottle, as the water reservoir forms a breeding ground for infection for bacteria such as *Pseudomonas aeruginosa* (Schobert and Tielen, 2010).

5.5.2. *Precautions and contraindications related to abdominal injuries*

5.5.2.1. *Adult patients*

- The patient should receive analgesia at least half an hour prior to the physiotherapy treatment session.
- Use caution when changing the sedated patient's position in bed or when mobilising a patient around the ICU or in the ward to ensure that no drainage tubes are pulled out accidentally.
- Use manual chest clearance techniques with caution over the anterior basal lung segments, as the patient might experience pain and discomfort from the laparotomy incision site and swelling over the abdominal area after surgery.
- Chest percussions have been shown to cause alveolar collapse in spontaneously breathing patients; therefore it should be interspersed with frequent periods of deep breathing with inspiratory hold. In ventilated patients it should be interspersed with MHI or ventilator hyperinflation

breaths to increase lung volumes and re-expand areas that might have collapsed during treatment (Guimaraes and Zin, 2008).

- Support any surgical wounds manually or with the use of pillows or rolled-up towels placed over the wound when coughing to enhance the effectiveness of the patient's cough.
- Patients who are nursed in the ICU with an open abdomen (damage control surgery) should not be sat up in bed immediately after surgery. A 25° head-up tilt to prevent aspiration is acceptable (Mietto *et al.*, 2013). These patients should only be sat up and mobilised out of bed once permission had been obtained from the trauma surgeon. The use of an abdominal binder (Fig. 5.12) is recommended in order to provide external support to the abdominal organs.
- After surgical closure of a prolonged open abdomen there is a risk for the development of abdominal compartment syndrome. In this situation, turning of the patient in bed for chest physiotherapy should be limited until the abdominal pressure has decreased to an acceptable level; discussion with the attending trauma surgeon will guide daily management.

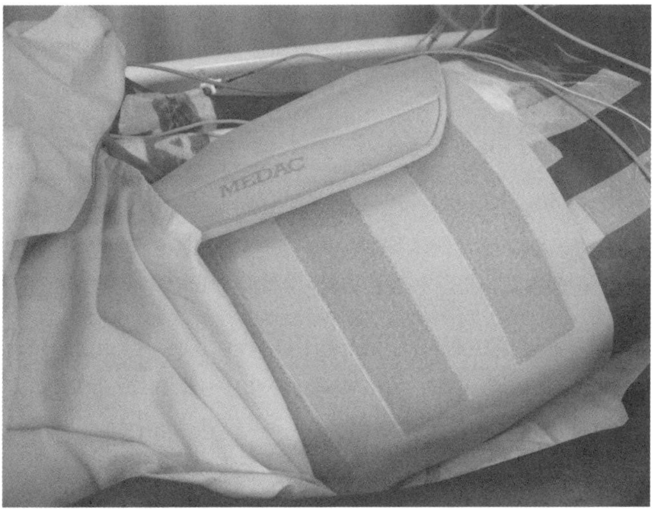

Fig. 5.12: Abdominal binder.

- Adequate time (minimum of six weeks) should be allowed for wound healing after abdominal closure before strengthening exercises are prescribed for the rectus abdominis and transverse oblique muscles.

5.5.2.2. *Paediatric patients*

- The same precautions and contraindications outlined above apply to a paediatric patient with blunt or penetrating abdominal injuries, but MHI should generally not be used.
- If MHI is considered essential, care should be taken to inflate to normal levels, according to patient weight, instead of hyperinflating, to prevent volutrauma. Peak inspiratory pressure should be monitored and generally be kept under 30 cm H_2O to minimise the risk of barotrauma.

5.5.3. *Precautions and contraindications related to thoracic injuries*

5.5.3.1. *Adult patients*

- The patient should receive analgesia at least half an hour prior to the physiotherapy treatment session.
- Manual chest shaking and chest vibrations should not be used over chest wall areas where rib fractures are present. Gentle manual chest percussion may be used over single rib fractures provided that the patient received sufficient analgesia prior to treatment and can tolerate the treatment. The use of a mechanical vibromat over the chest wall instead of manual chest therapy techniques, especially over flail rib segments, is suggested in order to prevent damage to the underlying lung tissue. The physiotherapist should monitor the patient's response to treatment closely.
- The physiotherapist should support any surgical wounds manually or with the use of pillows or rolled-up towels when the patient coughs in order to enhance the effectiveness of the cough effort.
- Caution should be used when a patient who has suffered from pulmonary contusion presents with a platelet count less than 50,000 cells/mm^3 and haemoptysis. The ICU physician or attending doctor should be consulted before such a patient receives chest physiotherapy treatment.

If the use of chest clearance techniques is granted, a mechanical vibromat should be used until the acute phase of haemoptysis has resolved.
- Manual chest clearance techniques are contraindicated in the presence of acute pulmonary oedema. Surfactant is often coughed up from the lungs during acute pulmonary oedema and not pulmonary secretions. As surfactant is removed from the lung fields, atelectasis develops and hypoxaemia progressively worsens.
- Care should be taken when using manual chest clearance techniques around the insertion site of ICD tubes so as not to cause excessive pain or discomfort.
- The ICD bottle should be kept below the level of insertion into the chest wall during a physiotherapy treatment session. If there is a need to lift the bottle above the chest wall insertion site, the tube should be temporarily clamped to prevent drainage of fluid back into the pleural cavity.
- During mobilisation the ICD bottle should be carried by its strings (or in a pillow case or equivalent if strings are not available) and held close to the body to prevent it from catching on objects in the ICU or ward environment (Fig. 5.13).
- In the event of the ICD tube pulling out of the chest wall, the patient should be instructed to exhale completely and cover the wound on the chest wall firmly with their hand to prevent air from the atmosphere from entering the chest cavity. The patient should then call for assistance from the nursing personnel.
- In the event of the ICD bottle breaking, the patient should be instructed to kink the tube closed to prevent air from the atmosphere from entering the chest cavity. They should then call immediately for assistance from the nursing personnel.
- After a sternotomy procedure has been done the physiotherapist should advise the patient that any upper limb activities above 90° shoulder elevation or abduction should be done bilaterally for the first six weeks. No forced shoulder movements should be performed. This is to minimise disruption of the bone union at the sternal surgical site.
- After a sternotomy the patient should be taught that when sitting up over the side of the bed, they should use their arms as little as possible and rather cross their arms over the chest to support the sternum, turn onto their side and slide their legs over the side of the bed to sit up.

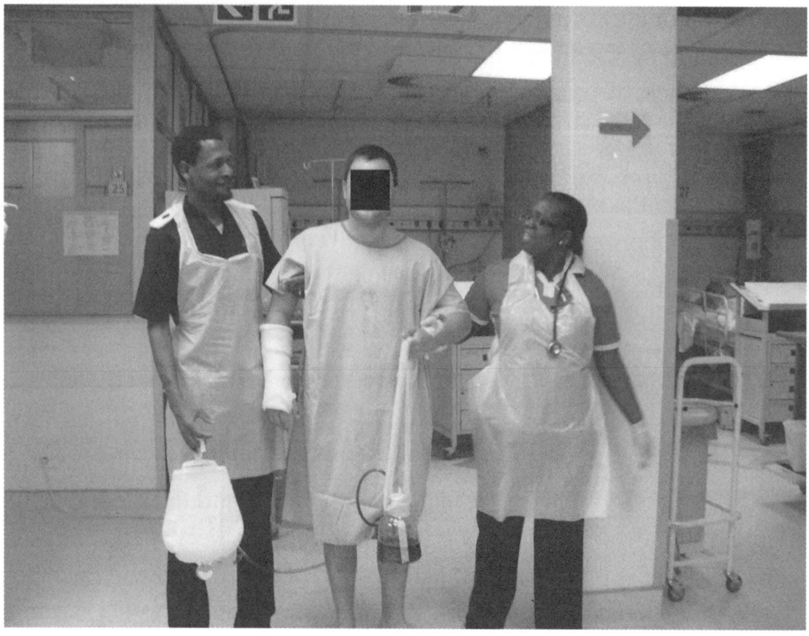

Fig. 5.13: Early mobilisation of patient with rib fractures and haemothorax (managed with ICD) in the ICU.

- In the case of sternotomy, support should be applied over the sternum when the patient coughs to clear retained secretions or during sneezing.
- General advice given to patients after a sternotomy procedure in relation to participation in ADL includes:
  - no opposing arm movements for the first six to eight weeks after surgery;
  - no driving for the first six weeks after surgery;
  - no heavy lifting or carrying of heavy objects for the first 12 weeks postoperatively; and
  - a return to sporting activities such as golfing, jogging and swimming by six to eight weeks postoperatively only after consultation with the surgeon (Paz and West, 2009).

Surgeons may, however, have their own preferred protocol to guide patients in participation in ADL, which necessitates good communication between the physiotherapist and surgeon for optimal patient self-reliance.

5.5.3.2. *Paediatric patients*

- Before treating a child who has sustained a thoracic injury, it is essential that any spinal injury has been excluded. One study of over 80 children with spinal injuries showed that 6% also had thoracic trauma (Turgut *et al.*, 1996). Therefore, spinal precautions must be maintained until clinical or radiographic clearance has been obtained from the orthopaedic surgeon or neurosurgeon.
- Physiotherapists must also be aware that even a severely contused lung may have no visible external bruising (Bliss and Silen, 2002).
- Similar precautions and contraindications as described above apply to paediatric patients with blunt or penetrating thoracic injuries.
- Education of the child's caregiver or parents regarding precautions related to the ICD, coughing with wound support and activity limitations following sternotomy is important to maximise treatment outcomes.

5.6. Physiotherapy Interventions

Physiotherapy management of the critically ill patient is often a daunting concept for physiotherapy students, newly-qualified physiotherapists and physiotherapists who don't regularly work in the ICU setting. In order to alleviate some of these anxieties, and to provide some standardisation to the physiotherapeutic management of critically ill patients, step-wise intervention protocols were published by Morris *et al.*, (2008) and Hanekom *et al.*, (2011). Although these protocols were written for the general ICU population and not specifically for patients with traumatic injuries, many of the principles of management remain the same and can be implemented for the patient recovering from blunt or penetrating abdominal or thoracic injuries.

In the acute stage early after injury, when the patient is sedated and uncooperative, physiotherapy management primarily focuses on the support of the respiratory system, followed by prevention of neuromusculoskeletal complications associated with immobility. As the patient's condition stabilises and they wake up from sedation in the ICU and become more cooperative, active rehabilitation is immediately commenced. The discussion of physiotherapy interventions provided below will therefore start with respiratory system followed by musculoskeletal system management. Recommendations provided here are based on evidence as well as expert opinion in the absence of research evidence.

5.6.1. *Respiratory system management*

5.6.1.1. *Oxygenation*

Oxygenation is most improved in the upright standing position, as in this position functional residual capacity (FRC) is optimal, as discussed in Chapter 4. Oxygenation may be improved for intubated as well as spontaneously breathing patients with abdominal or thoracic injuries by utilising body position changes to enhance V/Q matching.

5.6.1.1.1. Uncooperative sedated and intubated patient

The upright standing position is not feasible during the early stages of the patient's admission to the ICU and therefore positions such as 45–60° head-up high supported sitting positions may need to be used instead (only 25° for patients with open abdomens) for V/Q matching.

5.6.1.1.2. Cooperative intubated patient

Sitting over the edge of the bed (provided that precautions have been cleared with the surgeon) should be encouraged as well as sitting out in a chair by the bedside, as these positions increase FRC more than positions in bed and results in improved oxygenation (Frownfelter and Dean, 2006).

5.6.1.1.3. Spontaneously breathing patient

As the patient's condition continues to improve, upright standing and walking away from the bedside should be encouraged several times per day to optimise FRC and oxygenation (Frownfelter and Dean, 2006).

5.6.1.2. *Humidification*

5.6.1.2.1. Intubated patient

Humidification can be administered to intubated patients in the form of a heat–moisture exchanger attached to the ventilator circuit. If, however, the patient is ventilated for more than one week or if secretions become infected and more difficult to remove effectively from the airways, humidification in the form of a heated water humidifier is recommended (AARC, 2003). Patients with chronic lung disease, as co-morbidity, should always be treated with heated humidification applied through the ventilator circuit (AARC, 2003).

5.6.1.2.2. Spontaneously breathing patient

Humidification of a spontaneously breathing patient's airways can be achieved through heated humidified oxygen mask or intermittent nebulisation using 0.9% sodium chloride (NaCl) solution. This solution can be administered through a small volume (jet) nebuliser using a face mask or a mouth piece. Hypertonic saline solution may be used for patients with underlying chronic respiratory diseases such as cystic fibrosis (Elkins and Dentice, 2012). Hypertonic saline may cause bronchospasm, so close observation of the patient during treatment is important.

5.6.1.3. *Management of pulmonary secretions*

5.6.1.3.1. Intubated patient

For an intubated and mechanically ventilated patient with abdominal or thoracic trauma, pulmonary secretion mobilisation and removal can be achieved through the use of modified postural drainage positions, manual chest clearance techniques (within the limitation of precautions and contraindications described in Section 5.5), suction and MHI. The reader is referred to Chapter 4 (Section 4.2) for information on precautions and contraindications that should be considered prior to using these techniques, as well as how to effectively perform each technique.

During airway suction, 0.9% NaCl may be instilled in small amounts down the artificial airway in an attempt to stimulate a cough to enhance secretion clearance; however, close monitoring of the patient's peripheral oxygen saturation during saline instillation is advised. Saline instillation should not be a routine procedure during suction but should only be undertaken in the presence of viscous secretions which are difficult to clear. It is important to note that normal saline does not mix with mucus and therefore does not thin mucus but merely serves to stimulate a cough effort to assist with clearance of secretions (Halm and Hagel, 2008).

Key Messages

The position of the ETT should be monitored during treatment. Signs of an ETT that has migrated above the vocal cords include:

- Audible throat sounds when the patient coughs.
- Presence of bronchial breath sounds in the upper lobe segments of the right and left lung fields on auscultation.
- Noticeably decreased breath sounds in the basal lung segments of both lungs on auscultation.

The use of open suction versus closed suction has been a topic of many debates in the clinical setting. Two systematic reviews found that there was no significant difference between the two methods in relation to the risk for the development of ventilator-associated pneumonia, length of stay in the ICU, mortality, haemodynamic instability, oxygen saturation or cost (Pedersen *et al.*, 2009; Subirana *et al.*, 2010). This has also been shown to be true in the paediatric age group (Morrow and Argent, 2008; Morrow *et al.*, 2012).

5.6.1.3.2. Spontaneously breathing patient

The spontaneously breathing patient with abdominal or thoracic injuries may be shown how to perform the active cycle of breathing technique (ACBT) in order to assist with secretion mobilisation and clearance. The reader is referred to Chapter 4 (Section 4.2.1.2.) for information on how to perform ACBT. Encouragement to huff (forced expiratory technique), cough and expectorate retained secretions is vitally important. Some patients who breathe spontaneously may be too weak or in too much pain to clear secretions effectively with ACBT alone. These types of patients will benefit from the addition of postural drainage or modified postural drainage positions and manual chest therapy techniques (applied within the limitations of precautions and contraindications discussed in Section 5.5), together with ACBT. Mobilisation around the ward and active exercises further assists with secretion mobilisation and clearance.

5.6.1.4. *Lung capacity and volumes*

5.6.1.4.1. Intubated patient

Lung capacity in the form of FRC may be improved through the use of positive expiratory pressure (PEP). Positive expiratory pressure assists with splinting open the peripheral airways, enlarging FRC and in so doing increasing the surface area available for gas exchange, hence leading to improved oxygenation. Continuous PEP is administered to the intubated patient through the positive end-expiratory pressure (PEEP) setting on the ventilator. The advantage of PEEP is that the alveoli remain distended for prolonged periods, increasing surfactant production in those alveoli that were previously collapsed (Stokke, 1976; Soni and Williams, 2008).

Techniques such as regular body position changes in bed as well as MHI can be used to improve inspiratory lung volumes in patients who are intubated and mechanically ventilated. The reader is referred to Chapter 4 (Section 4.2.6.1.) for information on precautions and contraindications that should be considered prior to the use of MHI. Information is also provided on how to effectively perform MHI. If lung volumes are reduced in the lower lobe segments of the left lung, MHI performed with the patient in the supine position may not be successful in re-inflating these lung segments (Van Aswegen *et al.*, 2013) (see discussion in Chapter 4, Section 4.2.6.1.1.). Manual hyperinflation also reduces airway resistance and assists with the improvement of lung compliance (Paratz *et al.*, 2002; Choi and Jones, 2005).

As soon as the intubated patient regains consciousness, ACBT can be initiated, with emphasis on the thoracic expansion exercises component to encourage collateral ventilation through the peripheral airways and thereby improve lung volumes. The patient should be encouraged to observe and increase lung volume changes produced on the ventilator screen (biofeedback) during the thoracic expansion exercises component of ACBT to further emphasise lung expansion.

Body position changes that involve moving from supine to sitting and upright standing also lead to improvements in FRC, as discussed previously. These body position changes can be implemented as soon as the intubated patient is awake and cooperative.

5.6.1.4.2. Spontaneously breathing patient

Spontaneously breathing patients may improve lung volumes by performing techniques such as ACBT, incentive spirometry, intermittent positive pressure breathing (IPPB), active exercises and mobilisation. The reader is referred to Chapter 4 (Section 4.2) for information on how to perform these techniques safely and effectively.

Care should be taken during the use of incentive spirometry to encourage lateral costal deep breathing in order to correct the patient's breathing pattern from apical to diaphragmatic breathing (Fig. 5.14). The American Association for Respiratory Care (AARC) recommends that incentive spirometry be used in combination with deep breathing, directed coughing and early mobilisation to increase its effectiveness in improving lung volumes (AARC, 2011).

In a systematic review on the use of incentive spirometry for the prevention of PPC in adults after upper abdominal surgery, Guimaraes *et al.* (2009) stated that no evidence could be found to support the use of

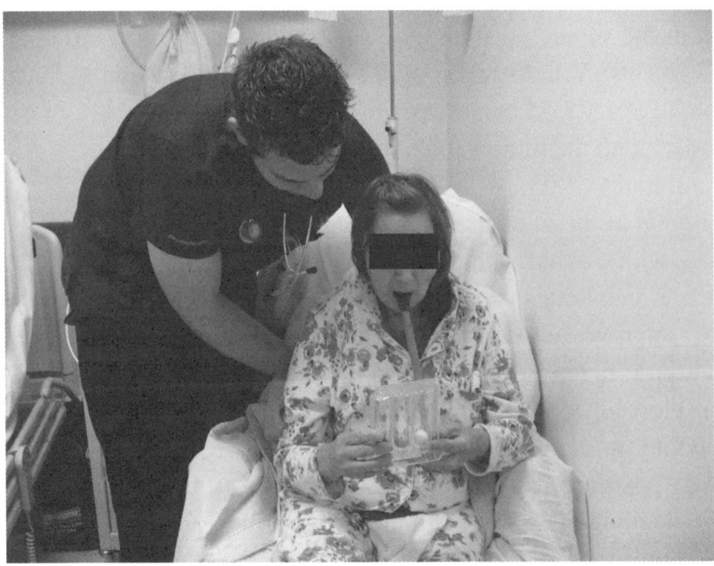

Fig. 5.14: Patient after thoracic surgery using incentive spirometry while physiotherapist encourages basal lung expansion.

incentive spirometry to prevent PPC. However, the authors acknowledged that the results of their review were limited by the low methodological quality of the included trials. The majority of the included trials did not assess the same outcomes and therefore results across trials could not be pooled for meta-analysis (Guimaraes *et al.*, 2009). Incentive spirometry remains a popular treatment technique among physiotherapists in cardiorespiratory care, but a lack of research evidence to support its use must be acknowledged. There is a need for well-designed randomised controlled trials on the use of incentive spirometry to prevent or reduce pulmonary complications in patients who suffered blunt or penetrating abdominal or thoracic trauma.

The only recent study published on the use of IPPB in thoracic surgery was that by Ludwig *et al.*, (2011). They administered 15–20 mmHg pressure to patients following lung resection surgery to see if the addition of IPPB to standard physiotherapy care would result in an improvement in lung function postoperatively. They reported similar pre- and post-operative lung function results in both the control and experimental groups and were unable to show any additional benefit of IPPB to standard physiotherapy care for their patient population (Ludwig *et al.*, 2011). No recent systematic reviews on the use of IPPB in patients after upper abdominal or thoracic surgery could be found and therefore the lack of evidence to support the use of IPPB in this patient population should be acknowledged. Similarly, there is a need for well-designed randomised controlled trials on the use of IPPB in the prevention or reduction of pulmonary complications in patients who have suffered blunt or penetrating abdominal or thoracic injuries.

Non-invasive continuous positive airway pressure (CPAP) ventilation has been used on spontaneously breathing patients postoperatively to increase FRC and prevent the onset of PPC such as atelectasis and pneumonia. Ferreyra *et al.*, (2008) conducted a meta-analysis on the use of CPAP to decrease the risk of PPC after elective abdominal surgery. They reported that CPAP significantly reduced the risk of the development of atelectasis (risk ratio 0.75) and pneumonia (risk ratio 0.33).

Continuous PEP may be administered through the use of a PEP mask. The reader is referred to Chapter 4 (Section 4.2.2.4.) for information on how to use a PEP mask safely and effectively during physiotherapy treatment. The PEP mask keeps the alveoli pressurised for the 10 breaths performed in a sequence, which also adds benefit compared to methods in which positive pressure is only maintained for a few seconds during expiration. Orman and Westerdahl (2010) investigated the use of PEP with chest physiotherapy in adult patients after abdominal and thoracic surgery. Their systematic review concluded that positive expiratory pressure in the form of a PEP mask or with the use of a bubble PEP bottle was not inferior to any other chest physiotherapy technique performed and had an effect similar to that of CPAP. They did, however, highlight the low methodological quality of the articles included in their review (Orman and Westerdahl, 2010). They recommended that the long-term effects of PEP on treatment outcomes in patients undergoing abdominal and thoracic surgery should be investigated.

Oscillating PEP may be administered to the patient through the use of a bubble PEP bottle or a flutter device. The reader is referred to Chapter 4 (Section 4.2.2.4.) for information about the safe and effective use of oscillating PEP devices.

5.6.1.5. *Respiratory muscle training*

Inspiratory muscle training for patients who undergo prolonged MV may be achieved by using ACBT with biofeedback (as described above). Progression can be achieved by applying gentle manual resistance to the diaphragm while the patient is performing ACBT (caution should be used in the presence of a laparotomy incision) and by gradually increasing the time dedicated to strength training during a single treatment session. Throughout each session careful monitoring of the patient's response to training should be performed by monitoring changes in respiratory rate and peripheral oxygen saturation. Care should be taken not to overexert the patient as this delays the progression of weaning from MV.

Another method of inspiratory muscle training is the temporary reduction in the level of pressure support or the trigger sensitivity delivered to the patient through the ventilator. The reader is referred to Chapter 4 (Section 4.2.1.5.) for information on how to perform these interventions. This approach to inspiratory muscle training should be discussed with the attending physician in the ICU and care should be taken to reset the pressure support or trigger sensitivity to the pre-treatment level at the end of each treatment session.

A spring-loaded inspiratory muscle trainer device (Fig. 5.15A) can also be used for inspiratory muscle training if available in the local ICU (Chapter 4, Section 4.2.1.5.1.1. as this is specific to spring loaded device). The encouragement of basal lung segment expansion is important while the patient trains with this device (Fig. 5.15B).

One case study has described the use of high-intensity inspiratory muscle training as part of the longer-term rehabilitation of an adult patient following a near-fatal thoraco-abdominal gunshot wound and symptoms of severe dyspnoea on exertion (Hill *et al.*, 2011). An average of five sessions of inspiratory muscle training was completed each week for 10 weeks. His maximum forced inspiratory flow increased by 48% and, although dyspnoea scores were not presented, his main complaints when exercising changed from dyspnoea to leg fatigue.

5.6.1.6. *Paediatric considerations*

Caregivers and their children should be informed about the need for and nature of physiotherapy interventions at an appropriate developmental level for the child. To the authors' knowledge there are currently no clinical studies into the effects or optimal methods of physiotherapy for children following thoracic and abdominal surgery; therefore recommendations are based on expert opinion derived from physiological and anatomical

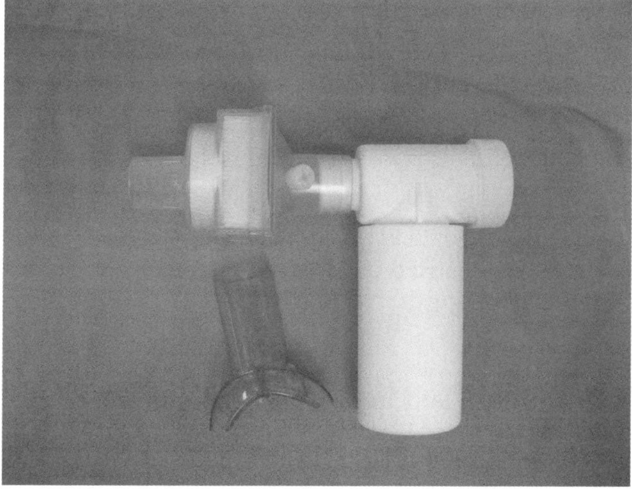

Fig. 5.15A: PowerBreathe® device.

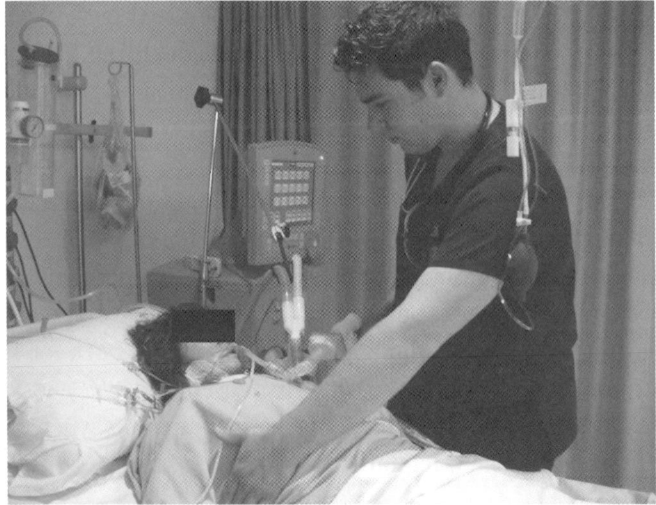

Fig. 5.15B: Patient performing deep basal breathing while attached to heat moisture exchanger and the PowerBreathe® device.

considerations. Generally, similar techniques can be used for the young and old, but these need to be adapted and tailored according to the patient's age and developmental level and acuity of presentation.

Most children will move and cough spontaneously if they are able to do so and it is pain free. Therefore, analgesia is probably the single most important consideration in optimising pulmonary and general function in children following a traumatic injury. In addition, the hospital, and particularly the paediatric ICU, is a frightening place for a young child, who may be without their family, with many of the interventions being painful, unfamiliar and unpleasant. These factors must be considered when choosing a treatment modality and, where possible and appropriate, the opportunity for autonomy (patient choice) should be given. The experience of physiotherapy for traumatised children should be as positive as possible, and at the very least pain free.

5.6.1.6.1. Intubated sedated and uncooperative child

The ventilated child may require mainly passive chest physiotherapy involving positioning to drain secretions and optimise V/Q matching (modified postural drainage with the head raised or flat but not inverted), manual therapy (vibrations, percussions or shaking) if permitted and endotracheal suctioning, provided the child is haemodynamically stable and there are no other contraindications (see Section 5.5). Endotracheal suctioning guidelines for infants and children are provided in a review paper by Morrow and Argent (2008).

Manual hyperinflation generally should not be used with young children and infants, particularly following any thoracic trauma, as children are physiologically more predisposed to developing pneumothoraces than adults (see Chapter 2). If a pneumothorax is already present with an ICD *in situ*, the use of MHI could lead to the formation of a bronchopulmonary fistula, by continually forcing air through the path of least resistance.

5.6.1.6.2. Spontaneously breathing child

Deep breathing and localised expansion exercises (Chapter 4, Section 4.2.1.) can be performed, even with very young children, through playful means such as bubble blowing (Fig. 5.16), with the hands placed on the thorax to allow sensory feedback and intercostal muscle stretch, when indicated, by end-expiratory pressure.

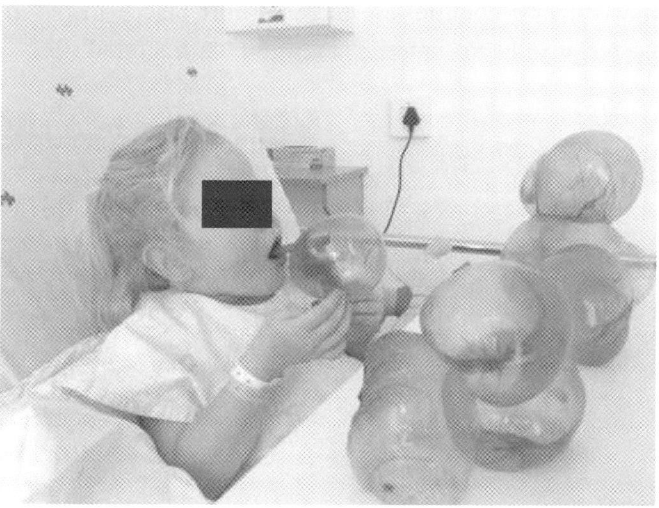

Fig. 5.16: Child doing deep breathing exercises with PEP by means of blowing games.

Incentive spirometry is useful in older children. Forced expiratory technique (huffing) can also be taught to quite young children who are able to mimic. Tracheal pressure to stimulate a cough should be avoided in any child with known or suspected airway injury, obstruction or inflammation, within a few days after extubation or where there are arrhythmias such as bradycardia. Tracheal rubs are also contraindicated in children less than nine months of age as the trachea is still very compliant and pressure may result in severe airway obstruction. In these cases, if a spontaneous cough is not elicited following treatment, and there are signs of secretion retention, a cough can be stimulated using nasopharyngeal, oropharyngeal or endotracheal suction (Chapter 4, Section 4.2.7.).

5.6.2. *Neuromusculoskeletal system management*

5.6.2.1. *Pain*

In addition to analgesic medication, pain relief for patients with rib fractures can be achieved through the use of kinesiotaping. Two methods of taping can be used. Figure 5.17A illustrates the square-shaped taping technique. The tape is applied around the area of the fracture, with the rib fracture in the centre of the square. Another taping method utilises the intercostal spaces (Fig. 5.17B): the tape should be applied with its base next to the vertebral column and three strands placed in the intercostal spaces (posterior to latero-anterior) between the fractured ribs.

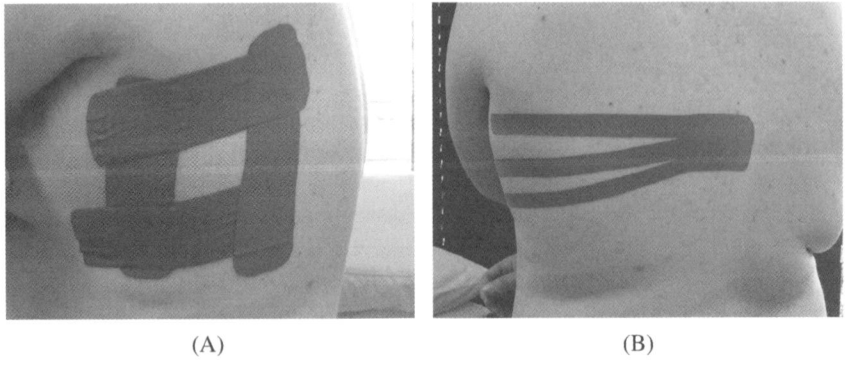

(A) (B)

Fig. 5.17: Kinesiotaping techniques for pain relief following rib fractures. (A) Square-shaped taping around a rib fracture; (B) Taping in intercostal spaces between fractured ribs.

Clinical benefits observed through the use of kinesiotaping include assistance with lymphatic drainage from the fracture site and resolution of skin discolouration and pain relief; however, no clinical trials have been conducted to date to provide evidence for the treatment effectiveness of kinesiotaping in the management of patients with chest wall injuries.

5.6.2.2. *Joint range of motion*

5.6.2.2.1. Uncooperative sedated and intubated patient

Daily passive ROM movements and passive stretches of all two-joint muscles should form part of the management of the musculoskeletal system while the patient is sedated. Passive cycling in bed to maintain or improve ROM may also be used for the sedated patient if the equipment is available in your local ICU. Benefits of a 20-minute daily passive cycling programme in addition to usual respiratory care in critically ill patients on prolonged MV were shown in terms of improvement in functional status, exercise endurance and duration of hospital stay (Burtin *et al.*, 2009).

5.6.2.2.2. Cooperative patient

Upper limb and trunk active ROM exercises are particularly important in the management of patients in the ICU and ward setting with an ICD *in situ* or after a thoracotomy. Such exercises should place particular emphasis on active end-of-range flexion, extension, abduction and rotation movements of the neck and shoulder girdle, as well as flexion, extension, side-flexion and rotation movements of the trunk, to prevent limitations in range and abnormal posture.

Key Message

The amount of blood that drains from the pleural space into the ICD bottle during physiotherapy treatment should be monitored closely. Excessive amounts of drainage in a single treatment session (> 200 ml) could indicate active bleeding in the pleural space. The trauma team should be alerted immediately.

5.6.2.3. *Muscle strength*

5.6.2.3.1. Uncooperative sedated and intubated patient

Neuro-muscular electrical stimulation (NMES) has been used by some physiotherapists for acutely ill, uncooperative patients in the ICU in an attempt to counteract musculoskeletal dysfunction such as muscle weakness and wasting. A systematic review of the effectiveness of NMES in addressing musculoskeletal dysfunction in critically ill patients was recently published (Maffiuletti *et al.*, 2013). Trials included in the review reported the application of NMES to various muscle groups including quadriceps, hamstrings, glutei, peroneus longi and biceps brachii. The method of application varied between the trials. The reviewers concluded that the addition of NMES to usual patient care in the ICU may prevent muscle weakness, but that further research was needed to determine if NMES could prevent muscle wasting associated with critical illness.

5.6.2.3.2. Cooperative intubated patient

As soon as consciousness is regained, active-assisted, active and active-resisted exercises should be encouraged to improve general muscle strength within the limits of the abovementioned precautions and contraindications. The reader is referred to Chapter 4 (Section 4.1) for exercise prescription guidelines for resistance training for patients in the acute and sub-acute stages after traumatic injury. Early active exercise following trauma and critical illness decreases pro-inflammatory and increases anti-inflammatory cytokine activity, which decreases inflammation, counteracts skeletal muscle protein catabolism and improves microcirculation (Kayambu *et al.*, 2013).

5.6.2.3.3. Spontaneously breathing patient

Progression of the strengthening exercises implemented during the intubation phase should be a rehabilitation priority, even if the patient is still in the ICU.

5.6.2.4. *Functional activities and mobilisation*

As soon as the patient regains consciousness in the ICU, functional activities such as rolling in bed, bridging, sitting up over the side of the bed, standing upright, stepping and walking should form part of their physiotherapy rehabilitation programme. The aims of these activities are to decrease the effects of immobility on the musculoskeletal system and to improve oxygenation and respiratory function. These activities should be commenced while the patient is still intubated and ventilated. Team work among members of the ICU interdisciplinary team is important to safely mobilise these patients out of bed. Devices such as standing hoists can be used to assist the deconditioned patient from a sitting to standing position. Electronic hoists or walking frames can be used to assist with transferring patients out of bed to a chair. Deconditioned patients may initially need assistance from more than one physiotherapist when practising sit-to-stand transfers from a chair in the ICU (Figs 5.18A and B).

Body position changes in adult intubated and ventilated patients after abdominal surgery (as described earlier) create positive changes in tidal volume, minute ventilation and respiratory frequency, and marching on

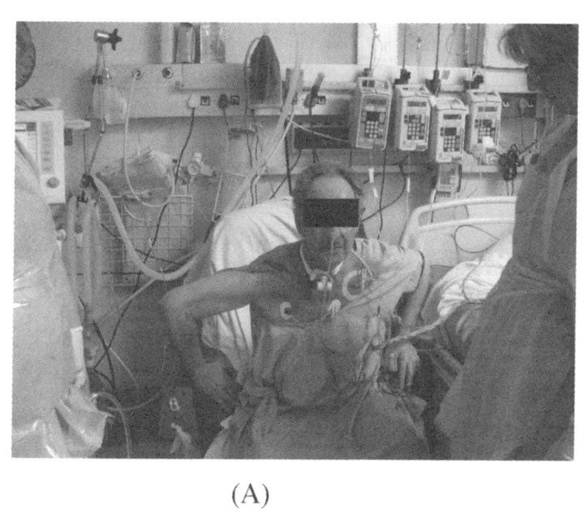

(A)

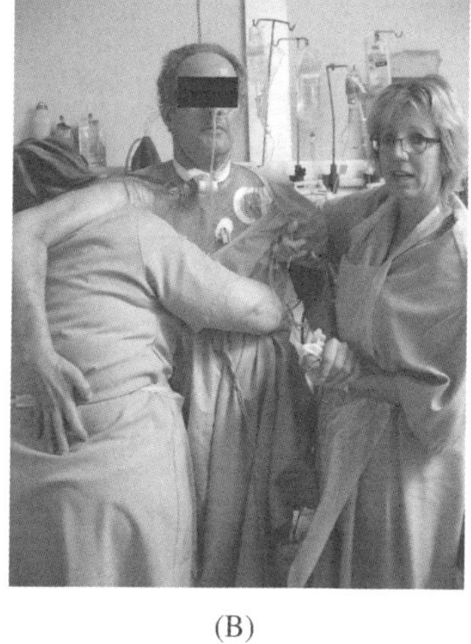

(B)

Fig. 5.18: A patient with multiple rib fractures, right-sided clavicle fracture, blunt abdominal trauma and prolonged ICU stay is stable enough on day 63 to practise sit-to-stand transfers from a chair. (A) The patient prepares to stand up from the chair by moving forwards and pushing through the arm rests of the chair; (B) Two physiotherapists assist the patient to stand up using a modified lifting technique on his right side to avoid traction on the fractured clavicle.

the spot by the bedside in the ICU may prevent lower limb muscle deconditioning (Zafiropoulos *et al.*, 2004).

Patients who are haemodynamically stable should be encouraged to sit out of bed in a chair as early as day one or two after surgery. Mobilisation of the patient should take the form of walking short distances away from the bedside (e.g. to the wash basin or the bathroom) regularly during the day. Early active mobilisation of patients in the ICU is safe and the few adverse events reported in the literature during mobilisation do not lead to extubation, complications that required additional treatment or increased cost or length of stay in the ICU or hospital (Li *et al.*, 2013). The physiotherapist should aim to increase the walking distance away from the bedside daily as a progression of mobilisation. If at this stage the patient is still intubated and a portable ventilator is not available, ventilation can be supplied through the use of an MHI circuit that is attached to the patient's endotracheal or tracheostomy tube and a portable oxygen cylinder during mobilisation. Recently, researchers from Australia found an association between delayed postoperative mobilisation and the development of PPC. They found that patients who underwent upper abdominal surgery and delayed mobilising away from the bedside were three times more likely to develop PPC than those who did manage to walk away from the bedside soon after surgery (Haines *et al.*, 2013).

5.6.2.5. *Exercise endurance*

Activities such as walking at a fast pace, cycling on a stationary bicycle in the ward or the hospital physiotherapy department, stair climbing, star-jumps and squatting should gradually be added to the patient's rehabilitation programme as their condition improves. The duration of these activities as well as the frequency of exercise per day should be increased in order to improve exercise endurance prior to discharge from the hospital. The reader is referred to Chapter 4 (Section 4.1) for aerobic exercise prescription guidelines for patients in the acute and sub-acute stages of hospitalisation. The patient should be able to perform more ADL independently and with less effort as their exercise endurance returns to pre-injury levels.

5.6.2.6. *Paediatric considerations*

Paediatric treatment, as with adults, is directed at early mobilisation when possible in order to optimise ventilation and perfusion and to prevent the numerous complications of immobility. Mobilisation occurs on a continuum from turning in bed, to sitting, to standing and walking (Fig. 5.19). The developmental level of the child as well as any associated injuries must be taken into account, with appropriate precautions in place when moving children who have sustained thoracic or abdominal trauma.

Bedridden children and infants will benefit from simple rolling games to reach toys, for example, or, if they are able to sit independently or with

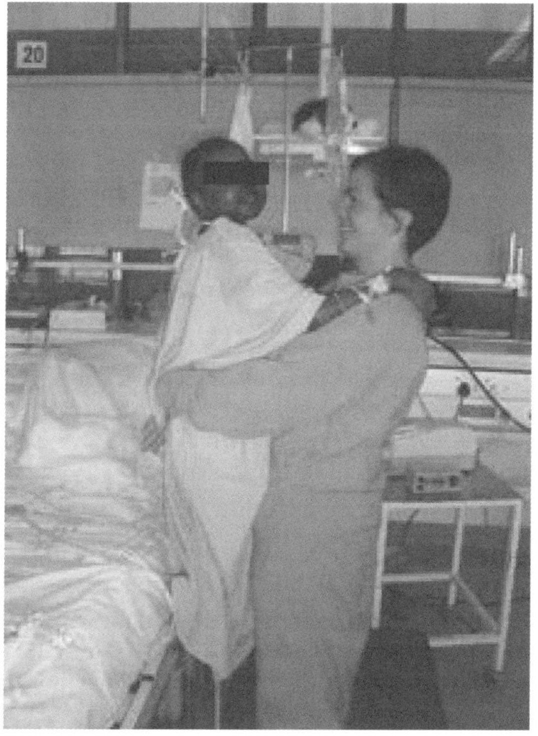

Fig. 5.19: One of the authors mobilising a ventilated 10-year-old child to standing in the paediatric ICU.

support, trunk rotational or flexion exercises using play will improve chest expansion and thoracic mobility as well as improve drainage via ICD. Upper extremity exercises are also essential, especially following thoracotomy or ICD insertion, to prevent loss of ROM at the shoulder and postural deformities such as scoliosis. This can again be accomplished through play in children (e.g. throwing or hitting a balloon or ball).

5.6.3. *Patient response to treatment*

The ultimate outcome measure for all patients with traumatic abdominal or thoracic injury should be function and to what degree they can return to their premorbid status. Some outcome measures may be more useful than others at particular stages of each patient's recovery. The reader is referred to Chapter 4 (Section 4.3) for a list of subjective and objective markers as well as outcome measurement tools to use during the evaluation of the effectiveness of treatment interventions given during patient rehabilitation.

5.7. Clinical Case Scenarios

5.7.1. *Adult clinical case scenarios*

5.7.1.1. *Case 1*

A 35-year-old man was held at gun point and robbed. The robbers proceeded to shoot him and he sustained injuries to the stomach, transverse colon, left hemi-diaphragm and lower lobes of the left lung. A laparotomy and thoracotomy were performed to stop the internal bleeding and repair the damaged organs. The damage control approach to surgery was used and the abdominal cavity was covered with gauze packs and OpSite® dressings but not surgically closed. Further surgery would be needed in the next few days to complete the repair of damaged organs. An ICD was placed through the left chest wall into the pleural cavity. The patient was then managed in the trauma ICU, where he was intubated, sedated and received full mechanical ventilator support.

- What infection control principles would you adhere to while working with this patient in the ICU environment?

- In light of the patient's injuries and condition, which precautions would you adhere to during physiotherapy treatment?

5.7.1.1.1. Discussion of case 1

5.7.1.1.1.1. *Infection control principles.* Aspects to consider around infection control should include thorough hand washing and cleaning of equipment brought to and removed from the patient's bedside, for example stethoscopes. Don a clean apron, gloves and protective eye gear before starting patient treatment. Be sure to maintain sterility when suction of the artificial airway is performed.

5.7.1.1.1.2. *Precautions to physiotherapy treatment.* Precautions to adhere to during treatment of this patient would include the following.

- Monitoring of the patient's haemodynamic status during position changes in bed, as the patient would have lost a lot of blood at the time of injury and in theatre so might become hypotensive.
- The physiotherapist should consider asking for additional analgesia to be given during physiotherapy treatment if the need for more pain control becomes apparent.
- Take care not to lift the ICD bottle above the level of insertion into the left chest wall during position changes in bed but clamp the ICD tubing temporarily for position changing.
- Be careful not to pull excessively on the lines attached to the patient during position changes in bed to prevent lines from pulling out.
- The physiotherapist should discuss with the surgeon any risks that the application of MHI might pose to damaging the repair site of the left hemi-diaphragm before the decision is made to use this modality during treatment.
- When the patient coughs during suctioning, the physiotherapist should apply manual support to the open abdomen to reduce discomfort and pain and improve the cough effort.
- The patient should only be sat to 25° head-up position to improve V/Q matching and prevent aspiration of nasogastric feed until the surgeon clears further mobilisation.

5.7.1.2. *Case 2*

A 70-year-old man had an argument with his daughter, who stabbed him through his left lateral chest wall. He was brought to the emergency department by other family members and a diagnosis of haemopneumothorax was made. An ICD was inserted in the left mid-axillary line to relieve the pressure from the thorax and he was transferred to the trauma ward.

On review of his file in the trauma ward, it is found that his past medical history consists of hypertension and a long smoking history. The patient states that he uses Salbutamol and Budesonide via a metered-dose inhaler at home. Arterial blood gas results on admission to the emergency department were pH 7.26, $PaCO_2$ 63.8 mmHg (8.5 kPa), PaO_2 41.9 mmHg (5.6 kPa), HCO_3 27.9 mmol/L and base excess -0.8 on room air. His vital signs in the trauma ward are:

- heart rate of 138 beats per minute;
- blood pressure of 170/103 mmHg;
- respiratory rate of 26 breaths per minute; and
- SpO_2 78% while receiving Atrovent and Berotec via nebulisation (face mask) at three litres per minute at the time of assessment.

On closer examination he presents with nasal flaring, apical breathing, use of accessory inspiratory muscles and an inability to speak in full sentences. Auscultation findings include coarse crackles widespread throughout both the left and right lungs with occasional expiratory wheezes but decreased breath sounds in the left lung compared to the right lung. His SpO_2 drops to 54% when he removes the nebuliser mask to expectorate thick green secretions, his heart rate increases to 147 beats per minute and respiratory rate increases to 35 breaths per minute. On palpation, subcutaneous emphysema is still present on the posterior chest wall region on the left and right sides. The ICD is draining blood-stained fluid and bubbles when the patient coughs. No follow-up chest x-ray is currently available.

- What chronic respiratory condition does this patient likely suffer from and how does the chest trauma influence his respiratory mechanics?
- How would you approach this patient's physiotherapy management?

5.7.1.2.1. Discussion of case 2

5.7.1.2.1.1. *Condition and respiratory mechanics.* This patient could suffer from chronic obstructive pulmonary disease due to his long smoking history and the fact that he uses bronchodilators and corticosteroids at home. Chronic obstructive pulmonary disease leads to premature airway collapse during expiration due to the destructive effects of chronic airway inflammation on the airway walls and lung parenchyma. This premature airway collapse results in air trapping in the distal airways. Chronic air trapping leads to pressure build-up in the lungs, and over time thoracic configuration changes to that of a barrel-shaped chest with a horizontal ribcage and flattened hemi-diaphragms. This leads to changes in respiratory dynamics characterised by prolonged expiration. The haemopneumothorax causes a temporary restrictive lung disorder due to collapse of the left lung under the pressure of the accumulated air and blood in the pleural space of the thorax. Both of these pathologies contribute to the patient's respiratory distress.

5.7.1.2.1.2. *Approach to physiotherapy management.* Initial management of this patient would focus on the following.

- Correction of the flow rate on the oxygen flow meter through which the nebuliser is driven. The flow rate should be set at six litres per minute to ensure adequate delivery of medication to the more distal parts of the tracheobronchial tree. This should ensure better response by the patient to the bronchodilator medication with less bronchospasm as a result.
- Humidification of his airways after the completion of bronchodilator therapy is essential to preserve mucociliary escalator function as much as possible. This can be achieved with the administration of nebulisation with 0.9% NaCl regularly during the day.
- Initial management of this patient should also include an attempt to decrease his respiratory distress. Methods such as positioning of the patient in high, supported sitting in bed positions can be used. High side lying on the left side may be uncomfortable due to the presence of the ICD tube and side lying on the right side may result in more respiratory distress due to the collapsed left lung and pressure in the thorax due to retained air and blood.

- Relaxation of the shoulder girdle should be encouraged, with gentle shoulder girdle exercises being performed to assist the patient to relax.
- As the shoulder girdle relaxes, the physiotherapist should demonstrate and educate the patient on diaphragmatic breathing through the use of the breathing control component of ACBT. All of these methods are employed in an attempt to reduce the patient's respiratory distress.
- The physiotherapist should discuss with the interdisciplinary team in the trauma ward the suitability for the use of non-invasive CPAP in order to reduce the patient's work of breathing. Discussions about the use of non-invasive CPAP should be held prior to the patient reaching a point of exhaustion, as this would be an indication for intubation and MV.

The next step in the management of this patient should be the identification of the cause for his clinical presentation (increased respiratory rate, tachycardia and low SpO_2).

- One of the causes could be pain which is not adequately controlled with the medication that he is currently receiving. His pain should be assessed with a pain scale. If his score is high, the physiotherapist should discuss with the interdisciplinary team possible adjustments to be made to the dosage of medication provided or the addition of other types of analgesic drugs to his existing drug prescription.
- Another cause for his clinical presentation could be an infective lung process that is in progress, as indicated by the thick green secretions that he is expectorating. Discussion with the interdisciplinary team should include taking another chest x-ray to identify if infective changes are present in the lung fields. Laboratory analysis of his sputum should also be done. The physiotherapist should obtain an adequate sputum sample from the patient to be sent to the laboratory for culture (to determine the type of bacteria) and sensitivity analysis (to identify the type of antibiotics to be prescribed).
- Lastly, his clinical presentation could be caused by a recurrence of the pneumothorax or by blood that is not draining adequately from the pleural space into the ICD bottle. Discussion between the physiotherapist and the interdisciplinary team should include a repeat chest x-ray to identify the placement of the ICD tube as well as the presence of a new pneumothorax. If the ICD tube is not in an optimal position to

drain blood from the pleural space, it should be repositioned by the trauma surgeon for optimal function of the ICD. If a new pneumothorax is diagnosed, a second ICD tube should be placed to drain the excess air from the pleural space. Only after correct placement of the ICD tube should physiotherapy treatment recommence.

Further physiotherapy management for this patient to loosen and clear retained secretions as his condition stabilises would include the following.

- Continuation of regular humidification of his airways with 0.9% NaCl solution through nebulisation.
- Active cycle of breathing technique would continue, with more emphasis placed on thoracic expansion exercises and forced expiratory technique (huffing) performed in a gentle manner to prevent premature closing of airways and coughing.
- Modified postural drainage positions (no head-down tilt) can be incorporated with ACBT as the patient is able to tolerate.
- A mechanical vibromat can be used to loosen secretions in specific lung segments if manual chest percussion and shaking is not well tolerated.
- The patient would be educated on how to use devices such as a flutter, bubble PEP bottle or a PEP mask correctly to assist with secretion clearance and to re-expand the collapsed left lung.
- Drainage of the haemopneumothorax and re-expansion of the left lung can be enhanced with the addition of mobilisation of the patient away from the bedside, with daily progression in the distance walked as well as the pace at which the patient walks.
- Active ROM exercises for the left and right shoulders as well as the trunk would be prescribed and the physiotherapist would ensure that active end-of-range motion is achieved for all movements. The patient would be encouraged to partake in the daily trauma ward group exercise class for all patients with ICDs.
- Exercise endurance can be improved with activities such as stair climbing and cycling on the stationary ward exercise cycle. The deep breathing that these activities elicit will assist with achieving optimal expansion of the left lung as well as the clearance of any additional retained secretions.
- Lastly, it is very important to re-assess his condition and needs on a daily basis and to adjust the approach to his rehabilitation accordingly,

to ensure optimal care is given to him and ensure a speedy recovery and discharge from the hospital.

5.7.2. *Paediatric case scenario*

A three-year-old girl was struck by a car whilst playing on the pavement outside her house. She was unconscious when the ambulance arrived, with shallow respirations. She was immobilised, her airway was cleared and supplementary oxygen was provided for transport to the tertiary paediatric hospital. On arrival in the paediatric ICU, her cervical spine was cleared and her level of consciousness rapidly improved. Her oxygenation deteriorated, however, and she required intubation and ventilation. Chest x-ray revealed a left-sided pulmonary contusion, with no effusion. Initially, secretions were largely fresh blood, but after a day nurses were suctioning out old blood and creamy secretions only. After three days she was extubated onto nasal prong oxygen. Her respiratory rate was 34 breaths per minute and there were scattered coarse crackles with reduced breath sounds over the left anterior chest. Chest wall movement was reduced on the left. She was reluctant to cough. There were no extra-thoracic injuries.

- What medication should you ensure has been given prior to treating this patient?
- What treatment modalities could you consider using?
- Are there any contraindications or precautions to treatment of this patient?

5.7.2.1. *Discussion*

5.7.2.1.1. Medication

It is essential to ensure that adequate analgesia has been given with sufficient time to take effect. A child in pain will not cough.

5.7.2.1.2. Treatment modalities

- Graded mobilisation should be implemented with support and encouragement. The child should be assisted to the sitting and then standing

positions (not necessarily in the same treatment session) and then progress to ambulation with and without support.
- In the sitting position, breathing exercises can be performed, including deep breathing exercises using play techniques (e.g. bubble blowing), which may also incorporate PEP therapy. Localised expansion exercises can be facilitated by placing the hands on the left hemithorax, with gentle pressure against inspiratory movement.
- Thoracic mobility exercises through play can be done while sitting or standing, depending on the child's ability. Examples include throwing balloons or pushing toy cars across the midline.
- Using mimicry, a child of three years old may be able to perform the forced expiratory technique or cough on command. Lack of expectoration is not an indication for suctioning, and nasal or oropharyngeal suctioning should only be considered if the spontaneous cough is inadequate or a secretion specimen is required.

5.7.2.1.3. Contraindications or precautions to treatment

- A tracheal stimulation should not be done on this patient to stimulate a cough, as she has recently been extubated and this may contribute to subglottic swelling.
- The child should be observed throughout the treatment session for signs of increased respiratory distress (e.g. increased tachypnoea, rib cage recessions, grunting, cyanosis or alar flaring) and rest periods accordingly.
- Oxygen saturation should be monitored throughout using a pulse oximeter.
- Percussions should not be used as a treatment modality, but vibrations could be used to mobilise secretions in side-lying positions if the active treatment is not effective.

5.8. Suggested Reading Material for Further Study

Clinical practice guideline for airway suctioning (AARC, 2010); paediatric endotracheal suctioning (Morrow and Argent, 2008); tracheostomy care protocols (St George's Hospital Tracheostomy Care Protocol (www.stgeorges.nhs.uk) and National Tracheostomy Safety Project (www.tracheostomy.org.uk)); assessment of function and activity in patients with critical illness (Elliott *et al.*, 2011).

5.9. Conclusion

Intentional and unintentional violence towards others or oneself has formed part of society for many decades and unfortunately is set to remain as such for the foreseeable future. The information provided in this chapter aimed to equip the physiotherapist who works in the acute care setting with basic knowledge of the interdisciplinary team management of patients who have suffered blunt or penetrating trauma to the abdomen or thorax. This information should enable the physiotherapist to provide high-quality evidence-based rehabilitative care to patients with similar injuries in the acute care setting in their own hospital. There is an urgent need for research into the effectiveness of a number of physiotherapy treatment modalities, which are frequently used in clinical practice, in the management of this specific patient population.

Bibliography

Adesanya, A.A., Da Rocha-Afodu, J.T., Ekanem, E.E., *et al.* (2000). Factors affecting mortality and morbidity in patients with abdominal gunshot wounds, *Injury,* **31**, 397–404.

American Association of Respiratory Care (AARC) Evidence-Based Clinical Practice Guidelines. (2003). Care of the ventilator circuit and its relation to ventilator-associated pneumonia, *Respir. Care,* **48**, 869–879.

American Association of Respiratory Care (AARC) Clinical Practice Guideline. (2010). Endotracheal suctioning of mechanically ventilated patients with artificial airways, *Respir. Care,* **55**, 758–764.

American Association of Respiratory Care (AARC) Clinical Practice Guideline. (2011). Incentive Spirometry, *Respir. Care,* **56,** 1600–1604.

American College of Surgeons Committee on Trauma. (2008). *Advanced Trauma Life Support® for Doctors: ATLS® Student Course Manual*, 8th edn., Hearthside Publishing Company, Chicago, MD.

Bansal, M.K., Maraj, S., Chewaproug, D., *et al.* (2005). Myocardial contusion injury: redefining the diagnostic algorithm, *Emerg. Med. J.,* **22**, 465–469.

Bastos, R., Calhoon, J.H., and Baisden, C.E. (2008). Flail chest and pulmonary contusion, *Semin. Thorac. Cardiovasc. Surg.,* **20**, 39–45.

Bliss, D., and Silen, M. (2002). Pediatric thoracic trauma, *Crit. Care Med.,* **30** [Suppl], S409–S415.

Brady, J.E., and Li, G. (2013). Prevalence of alcohol and drugs in fatally injured drivers, *Addiction,* **108**, 104–114.

Burtin, C., Clerckx, B., Robbeets, C., *et al.* (2009). Early exercise in critically ill patients enhances short-term functional recovery, *Crit. Care Med.,* **37**, 2499–2505.

Carrasco, C.E., Godinho, M., Barros, M.B.A., *et al.* (2012). Motor cycle crashes: a serious public health problem in Brazil, *World J. Emerg. Surg.,* **7** [Suppl], S5. [Online] Available at: http://www.wjes.org/content/7/S1/S5 [Accessed 15 November 2014].

Chidester, S., Rana, A., Lowell, W., *et al.* (2009). Is the 'seat belt sign' associated with serious abdominal injuires in pediatric trauma? *J. Trauma,* **67** [Suppl], S34–S36.

Choi, J.S.P., and Jones, A.Y.M. (2005). Effects of manual hyperinflation and suctioning on respiratory mechanics in mechanically ventilated patients with ventilator-associated pneumonia, *Aust. J. Physiother.,* **51**, 25–30.

Chughtai, T., Ali, S., Sharkey, P., *et al.* (2009). Update on managing diaphragmatic rupture in blunt trauma: a review of 208 consecutive cases, *Can. J. Surg.,* **52**, 177–181.

Cirocchi, R., Abraha, I., Montedori, A., *et al.* (2010). Damage control surgery for abdominal trauma, *Cochrane Database Syst. Rev.,* **1**, CD007438.

Cirocchi. R., Montedori. A., Farinella, E., *et al.* (2013). Damage control surgery for abdominal trauma, *Cochrane Database Syst. Rev.*, **3**, CD007438.

Clarke, G.M. (2003). 'Chest injuries', in Bersten, A.D., Soni, N., and Oh, T.E. (eds), *Oh's Intensive Care Manual*, 5th edn., Butterworth Heinemann, Edinburgh, pp. 719–729.

Cohn, S.M., and DuBose, J.J. (2010). Pulmonary contusion: an update on recent advances in clinical management, *World J. Surg.,* **34**, 1959–1970.

Coppola, C.P., and Gilbert, J.C. (2011). 'Abdominal trauma in pediatric critical care', in Fuhrman, B.P., and Zimmerman, J.J. (eds), *Pediatric Critical Care*, 4th edn., Elsevier Saunders, Philadelphia, PA, pp. 1528–1537.

Dandy, D.J., and Edwards, D.J. (2009). *Essential Orthopaedics and Trauma*, 5th edn., Churchill Livingstone Elsevier, Edinburgh.

De Groot, K.M., and Von Oppell, U.O. (2003). 'Penetrating chest trauma', in Mieny, J., and Mennen, U. (eds), *Principles of Surgical Patient Care*, 2nd edn., New Africa Books, Cape Town, pp. 715–724.

DuBose, J., Inaba, K., Okoye, O., *et al.* (2012). Development of posttraumatic empyema in patients with retained hemothorax: results of a prospective, observational AAST study, *J. Trauma Acute Care Surg.,* **73**, 752–757.

Elkins, M., and Dentice, R. (2012). Timing of hypertonic saline inhalation for cystic fibrosis, *Cochrane Database Syst. Rev.,* **2**, CD008816.

Elliott, D., Denehy, L., Berney, S., *et al.* (2011). Assessing physical function and activity for survivors of a critical illness: a review of instruments, *Austr. Crit. Care,* **24**, 155–166.

Evans, J.A., Van Wessem, K.J., McDougall, D., *et al.* (2010). Epidemiology of traumatic deaths: comprehensive population-based assessment, *World J. Surg.,* **34**, 158–163.

Feliciano, D.V. (2003). 'Abdominal vascular injury', in Feliciano, D.V., Moore, E.E., and Mattox, K.L. (eds), *Trauma Manual*, 4th edn., McGraw-Hill Professional, New York, NY, pp. 276–287.

Feliciano, D.V. (2004). 'Abdominal vascular injury', in Moore, E.E., Feliciano, D.V., and Mattox, K.L. (eds), *Trauma*, 5th edn., McGraw-Hill Professional, New York, NY, pp. 755–778.

Ferreyra, G.P., Baussano, I., Squadrone, V., *et al.* (2008). Continuous positive airway pressure for treatment of respiratory complications after abdominal surgery, *Ann. Surg.,* **247**, 617–626.

Fitzpatrick, D.C., Denard, P.J., Phelan, D., *et al.* (2010). Operative stabilization of flail chest injuries: review of literature and fixation options, *Eur. J. Trauma Emerg. Surg.,* **36**, 427–433.

Frownfelter, D., and Dean, E. (2006). *Cardiovascular and Pulmonary Physical Therapy: Evidence and Practice*, 4th edn., Mosby Elsevier, Philadelphia, PA.

Gaines, B.A. (2009). Intra-abdominal solid organ injury in children: diagnosis and treatment, *J. Trauma,* **67** [Suppl], S135–S139.

Gosselink, R., Bott, J., Johnson, M., *et al.* (2008). Physiotherapy for adult patients with critical illness: recommendations of the European Respiratory Society and European Society of Intensive Care Medicine Task Force on physiotherapy for critically ill patients, *Intensive Care Med.,* **34**, 1188–1199.

Guimaraes, F.S., and Zin, W.A. (2008). Thoracic percussion yields reversible mechanical changes in healthy subjects, *Eu.r J. Appl. Physiol.,* **104**, 601–607.

Guimaraes, M.M.F., El Dib, R.P., Smith, A.F., *et al.* (2009). Incentive spirometry for prevention of postoperative pulmonary complications in upper abdominal surgery: systematic review, *Cochrane Database Syst. Rev.,* **3**, CD006058.

Gunduz, M., Unlugenc, H., Ozalevli, M., *et al.* (2005). A comparative study of continuous positive airway pressure (CPAP) and intermittent positive pressure ventilation (IPPV) in patients with flail chest, *Emerg. Med. J.,* **22**, 325–329.

Haines, K.J., Skinner, E.H., and Berney, S. (2013). Association of postoperative pulmonary complications with delayed mobilisation following major abdominal surgery: an observational cohort study, *Physiotherapy,* **99**, 119–125.

Halm, M.A., and Hagel, K.K. (2008). Instilling normal saline with suctioning: beneficial technique or potentially harmful sacred cow? *Am. J. Crit. Care,* **17**, 469–472.

Hanekom, S.D., Gosselink, R., Dean, E., *et al.* (2011). The development of a clinical management algorithm for early physical activity and mobilisation of critically ill patients: synthesis of evidence and expert opinion and its translation into clinical practice, *Clin. Rehabil.,* **25**, 771–787.

Hauer, T., Huschitt, N., Kulla, M., *et al.* (2011). Bullet and shrapnel injuries in the face and neck regions: current aspects of wound ballistics, *HNO,* **59,** 752–764.

Herrera, P., and Langer, J.C. (2008). ‘Thoracic trauma in children’, in Mikrogianakis, A., and Valani, R. (eds), *The Hospital for Sick Children Manual of Pediatric Trauma*, Wolters Kluwer/Lippincott Williams & Wilkins, Philadelphia, PA, pp. 131–144.

Hill, K., Gain, K.R., McKay, S.W., *et al.* (2011). Effects of high-intensity inspiratory muscle training following a near-fatal gunshot wound, *Phys Ther.,* **91**, 1377–1384.

Hoth, J.J., Burch, P.T., and Richardson, J.D. (2002). Posttraumatic empyema, *Eur. J. Trauma,* **28**, 323–332.

Kacmarek, R.M., Stoller, J.K., and Heuer, A.J. (2013). *Egan’s Fundamentals of Respiratory Care*, 10th edn., Elsevier, St Louis, MO.

Kadish, H.A. (2006). ‘Thoracic trauma’, in Fleisher, G.R., Ludwig, S., and Henretig, F.M. (eds), *Textbook of Pediatric Emergency Medicine*, 5th edn., Lippincott Williams & Wilkins, Baltimore, MD, pp. 1433–1452.

Kayambu, G., Boots, R., and Paratz, J. (2013). Physical therapy for the critically ill in the ICU: a systematic review and meta-analysis, *Crit. Care Med.,* **41**, 1543–1554.

Keilin, R., Steng, A., Valadka, A.B., *et al.* (2003). ‘Indications for thoracotomy’, in Feliciano D.V., Moore, E.E., and Mattox, K.L. (eds), *Trauma Manual*, 4th edn., McGraw-Hill Professional, New York, NY, pp. 161–169.

Kirkpatrick, A.W., Laupland, K.B., Karmali, S., *et al.* (2006). Spill your guts! Perceptions of trauma association of Canada member surgeons regarding the open abdomen and the abdominal compartment syndrome, *J. Trauma,* **60**, 279–286.

Klein, J.R. (2011). *Pediatric Trauma: Pearls of Management*. [Online] Available at: http://www.ucsfcme.com/2011/slides/MEM11002/19KleinPedsTrauma.pdf [Accessed 1 April 2012].

Li, Z., Peng, X., Zhu, B., *et al.* (2013). Active mobilisation for mechanically ventilated patients: a systematic review, *Arch. Phys. Med. Rehabil.,* **94**, 551–561.

Livingstone, D.H., and Hauser, C.J. (2004). 'Trauma to the chest wall and lungs', in Moore, E.E, Feliciano, D.V., and Mattox, K.L. (eds), *Trauma*, 5th edn., McGraw-Hill Professional, New York, NY, pp. 507–538.

Ludwig, C., Angenendt, S., Martins, R., *et al.* (2011). Intermittent positive pressure breathing after lung surgery, *Asian Cardiovasc. Thorac. Ann.,* **19,** 10–13.

Maffiuletti, N.A., Roig, M., Karatzanos, E., *et al.* (2013). Neuromuscular electrical stimulation for preventing skeletal-muscle weakness and wasting in critically ill patients: a systematic review, *BMC Med.,* **11**, 137. [Online] Available at: http://www.biomedcentral.com/1741-7015/11/137 [Accessed 15 November 2014].

Maiden, N. (2009). Ballistics reviews: mechanisms of bullet wound trauma, *Forensic Sci. Med. Path.,* **5**, 204–209.

Mauffrey, C. (2005). Management of gunshot wounds to the limbs: a review. *The Internet Journal of Orthopedic Surgery*. [Online]. Available at: https://ispub.com/IJOS/3/1/10193. [Accessed 14 November 2014].

Melling, L., Lansdale, N., Mullaserry, D., *et al.* (2012). Penetrating assaults in children: often non-fatal near-miss events with opportunities for prevention in the UK, *Injury,* **43**, 2088–2093.

Mietto, C., Pinciroli, R., Patel, N., *et al.* (2013). Ventilator-associated pneumonia: evolving definitions and preventive strategies, *Respir. Care,* **58**, 990–1003.

Minei, J.P., Nathens, A.B., West, M., *et al.* (2006). II Guidelines for prevention, diagnosis and treatment of ventilator-associated pneumonia (VAP) in the trauma patient, *J. Trauma,* **60**, 1106–1113.

Mitchell, R.B., Hussey, H.M., Setzen, G., *et al.* (2013). Clinical consensus statement: tracheostomy care, *Otolaryngol. Head Neck Surg.,* **148**, 6–20.

Moore, M.A., Wallace, C., and Westra, S.J. (2009). The imaging of paediatric thoracic trauma, *Pediatr. Radiol.,* **39**, 485–496.

Morris, P.E., Goad, A., Thompson, C., *et al.* (2008). Early intensive care unit mobility therapy in the treatment of acute respiratory failure, *Crit. Care Med.,* **36**, 2238–2243.

Morrow, B., and Argent, A. (2008). A comprehensive review of pediatric endotracheal suctioning: effects, indications and clinical practice, *Pediatr. Crit. Care Med.,* **9**, 465–477.

Morrow, B.M., Mowzer, R., Pitcher, R., *et al.* (2012). Investigation into the effect of closed-system suctioning on the frequency of pediatric ventilator-associated pneumonia in a developing country, *Pediatr. Crit. Care Med.,* **13**, e25–e32.

National Institute for Health and Clinical Excellence (UK). (2009). *Rehabilitation after Critical Illness. NICE Clinical Guidelines No. 83*. NCBI Bookshelf. [Online] Available at: http://www.ncbi.nlm.nih.gov/books/NBK11653 [Accessed 14 August 2014].

Nayak, N.H. (2008). 'Trauma and shock', in Nayak, N.H. (ed.), *Guidelines to Practice of Emergency Medicine*, 2nd edn., Elsevier, Delhi, pp. 127–130.

Norton, J.A., Barie, P.S., Bollinger, R.R., *et al.* (2008). *Surgery: Basic Science and Clinical Evidence*, 2nd edn., Springer, Philadelphia, PA.

O'Connor, J.V., Byrne, C., Scalea, T.M., *et al.* (2009). Vascular injuries after blunt chest trauma: diagnosis and management, *Scand. J. Trauma Resusc. Emerg. Med.,* **17**, 42. [Online] Available at: http://www.sjtrem.com/content/17/1/42. [Accessed 14 November 2014].

Oikonomou, A., and Prassopoulos, P. (2011). CT imaging of blunt chest trauma, *Insights Imaging,* **2**, 281–295.

Orman, J., and Westerdahl, E. (2010). Chest physiotherapy with positive expiratory pressure breathing after abdominal and thoracic surgery: systematic review, *Acta Anaesthesiol. Scand.,* **54**, 261–267.

Panté, M.D., Andrew, N., and Pollak, M.D. (2010). 'Torso trauma', in American Academy of Orthopaedic Surgeons (eds), *Advanced Assessment and Treatment of Trauma*, Jones and Bartlett Learning, Sudbury, pp. 130–157.

Paramasivan, E., and Bodenham, A. (2007). Pleural fluid collections in critically ill patients, *Continuing Education in Anaesthesia, Critical Care & Pain,* **7**, 10–14.

Paratz, J., Lipman, J., and McAuliffe, M. (2002). Effect of manual hyperinflation on hemodynamics, gas exchange and respiratory mechanics in ventilated patients, *J. Int. Care Med.,* **17**, 317–324.

Paz, J.C., and West, M.P. (2009). *Acute Care Handbook for Physical Therapists*, 3rd edn., Saunders Elsevier, St. Louis, MO.

Pedersen, C.M., Rosendahl-Nielson, M., Hjermind, J., *et al.* (2009). Endotracheal suctioning of the adult intubated patient — what is the evidence? *Int. Crit. Care Nurs.,* **25**, 21–30.

Prinsloo, M., Laubscher, R., Neethling, I., *et al.* (2012). Fatal violence among children under 15 years in four cities of South Africa, 2001–2005, *Int. J. Inj. Contr. Saf. Promot.,* **19**, 181–184.

Pujalte, G.G., and Housner, J.A. (2008). Management of clavicle fractures, *Curr. Sports Med. Rep.,* **7**, 275–280.

Quinn, A.C., and Sinert, R. (2011). What is the utility of the focussed assessment with sonography in trauma (FAST) exam in penetrating torso trauma? *Injury,* **42**, 482–487.

Rippey, J.C., and Royse, A.G. (2009). Ultrasound in trauma, *Best. Pract. Res Clin. Anaesthesiol.,* **23**, 343–362.

Roberts, D.J., Zygun, D.A., Grendar, J., *et al.* (2012). Negative-pressure wound therapy for critically ill adults with open abdominal wounds: a systematic review, *J. Trauma Acute Care Surg.,* **73**, 629–639.

Saladina, R.A., and Lund, D.P. (2006). 'Abdominal trauma', in Fleisher, G.R., Ludwig, S., and Henretig, F.M. (eds), *Textbook of Pediatric Emergency Medicine*, 5th edn., Lippincott Williams & Wilkins, Baltimore, MD, pp. 1453–1462.

Schecter, S.C., Betts, J., Schecter, W.P., *et al.* (2012). Pediatric penetrating trauma: the epidemic continues, *J. Trauma Acute Care Surg.,* **73**, 721–725.

Schobert, M., and Tielen, P. (2010). Contribution of oxygen-limiting conditions to persistent infection of *Pseudomonas aeruginosa*, *Future Microbiol.,* **5**, 603–621.

Shukla, A.N., Ghaffar, Z.B.A., Auang, A.C., *et al.* (2008). Continuous paravertebral block for pain relief in unilateral multiple rib fracture: a case series, *Acute Pain,* **10**, 39–44.

Soni, N., and Williams, P. (2008). Positive pressure ventilation: what is the real cost? *B. J. Anaesth.,* **101**, 446–457.

Søreide, K., Krüger, A.J., Vårdal, A.L., *et al.* (2007). Epidemiology and contemporary patterns of trauma deaths: changing place, similar pace and older face, *World J. Surg.,* **31**, 2092–2103.

Stelfox, H.T., Crimi, C., Berra, L., *et al.* (2008). Determinants of tracheostomy decannulation: an international survey. *Crit. Care,* **12**, R26. [Online] Available at: http://ccforum.com/content/12/1/R26 [Accessed 14 November 2014].

Stokke, D.B. (1976). Review: artificial ventilation with positive end-expiratory pressure (PEEP): historical background, terminology and patho-physiology, *Eur. J. Intensive Care Med.,* **2**, 77–85.

Subirana, M., Solá, I., and Benit, S. (2010). Closed tracheal suction systems versus open tracheal suction systems for mechanically ventilated adult patients, *Cochrane Database Syst. Rev.,* **7**, CD004581.

Subramanian, S., Kellum, J.A., and Ronco, C. (2008). 'Acute renal failure', in Ronco, C., Bellomo, R., and Kellum, S. (eds), *Critical Care Nephrology,* 2nd edn., Saunders Elsevier, Philadelphia, PA, pp. 341–345.

Tai, N.R.M., and Boffard, K.D. (2003). Thoracic trauma: principles of early management, *Trauma,* **5**, 123–136.

Taio, G.M., Griffith, P.M., Szmuszkovicz, J.R., *et al.* (2000). Cardiac and great vessel injuries in children after blunt trauma: an institutional review, *J. Pediatr. Surg.,* **35**, 1656–1660.

Thim, T., Krarup, N.H.V., Grove, E.L., *et al.* (2012). Initial assessment and treatment with the airway, breathing, circulation, disability, exposure (ABCDE) approach, *Int. J. Gen. Med.,* **5,** 117–121.

Thomson, S.R. (2003). 'Trauma of the abdomen: blunt and penetrating', in Mieny, C.J., and Mennen, U. (eds), *Principles of Surgical Patient Care*, 2nd edn., New Africa Books, Cape Town, pp. 863–865.

Tovar, J.A. (2008). The lung and pediatric trauma, *Semin. Pediatr. Surg.,* **17**, 53–59.

Trauma.Org. (2013a). *Chest Trauma: Rib Fractures and Flail Chest*. Thoracic trauma. [Online] Available at: http://www.trauma.org/archive/thoracic/CHESTflail.html [Accessed 10 May 2013].

Trauma.Org. (2013b). *Chest Trauma: Pneumothorax — Open*. Thoracic trauma. [Online] Available at: http://www.trauma.org/archive/thoracic/CHESTopen.html [Accessed 10 May 2013].

Turgut, M., Akpinar, G., Akalan, N., *et al.* (1996). Spinal injuries in the pediatric age group: a review of 82 cases of spinal cord and vertebral column injuries, *Eur. Spine J.,* **3**, 148–152.

Van As, A.B. (2010). Paediatric trauma care, *Afr. J. Paediatr. Surg.,* **7**, 129–133.

Van Aswegen, H., Van Aswegen, A., Du Raan, H., *et al.* (2013). Airflow distribution with manual hyperinflation as assessed through gamma camera imaging: a crossover randomised trial, *Physiotherapy,* **99**, 107–112.

Van der Vlies, C.H., Olthof, D.C., Gaakeer, M., *et al.* (2011). Changing patterns in diagnostic strategies and the treatment of blunt injury to solid abdominal organs, *Int. J. Emerg. Med.,* **4**, 47. [Online] Available at: http://www.intjem.com/content/4/1/47 [Accessed 08 November 2014].

Van Vugt, R., Deunk, J., Brink, M., *et al.* (2011). Influence of routine computed tomography on predicted survival from blunt thoracoabdominal trauma, *Eur. J. Trauma Emerg. Surg.,* **37**, 185–190.

Vikram, K. (2011). *Exploratory Laparotomy*. Medscape. [Online] Available at: http://www.emedicine.medscape.com/article/1829835-overview [Accessed 08 May 2013].

Vilallonga, R., Pastor, V., Alvarez, L., *et al.* (2011). Right-sided diaphragmatic rupture after blunt trauma. An unusual entity, *World J. Emerg. Surg.,* **6**, 3. [Online] Available at: http://www.wjes.org/content/6/1/3 [Accessed 15 November 2014]

Smith, R. (2013). 'Trauma care: thoracic injuries', in Dolan, B., and Holt, L. (eds), *Accident and Emergency: Theory into Practice*, 3rd edn., Baillière Tindall Elsevier, Edinburgh, pp. 121–136.

Yamamoto, L., Schroeder, C., Morley, D., *et al.* (2005). Thoracic trauma: the deadly dozen, *Crit. Care Nurs. Q.,* **28**, 22–40.

Zafiropoulos, B., Alison, J.A., and McCarren, B.M. (2004). Physiological responses to the early mobilisation of the intubated, ventilated abdominal surgery patient, *Aust. J. Physiother.,* **50**, 95–100.

Zamakhshary, M., and Wales, P.W. (2008). 'Abdominal and pelvic trauma', in Mikrogianakis, A., and Valani, R. (eds), *The Hospital for Sick Children Manual of Pediatric Trauma*, Wolters Kluwer/Lippincott Williams & Wilkins, Philadelphia, PA, pp. 145–159.

Zargar, M., Khajia A., and Karbakhsh, D.M. (2007). Thoracic injury: a review of 276 cases, *Chin. J. Traumatol.*, **10**, 259–262.

Chapter 6

Burn Injuries

Written by S. Hanekom, M. Wilson, B.M. Morrow and H. van Aswegen

The skin performs an important role as a physical barrier by protecting the body against fluid loss, mechanical damage and infection, as well as assisting with temperature regulation. However, the most important function of the skin is that it gives each individual their own identifying characteristics. The physical and emotional trauma that result from burn injuries are complex and can result in life-long psychological and physical disability. Burn injuries have been described as a global public health problem that affects both developing and developed countries (Atiyeh *et al.*, 2009a; Peck, 2011, 2012). Burn injuries rank in the top 15 leading causes of the burden of disease globally. They are the fourth leading cause of traumatic injuries worldwide, following motor vehicle accidents, falls and interpersonal trauma. Morbidity and mortality vary with age and region (Atiyeh *et al.*, 2009b; Peck, 2011, 2012).

This chapter covers:

- The causes and mechanisms of burn injuries.
- Types of burn injuries.
- The systemic effects of a burn injury.
- The classification of burn injuries.

(Continued)

(*Continued*)

- The medical and surgical management of a patient who has sustained a burn injury.
- Physiotherapy aims for the management of a patient who sustained a burn injury in the intensive care unit and burns ward.
- The contraindications and precautions related to the physiotherapy management of a patient with burn injuries.
- Physiotherapy interventions for patients who have suffered burn injuries.
- Adult and paediatric clinical case scenarios.

6.1. Causes and Mechanisms of Burn Injury

The worldwide incidence of fire-related injuries was estimated to be 1.1 per 100000 populations in 2004 (Forjuoh, 2006). The most vulnerable groups for burn injuries are children, women and the elderly. Lack of supervision of children, frailty and co-morbid illnesses of the elderly, clothing made of flammable materials, parental illiteracy, congested housing, pre-existing impairment of a child and low socioeconomic status are important risk factors for burn injuries (Atiyeh *et al.*, 2009a; Parbhoo *et al.*, 2010; Peck, 2011; Balan and Lingam, 2012).

6.1.1. *Injury in adults*

Most burn injuries are preventable. Burn injuries are more prevalent in the domestic setting for women and children. Cooking has been identified as the most common activity that poses a risk for burn injury, particularly in lower-income countries, in which there is exposure to open flames and non-electric appliances used for cooking, heating and lighting. The elderly are particularly at risk (Peck, 2011). This is due to the deterioration in judgement and coordination. Medication use by the elderly may lead to alterations in cognition and balance, which places them at further risk of injury. The elderly are more likely to sustain an injury inside the house if they smoke or because they tend to use heating devices more frequently than younger adults. Adult men are more likely to be injured in outdoor and work locations (Peck, 2011).

The majority of burn injuries worldwide are unintentional. Less than 5% are deliberate self-burnings or the result of abuse, with regional exceptions (Peck, 2012). Assault, usually by a spouse, is most often caused by throwing caustic chemicals or flammable liquids at the victim's face or genitalia or by the ignition of clothing (e.g. dowry deaths in India) (Shaha and Mohanthy, 2006; Kumar *et al.*, 2013). In locations with seasonal variations of temperature, burns occur more frequently in the colder winter months. Clothing ignition, such as bedclothes and loose-fitting cotton garments, is a common cause of unintentional and intentional severe flame burns. Work-related injuries account for 20–25% of all serious burns, with the most common being fire or flame and scald. Food service industries (e.g. restaurants that use deep fryers) are responsible for 12% of work-related injuries (Dissanaike and Rahimi, 2009; Dissanaike *et al.*, 2009; Teo *et al.*, 2012).

6.1.2. *Injury in paediatrics*

Infants in Africa have an incidence of fire-related burns that is three times the world average for this age group (Peck, 2011). In children younger than three years, scalds are responsible for most of the burns (Lowell *et al.*, 2008). Scald burns usually occur when a child accidentally pulls a container with hot liquid onto themselves. It may also result from bathtub submersion injuries, usually by an unattended child. In older children, flame burns are more common. Young children are particularly vulnerable to thermal injury, partly due to a lack of discernment about what could be hazardous. In addition, the relative immobility of infants means that they may not be able to move away from the hot substance or surface, which can result in a deeper burn (Birchenough *et al.*, 2008). Burns account for 10% of all cases of child abuse (Parbhoo *et al.*, 2010). Contact with heated objects including cigarettes, irons, curling irons, hair dryers and heated kitchen utensils are commonly used in abuse cases (Van Niekerk *et al.*, 2004; Parbhoo *et al.*, 2010).

Many people place infants in 'baby walkers' or 'walking rings' before they are able to walk, and often even before they are able to stand independently or with support. This device affords infants mobility beyond their natural capability and gives them greater reach, with a consequently greater risk of injury. The increased access to environmental hazards, such as oven doors, kettles and cooking pots on floor-standing stoves, poses the risk of severe burn injuries (Cassell *et al.*, 1997; Smith *et al.*, 1997). One study reported that over 6% of children hospitalised for burn injuries at a children's hospital sustained their injuries in a walker (Johnson *et al.*, 1990). Children burned while in a walker have been shown to sustain a greater body surface area injured than those with burns from abuse, neglect or other accidents (Johnson *et al.*, 1990). It has been suggested that walkers expose infants to unnecessary hazards, including potentially serious burns, with apparently no known benefit to development. The use of baby walkers has been discouraged by many professionals in the paediatric field. More recently, risk factors related to burn injuries in infants and children have been linked with a low educational level of the parents, young mothers (younger than 20 years), having more than three children per family and epilepsy (Peck, 2011).

6.2. Types of Burn Injuries

A burn is a traumatic injury to the skin or other organic tissue primarily caused by thermal or other acute exposures. Burns occur when some or all of the cells in the skin or other tissues are destroyed by heat, cold, electricity or caustic chemicals. Burns are acute wounds caused by an isolated, non-recurring insult and the majority of burn injuries progress rapidly through an orderly series of healing steps. Flame injuries are the most common causes of burns. This is followed by scalding, contact with a hot object, electrical and chemical injuries (Sheridan, 2002).

The following types of burn injuries are discussed in this section:

- chemical,
- electrical,
- inhalation, and
- thermal.

6.2.1. *Chemical burns*

Chemical burn injuries may occur as a result of assault, attempted suicide or may be work-related. In work-related injuries the extremities are mostly involved, whereas in the case of assault or attempted suicide the head, neck and trunk are mostly affected (Olaitan and Jiburum, 2008; Tahir *et al.*, 2012; Li *et al.*, 2013). Injury to the skin and underlying structures is caused by a wide range of corrosive reactions. This includes alteration of pH, disruption of cellular membranes and direct toxic effects on metabolic processes. Injury severity is determined by the duration of exposure and the nature of the agent. Tissue coagulation will result from acid contact, while alkaline burns results in liquefactive necrosis. Systemic absorption of some chemicals is life threatening (Palao *et al.*, 2010). Complications associated with chemical burns include respiratory failure, septicaemia, renal failure, blindness, axillary contractures and hypertrophic scarring, to name a few, and often lead to a prolonged hospital stay (Olaitan and Jiburum, 2008).

6.2.2. *Electrical burns*

Electrical injury occurs mostly in electricians, construction workers and children playing at home. Electrical injury has a mortality rate as high as 58% (Saracoglu *et al.*, 2014). Electrical injury is classified as high-voltage, low-voltage, electric arc or lightning strike (Table 6.1). Electrical energy is converted to thermal injury as the current passes through body tissues with different levels of conductivity. Patient presentation differs from no external evidence of burn injury with major internal organ injuries to skin burns with no significant internal organ injury (Herrera *et al.*, 2010; Salehi *et al.*, 2014). The degree of injury sustained due to electrical current is influenced by the magnitude of the energy delivered, resistance encountered by bodily tissues (dependent on water content of tissues), type of current and current pathway, as well as the duration of contact. Tissues with high water content offer low resistance to electrical current flow (Herrera *et al.*, 2010). Patients with total body surface area (TBSA) burns greater than 50% have an 18.8 times greater risk of mortality (Saracoglu *et al.*, 2014). Patients who have suffered electrical burns need

Table 6.1: Classification of electrical burns and complications associated with each type of burn*.

Electrical injury	Definition	Complications
High voltage	Electrical current greater than 1000 volts. Most debilitating of all electrical injuries.	• Cardiac arrest • Cardiac dysrhythmias • Muscle necrosis (escharotomy, fasciotomy) • Amputation of extremities and digits • Fractures • Traumatic brain injury • Peripheral mono- or polyneuropathy • Exposed tendons • Sepsis • Pigmented urine (indicates muscle damage) • Renal failure • Cataract formation
Low voltage	Electrical current less than 1000 volts. Most common sources are electrical appliances in the home.	• Fewer complications than high voltage injuries • Fasciotomy • Amputation
Electric arc	Flash-type injury in which the current does not pass directly through the body. Lowest mortality rate of all electrical injuries.	• Fasciotomy • Seldomly amputation
Lightning strike	Injury results from sudden, short-duration, high-intensity electrical energy. It is associated with blunt trauma due to violent tetanic muscle contraction and large fluctuations in temperature during lightning strike.	• Cardiac arrhythmia • Cardiac and respiratory arrest (more frequently than high voltage injury) • Blunt head trauma • Spinal cord injury • Solid intra-abdominal organ injury • Fractures (long bones, orbit, scapula and vertebrae) • Rupture of tympanic membrane • Corneal burns • Cataracts • Peripheral neuropathy • Impaired mental ability

*Sources: Whitcomb *et al.* (2002); Arnoldo *et al.* (2004); Russell *et al.* (2013).

close monitoring for cardiac arrhythmias. Tissue oedema may lead to the development of compartment syndrome and reinforces the need for close patient monitoring after electrical burns (Kasten *et al.*, 2011).

Patients who have suffered lightning strikes need to be treated as any other trauma patient with regard to primary and secondary surveys and definitive care. Although the duration of lightning strike is often short, it can cause electrical conduction disturbances within the body and lead to cardiac arrest due to asystole. The extent of the injuries sustained may not be visible and therefore patients need close monitoring (Whitcomb *et al.*, 2002). Lichtenberg features may be visible on the patient's skin. This refers to ferning or feathering patterns on the skin and is not associated with permanent injury (Russell *et al.*, 2013).

6.2.3. *Inhalation burns*

Inhalation injury is defined as the aspiration of superheated gasses, steam, hot liquid and toxic products of incomplete combustion. Inhalation burns are a predictor of injury severity, need for ventilation and mortality (Osler *et al.*, 2010; Kasten *et al.*, 2011). Inhalation injuries will increase the risk of death by 20% irrespective of the victim's age and the extent of the burn injury (Osler *et al.*, 2010). There are three phases of inhalation injury (upper airway thermal injury, lower airway and lung parenchyma chemical injury and systemic toxicity), which are discussed below.

6.2.3.1. *Upper airway injury*

Thermal injury is usually limited to the oropharyngeal area due to the poor conductivity of dry air, rapid heat dissipation of the smoke-filled air and reflex closure of the glottis. Animal experiments have shown that at 142°C, inhaled air cools to 38°C by the time it reaches the carina. The thermal injury results in mucosal oedema; this peaks at 24 hours after the initial insult and resolves within the first week. This oedema can cause upper airway obstruction and will develop independent of fluid resuscitation. Steam can burn the airway below the glottis due to the high conductivity of moist air (Mlcak *et al.*, 2007). Because the paediatric airway is much smaller than that of an adult, it may be more rapidly and readily occluded as a result of oedema after thermal injury (Sheridan, 2002).

6.2.3.2. *Lower airway and lung parenchyma injury*

The lower respiratory tract is mostly damaged by steam inhalation, but toxic chemicals (aldehides, oxides of sulphur and nitrogen) produced in fires may also injure the lower airways with chemical burns. Inhalation of the toxic products resulting from incomplete combustion destroys the epithelial layer of the airways, resulting in airway sloughing. In reaction to the damaged epithelium, mucosal oedema develops, causing airway obstruction. The release of oxygen free radicals and inflammatory mediators contribute to the development of pulmonary oedema, which may occur within two days after injury (Church *et al.*, 2006). In addition, hyper-secretion of mucus and epithelial ciliary damage decreases the effectiveness of the mucociliary clearance system. As a result, patients present with excessive amounts of secretions which further increase airways obstruction. This, coupled with surfactant inactivation due to destruction of type II pneumocytes, could result in atelectasis. Ultimately, ventilation/perfusion (V/Q) mismatch develops as the alveolar injury progresses, while there is an increase in lung and bronchial blood flow (Demling, 2008). A clinical picture consisting of a decrease in lung compliance, hypoxia and hypercarbia develops. If not managed effectively, pneumonia may develop any time between four days and four weeks after inhalation injury (Demling, 2008).

Key Message

The physiotherapist must be aware that bronchospasm is a common problem for young children after inhalation injury.

6.2.3.3. *Systemic toxicity*

The inhalation of toxic gases causes extensive damage to cellular functioning. Carbon monoxide is produced during combustion and, when inhaled, carbon monoxide decreases the ability of oxygen to bind to haemoglobin due to its high affinity for haemoglobin. This results in decreased oxygen delivery to organs, thereby impairing cellular respiration. In addition, carbon monoxide also binds to the enzyme *cytochrome oxidase* and inhibits mitochondrial function at a cellular level. Carbon monoxide poisoning should be suspected if the inhalation injury took place in an enclosed area and the patient is unconscious. The symptoms of carbon monoxide poisoning include increased muscle tone, nausea and vomiting, headache, hyperventilation, hypotension and coma (Demling, 2008).

Combustion of plastics, polyurethane, wool, silk, nylon, rubber and paper products can all lead to the production of cyanide gas. Cyanide interferes with cellular metabolism by binding the ferric ion in cytochrome a3. Anaerobic metabolism ensues, with the development of lactic acidosis and decreased oxygen utilisation. Cyanide poisoning should be suspected in burn patients who present with persistent lactic acidosis despite adequate fluid resuscitation (Huzar *et al.*, 2013). The extent of the damage caused during inhalation injury is related to duration of exposure and the nature of the materials aspirated.

6.2.4. *Thermal burns*

The depth of the burn injury is related to contact temperature, duration of contact with the external heat source and the thickness of the skin. Because the thermal conductivity of skin is low, most thermal burns involve the epidermis and part of the dermis. The most common thermal burns are associated with flames, hot liquids, hot solid objects and steam. The depth of the burn largely determines the healing potential and the need for surgical grafting and will be discussed in Section 6.4 (Sheridan, 2002; Church *et al.*, 2006).

Cold temperatures can cause burn injury. In cold exposure, damage to the skin and underlying tissues occurs when ice crystals puncture the cells or when the crystals create a hypertonic tissue environment. As a result, blood flow can be interrupted, causing haemo-concentration and intravascular thrombosis with tissue hypoxia (Sheridan, 2002).

6.3. Systemic Effects of a Burn Injury

6.3.1. *Burn shock*

In the first 24 hours following a major burn incident (excess of 20% body surface area (BSA) involved) the functioning of the body is affected.

Systemic inflammatory response develops due to the release of cytokines and other mediators into the bloodstream. As a result the capillary permeability increases, which allows for a 'seeping' of protein-rich fluid into the intravascular compartment with resultant build up of interstitial oedema in various organs and soft tissues; often referred to as 'third-spacing' of fluid. In addition, peripheral and splanchnic vasoconstriction occurs due to the release of catecholamines, vasopressin and angiotensin. Myocardial contractility may also be reduced (refer to Chapter 1 (Section 1.2) for information on shock). Bronchospasm can occur during this initial phase even in the absence of inhalation injury. Adequate fluid resuscitation is crucial to the survival of the patient during this phase of injury. The effective management of patients in this early phase has improved the survival of burn patients (Mosier *et al.*, 2013).

Children have nearly three times the BSA to body mass ratio of adults, resulting in proportionally higher fluid losses in children than in adults. Therefore, children have relatively greater fluid resuscitation requirements and more evaporative water loss than adults (Sharma and Parashar, 2010).

6.3.2. *Immune system responses*

Patients with extensive burn injuries are at a significantly increased risk for developing severe sepsis. This is due to the loss of the cutaneous protective barrier, suppression of specific and non-specific immune systems, hyper-catabolism and the placement of invasive lines, which is essential for the effective monitoring and nursing of the patient (refer to Chapter 1 (Section 1.2.3.) for information on sepsis and septic shock).

6.3.3. *Metabolic responses*

There is an increased metabolic response rate as a result of burn injury. Metabolic rates increase up to three times the normal value and this increased rate can remain up to one year after the closure of a burn wound. Hyper-catabolism has been linked to an increased risk for sepsis, difficulty in wound closure and a decrease in lean body mass (Chan and Chan, 2009). Increased levels of circulating catabolic hormones result in decreased protein synthesis and a rapid breakdown of visceral and skeletal muscle. Increased osteoclastic activity can also make patients more susceptible to fractures. In children with burns that exceed 40% of BSA, a 5.8% incidence of fractures has been reported. The authors speculated that increased osteoclastic activity, decreased vitamin D levels, inadequate protein intake and decreased weight-bearing activity after burn injury were to blame (Mayes *et al.*, 2003).

6.3.4. *Thermoregulatory system*

The thermoregulatory system resets to a higher baseline temperature of around 38.5°C after burn injury. Adult patients suffer from hyperthermia due to the metabolic response to systemic inflammation or an infective process. Cellular injury and death may ensue if hyperthermia is sustained above 40°C (Nachiappan *et al.*, 2012).

The large BSA to body mass ratio of the child, in addition to the thinner skin and subcutaneous layers, predisposes the child to hypothermia, which is important to avoid. In very young children, temperature regulation is partially based on non-shivering thermogenesis, which further increases metabolic rate, oxygen consumption and lactate production. The thin skin in young children may make the initial burn depth assessment difficult (Sharma and Parashar, 2010).

6.4. Classification of Burn Injuries

The skin consists of two main layers, namely the epidermis and dermis. A basement membrane connects the epidermis to the dermis and the dermis is attached to the underlying bone and muscles through a hypodermis (does not form part of the skin). Table 6.2 lists the composition and functions of the layers of the skin.

Burn wounds are classified according to the depth of tissue injury and the extent of the burns.

6.4.1. *Depth of tissue injury*

Burn wounds are not usually uniform in depth and many have a mixture of deep and superficial components. A precise classification of the burn

Table 6.2: Composition and functions of the epidermis and dermis.

Skin layer	Composition	Function
Epidermis	• Keratinocytes • Melanocytes	• Provides a protective cover for the body against infiltration by micro-organisms • Assists with temperature regulation of the body through controlled water loss
Dermis	• Collagen fibrils • Elastic fibres • Nerve endings • Hair follicles • Sweat glands • Sebaceous glands • Lymphatic and blood vessels	• Protects the body against injury from external forces • Provides sense of touch and heat • Nourishes and removes waste from epidermal and dermal cells

wound may be difficult and may require up to three weeks for a final determination. Thin skin, particularly on the volar surfaces of the forearms, medial thighs, perineum and ears, sustains deeper burn injuries than suggested by initial appearance. It is best to assume there are no shallow burns in these areas. Children under the age of five and adults over the age of 55 are also more susceptible to deeper burns because of thinner skin.

The traditional classification of burns as first, second, third or fourth degree is now replaced by a system that reflects the need for surgical intervention. Current designations of burn depth are superficial, superficial partial thickness, deep partial thickness and full thickness. The term fourth degree is still used to describe the most severe burns. These are burns that extend into the muscle, bone and joints.

6.4.1.1. *Superficial burns*

Superficial or epidermal burns involve only the epidermal layer of the skin. They do not blister but are dry, painful, red and blanch with pressure. Over the following two to three days the pain and erythema subside. By day four, the injured epithelium peels away from the newly healed epidermis. Such injuries are generally healed in six days without scarring. This process is commonly seen with sunburns (Rice and Orgill, 2012).

6.4.1.2. *Partial thickness burns*

Partial thickness burns involve the epidermis and portions of the dermis. They are characterised as either superficial or deep (Kasten *et al.*, 2011; Rice and Orgill, 2012).

6.4.1.2.1. Superficial partial thickness burns

These burns characteristically form blisters between the epidermis and dermis within 24 hours and are painful, red, weeping and blanch with pressure. Burns that initially appear to be only epidermal in depth may be determined to be partial thickness 12–24 hours later. These burns generally heal in seven to 21 days; scarring is unusual, although pigment changes may occur. A layer of fibrinous exudates and necrotic debris may accumulate on the surface, which may predispose the burn wound to heavy bacterial colonisation and delayed healing. These burns typically heal without functional impairment or hypertrophic scarring.

6.4.1.2.2. Deep partial thickness burns

These burns extend into the deeper dermis and are characteristically different from superficial partial thickness burns. Deep burns damage hair follicles and glandular tissue. They are painful to pressure only, almost always blister, are wet or waxy dry and have variable mottled colorization from patchy cheesy white to red (Fig. 6.1). They do not blanch with pressure. If infection is prevented and wounds are allowed to heal spontaneously without grafting, they will heal in three to nine weeks. These burns invariably cause hypertrophic scarring (see Section 6.8.5.3.), particularly in children (Sheridan, 2002). If they involve a joint, joint dysfunction is expected even with aggressive physical therapy. A deep partial thickness burn that fails to heal in three weeks is functionally and cosmetically equivalent to a full thickness burn. Differentiation from full thickness burns is often difficult.

6.4.1.3. *Full thickness burns*

Full thickness burns extend through and destroy the epidermis, all layers of the dermis and often injure the underlying subcutaneous tissue. If a

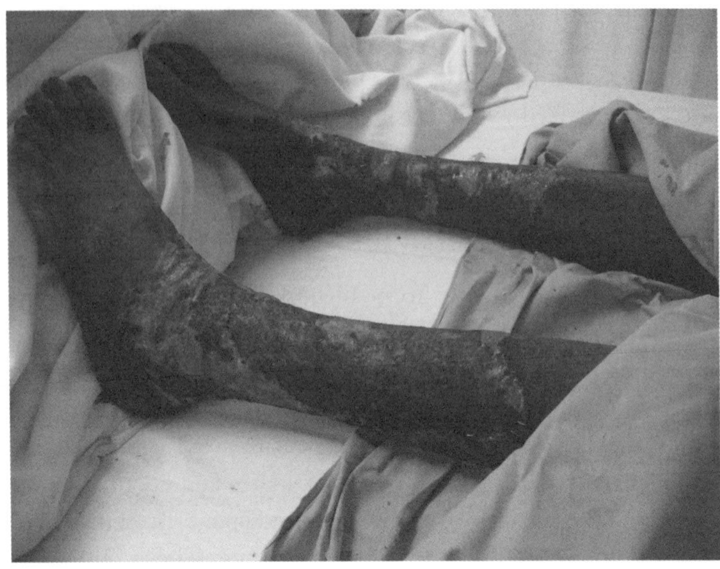

Fig. 6.1: A patient with deep partial thickness and full thickness burns to the legs as a result of exposure to hot tar. Skin grafting has been performed to enhance wound healing.

burn is deep and circumferential then eschar (dead and denatured dermis) will form. With oedema and increased pressures there can be compression of the neurovascular structures. This compression acts like a tourniquet and compromises the viability of structures distal to the eschar (limb or torso) (Fig. 6.2). Full thickness burns are usually anaesthetic or hypoaesthetic. Skin appearance can vary from waxy white to leathery grey to charred and black. The skin is dry, inelastic and does not blanch with pressure. Hairs can easily be pulled from hair follicles. Vesicles and blisters do not develop.

The eschar eventually separates from the underlying tissue and reveals an unhealed bed of granulation tissue. Without surgery, these wounds heal by wound contracture with epithelialisation around the wound edges. Scarring is severe with contractures and complete spontaneous healing is not possible (Rice and Orgill, 2012).

Fourth degree burns are deep and potentially life-threatening injuries that extend through the skin into underlying tissues such as fascia, muscle or bone (Rice and Orgill, 2012). Contractures potentially result in significant

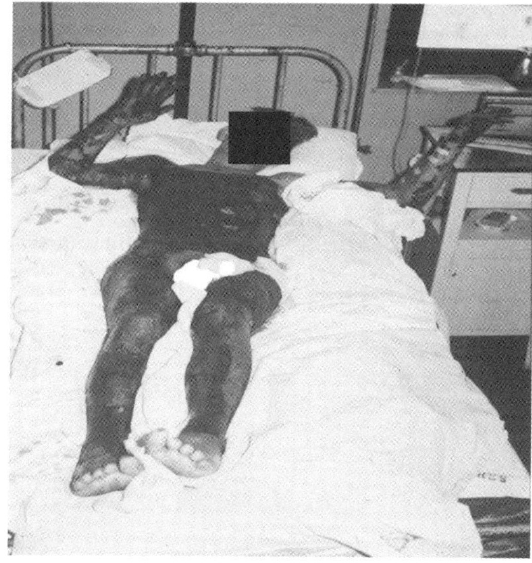

Fig. 6.2: A patient with eschar covering full thickness burns.

loss of function. Contractures commonly occur in the neck, the web spaces and flexor surfaces of the hand, the ante-cubital space of the arm, axilla, popliteal space of the knee and the hip flexor surfaces (Birchenough *et al.*, 2008). In children, contracture bands may impede the growth of both bony and soft tissue structures (Sheridan *et al.*, 1999).

6.4.2. *Extent of burn wounds*

The extent of the burn wounds are expressed as a percentage of the TBSA involved in the injury. This is necessary to guide therapy (Freiburg *et al.*, 2007). The two commonly used methods of assessing TBSA are the rule of nines and the Lund Browder chart. The Lund Browder chart is the most accurate method for estimating TBSA for both adults and children as it takes into account the relative percentage of BSA affected by growth. Children have proportionally larger heads and smaller lower extremities, so the percentage BSA is more accurately estimated using the Lund Browder chart (Panté *et al.*, 2010; Alharbi *et al.*, 2012). For adult assessment, the most expeditious method to estimate TBSA is the rule of nines (Fig. 6.3).

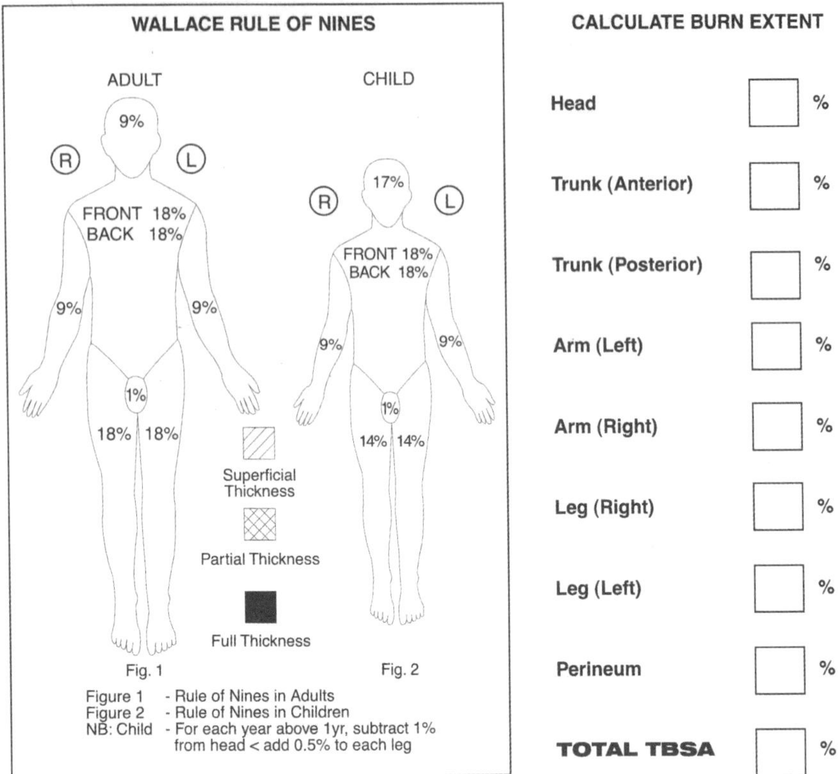

Fig. 6.3: Example of rule of nines chart used in the emergency department to calculate percentage of TBSA involved by burn injury.

The revised Baux score has been developed as a tool for the assessment of mortality risk for burn injured patients (Osler *et al.*, 2010). This score considers the effect of inhalation burn, in addition to age and TBSA, on patient survival (refer to Section 6.10 for suggested further reading on the revised Baux score). Overestimation by health care providers of the percentage TBSA involved remains problematic and newer methods to calculate burn surface area are being investigated. These methods include computerised imaging, two- and three-dimensional graphics and body contour reproductions. Research is underway to establish whether these newer methods will improve accuracy in initial wound assessment (Kasten *et al.*, 2011).

6.5. Medical and Surgical Management

Advances in the medical and surgical management of patients with burn injury have improved the mortality and morbidity. The medical and surgical management of patients with burn injuries is divided into:

- primary survey and resuscitation of vital functions;
- detailed secondary survey as adjunct to the primary survey; and
- definitive care.

6.5.1. *Primary survey and resuscitation of vital functions*

On admission to the emergency department, the adult or paediatric patient with burn injury will undergo initial assessment and treatment according to the 'airways, breathing, circulation, disability, exposure' (ABCDE) approach to basic life support, as described in Chapter 5 (Section 5.3.1.). Components of the ABCDE approach that are especially important for patients with burn injuries include the following (Alharbi *et al.*, 2012).

- *Airway* patency. If soot is present in the mouth, early intubation should be considered even if the patient is breathing normally, as mild pharyngeal oedema can rapidly progress to upper airway obstruction (Latenser, 2009).
- Presence or absence of *breathing*. In the case of stridor, immediate airway intubation is indicated.
- Injuries by *exposing* the patient through the removal of clothes in order to visualise the skin and identify injuries. The patient's clothes are removed but the patient is kept warm in order to prevent the onset of hypothermia. The room temperature should be kept between 28°C and 32°C in order to keep the patient's core temperature above 34°C. This is particularly important in the management of children with thermal injuries.

The type of radiological investigations performed and the care provided to the patient is similar to that described in Chapter 5 (Section 5.3.1.). Nasogastric tube placement is undertaken for patients with 20% or greater TBSA burns.

6.5.2. *Secondary survey as adjunct to primary survey*

The secondary survey may take place in the emergency department or in the burn unit. It is a 'head-to-toe' evaluation of the patient, which involves taking a detailed history of the patient as well as a complete neurological and physical examination including the abdomen, cornea, ears (especially with explosion trauma), genital region, lower and upper limbs. The history should include mechanism of injury, time of injury, consideration of abuse (especially if the patient is a child) and lastly, possibility of carbon monoxide intoxication (based on presence of soot in the mouth and nose and on a history of burns in a closed area) (Alharbi *et al.*, 2012).

Care and treatment provided to the patient during the secondary survey is similar to that described in Chapter 5 (Section 5.3.2.).

6.5.3. *Definitive care*

Definitive care is initiated after completion of the primary and secondary surveys. Definitive care has been broken down into care provided over the first 24 hours, surgery and wound management. Each of these is discussed below.

6.5.3.1. *Care provided over the first 24 hours*

6.5.3.1.1. Fluid replacement

The Parkland formula is a formula used to calculate a patient's fluid replacement requirements over the first 24 hours following burn injury in order to ensure they remain haemodynamically stable. It is the most widely used resuscitation guideline and has been renamed the consensus formula (Blumetti *et al.*, 2008; Latenser, 2009; Alharbi *et al.*, 2012). The amount of ringer's solution to be administered is calculated using the consensus formula, 4 ml/kg/%TBSA burn. One half of the amount is administered during the first eight hours following injury and the other half is divided equally and administered over the next 16 hours. The formula is regarded as an excellent starting point for fluid resuscitation (Blumetti *et al.*, 2008). Some patients may need more fluid volume than that predicted with the formula, especially those with burn inhalation injury, electrical burns or history of alcohol or illicit drug use; therefore close monitoring of each individual patient to assess whether their fluid needs are being met is of great importance (Latenser, 2009). Monitoring includes regular measurements of arterial blood pressure, heart rate and urine output. A heart rate less than 110 beats per minute indicates adequate fluid volume administration (Latenser, 2009). The aim of fluid replacement therapy is to maintain a urine output of 0.5 ml/kg/hour in adults and an output of 0.5–1 ml/kg/hour in patients who weigh less than 30 kg (Blumetti *et al.*, 2008; Latenser, 2009; Alharbi *et al.*, 2012). Invasive cardiac monitoring may become necessary for patients with severe injury in order to determine preload on the heart.

Ringer lactate, ringer acitate or balanced electrolyte solutions may be used for fluid replacement therapy over the first 24 hours of admission. The use of colloids and other blood products is not recommended during this time period as these have been shown to prolong tissue oedema and increase the risk for mortality (Latenser, 2009; Alharbi *et al.*, 2012).

6.5.3.1.2. Calorie intake

Patients with burns have a markedly increased caloric requirement because of the development of a hypermetabolic response after injury as a result of the burn itself, catecholamine release, pain and anxiety, surgical interventions and tissue metabolic demands. Delivery of appropriate nutrition (including protein and carbohydrate) to a patient with burn injuries is vital for wound healing, management of inflammation, suppression of the hypermetabolic response and reduction of sepsis-related morbidity and mortality (Kasten *et al.*, 2011). The patient's caloric needs are determined using the Harris Benedict equation or the Curreri formula (Alharbi *et al.*, 2012). Adult patients with 20% TBSA burn or greater will be fed through enteral feeding tubes (nasojejunal or orojejunal) to ensure adequate nutrition is supplied to meet the patient's energy needs (Hall *et al.*, 2012). In general, a child with a burn greater than 20–30% TBSA will require placement of a nasoduodenal feeding tube to provide the required caloric supplementation (Sharma and Parashar, 2010).

6.5.3.1.3. Routine interventions

Routine interventions include screening for bacterial colonisation. This is done using cotton swabs that are swiped over different bodily areas such as the mouth, nose, burn and inguinal areas. Re-evaluation of the TBSA and depth of burn wounds is performed after the patient is washed. At this stage determination of indications for emergent surgery (debridement, escharotomy or skin grafting) is done. Circumferential burns over the abdomen may lead to organ hypoperfusion and could lead to burn-induced compartment syndrome. Abdominal compartment syndrome can lead to impairment in renal function, gastrointestinal ischaemia, and poor perfusion of the cardiac and pulmonary systems (Latenser, 2009). Compartment syndrome may also develop in extremities with circumferential burns. Intra-abdominal pressure should be monitored regularly for the early identification of the development of compartment syndrome.

6.5.3.1.4. Laboratory tests

Laboratory tests that are ordered for patients with burn injuries within the first 24 hours of admission are listed in Table 6.3.

Urea, electrolytes, myoglobin and urine culture are performed to assess renal function and to identify renal injury. Prothrombin time, partial thrombin time and international normalised ratio are done to establish the patient's blood clotting profile. Creatine kinase and C-reactive protein are

Table 6.3: Routine laboratory tests performed following burn injury.

- Complete blood count
- Arterial blood gas
- Urea and electrolytes
- Prothrombin and partial thrombin time
- International normalised ratio
- Creatine kinase and C-reactive protein
- Blood glucose
- Albumin, thyroid and myoglobin
- Sputum culture and sensitivity
- Urine culture

inflammatory markers, indicative of the patient's immune response to injury (Alharbi *et al.*, 2012).

6.5.3.1.5. Impaired respiration and inhalation injury

Circumferential burns of the neck or chest pose the threat of airway and ventilation compromise. Burns of the neck area, especially in children, can result in eschar, which compresses and obstructs the airway. Early removal of eschar could decrease the external pressure exerted on the trachea, thereby protecting the airway. Circumferential burns in the chest area restrict natural chest wall movement and lead to increasing ventilatory demands for good gaseous exchange. This is a surgical emergency. Signs that may indicate respiratory compromise in a patient with severe chest wall burns are listed in Table 6.4.

Smoke inhalation injury should be suspected when a patient presents with singed nasal hair, soot in the mouth, history of suppressed level of consciousness and confinement in an enclosed space (with or without facial burns), change in voice and expectoration of carbonaceous sputum (Dries and Endorf, 2013). Fibre-optic bronchoscopy is used to determine the extent of damage to the airways. Typical bronchoscopy findings in patients with inhalation injury are listed in Table 6.5.

Chest x-ray and computed tomography (CT) may be insensitive to the diagnosis of inhalation injury early in the patient's admission due to a relatively normal lung and airway appearance (Kasten *et al.*, 2011). Indications for intubation in patients with inhalation injuries are listed in Table 6.6 (Mlcak *et al.*, 2007).

Table 6.4: Signs of respiratory compromise in a patient with severe chest burns.

- Visible eschar on the chest wall
- Increased respiratory rate in a spontaneously breathing patient
- Wheezing
- Voice hoarseness
- Reduced tidal volumes in a ventilated patient, with visibly increased work of breathing to maintain adequate oxygenation
- Decreased chest wall excursion

Table 6.5: Typical bronchoscopy findings that confirm the diagnosis of inhalation injury.

- Carbonaceous deposits below the glottis
- Extensive airway oedema
- Bronchial mucosal erythema
- Bronchial mucosal haemorrhage
- Bronchial mucosal ulceration

Table 6.6: Indications for intubation in patients with inhalation injury.

- Stridor
- Hypoxaemia or hypercapnia
- Facial burns and lowered level of consciousness
- Facial burns and full thickness burns to the neck
- Full thickness burns to the lips and nose
- Oropharyngeal oedema
- Carboxyhaemoglobin >20%

Medication recommended for patients with inhalation injury include anti-inflammatory and anti-coagulant drugs, bronchodilator therapy, inhaled nitric oxide (to improve pulmonary blood flow) and heparin sulphate combined with N-acetylcysteine. This regimen has been reported by some to reduce mortality from inhalation injuries in adult and paediatric patients (Church *et al.*, 2006; Mlcak *et al.*, 2007; Alharbi *et al.*, 2012); however, one case report has stated that coagulopathy developed in a patient exposed to inhaled heparin and N-acetylcysteine (Dries and Endorf, 2013). The majority of patients with inhalation injury are at risk of developing ventilator-associated pneumonia (VAP) (Latenser, 2009). Strategies for the prevention of VAP such as elevation of the head of the bed to 30°, regular oral care and body position changes should be part of standard care in the ICU (Latenser, 2009). Physiotherapeutic interventions like therapeutic coughing, humidification of inhaled gases, chest physiotherapy, airway suctioning and early mobility are indicated to effect facilitation of the removal of retained secretions (see Section 6.8).

In patients with suspected carbon monoxide intoxication as a result of inhalation injury, the levels of carboxyhemoglobin are evaluated with arterial blood gas analysis. A level greater than 3% in non-smokers or 10% in smokers confirms the diagnosis (Dries and Endorf, 2013). Oxygen therapy at 100% is commenced in the form of a non-rebreathing oxygen mask or through an artificial airway to speed up elimination of carbon monoxide from the lungs. Hyperbaric oxygen therapy is often advocated to further enhance clearance of carbon monoxide, but outcomes from this therapy remain controversial (Dries and Endorf, 2013). Complications associated with hyperbaric oxygen include air embolism, barotrauma, tympanic membrane disruption and seizures (Dries and Endorf, 2013).

6.5.3.1.6. Pain management

Pain originates from various sources in patients with burn injury. Pain management for patients with burn injury therefore becomes quite complex. Pain originates from the site of injury as a direct result of injury to and stimulation of nociceptors in the dermis and epidermis (De Castro *et al.*, 2013). Pain is also generated from the local inflammatory response to injury, which is activated a few minutes after injury. Numerous chemical irritants are released into the area and sensitise and stimulate the nociceptors. This leads to primary hyperalgesia, which means the injured area remains painful and sensitive to mechanical and thermal stimuli (De Castro *et al.*, 2013). Secondary hyperalgesia develops in the tissues that surround the burn site. As the inflammatory response subsides over time, a change in pain quality is observed. Where nociceptors are destroyed as a result of severe burn injury, insensitivity to pain may be noted initially; however, neuropathic pain may develop in these areas as nerve tissue regenerates in a disorderly fashion. Neuropathic pain develops in over half of patients with severe burn injury and is chronic in nature (De Castro *et al.*, 2013). Pain also originates from procedures such as placement of lines or cleaning of wounds. Effective pain management is crucial for the successful management of patients following burn injuries. Ineffective pain management may result in the patient distrusting the interdisciplinary team and has a negative impact on early patient rehabilitation. It may also lead to the development of psychiatric disorders such as depression and post-traumatic stress disorder (De Castro *et al.*, 2013).

Patients may experience four patterns of pain; for example, background pain (constant pain at rest and during movement), breakthrough pain (episodes of intense and sudden pain), pain produced by procedures and postoperative pain (De Castro *et al.*, 2013). During the first 24 hours following burn injury, analgesic therapy is administered, monitored and regularly adjusted as needed. The dose and type of analgesia given is dependent on the size of the burn, depth, patient age and the presence of other traumatic injuries (Alharbi *et al.*, 2012). Background pain is usually managed in the acute phase, with a continuous infusion of opioids (with or without patient-controlled analgesia), oral long-term opioids, non-steroidal anti-inflammatory drugs and anxiolytics (De Castro *et al.*, 2013). Procedural pain is managed with opioids (remifentanil, fentynal or alfentanil) and anaesthetics (ketamine). The pharmacological management of neuropathic pain is achieved through administration of opioids (tramadol), anticonvulsants (gabapentin) and antidepressants (amitriptyline) (De Castro *et al.*, 2013). The reader is referred to Section 6.8.2 for information on the non-pharmacological management of pain in patients with burn injury.

6.5.3.2. *Surgery*

Dead tissue is an excellent medium for the growth of bacteria, so it needs to be removed as quickly and thoroughly as possible in patients who have sustained burn injury. Evidence shows that early burn wound excision (between days two and seven of admission) leads to decreased mortality and length of hospital stay in patients aged 30 years or younger (Kasten *et al.*, 2011).

6.5.3.2.1. Debridement

Deep cleaning and removal of dead tissue and contaminants from burn wounds is called debridement. Some units make use of burns baths or shower the patient in the cubicle even in the ICU setting. Autolytic, enzymatic or surgical means can be used to perform debridement and are discussed below (Alharbi *et al.*, 2012).

6.5.3.2.1.1. *Autolytic debridement.* This type of debridement is usually performed on more superficial burns, but also if the patient is unable to tolerate a more aggressive form of debridement (such as the elderly or those with co-morbidities). Dressings such as hydrogels or hydrocolloids (which are moist) are used to retain wound fluids and allow the body to get rid of dead tissue on its own. Autolytic debridement is not suitable for infected wounds but can be used in moist wounds. Wounds generally heal without grafting (Edwards, 2010).

6.5.3.2.1.2. *Enzymatic debridement.* Enzymatic debridement is useful for burn wounds where surgical debridement is often technically difficult, such as the hands (Krieger *et al.*, 2012). Various kinds of chemicals are applied to the wound bed. These chemicals dissolve the dead tissue and prepare the burn area for healing or grafting.

6.5.3.2.1.3. *Surgical debridement.* This type of debridement is usually carried out in the operating theatre under general anaesthetic or at the patient's bedside. Dead tissue is surgically excised with a scalpel or with laser therapy. Surgical debridement can be very extensive and aggressive, involving many body areas simultaneously. This is also the preferred method if sepsis has entered the bloodstream (positive blood cultures) or if there is deep tissue damage, for example in the case of a deep thermal or electrical burn. The application of methylene blue to burn wounds to facilitate precise surgical debridement has been described in the literature (Dorafshar *et al.*, 2010). This technique assists the surgeon to distinguish between viable and non-viable tissue and epithelialised and non-epithelialised areas. An alternative to standard scalpel debridement is the Vesajet® system. This is a water jet surgical tool that has been used successfully in the debridement of superficial partial thickness and mid-dermal partial thickness wounds of the face, hands and feet (Rennekampff *et al.*, 2006).

6.5.3.2.1.4. *Repeat debridement procedures.* Flammable liquid burns, hot oil, electrical and chemical burns all have a high potential for becoming infected. It may be necessary to debride such wounds more than once to ensure proper cleansing of the wound bed in order to promote healing. This is especially important when preparing the burn wound for grafting. In reality the patient may have a debridement every 24 or 36 hours. With deep debridement there may be extensive bleeding, which has the potential to make the acutely ill patient even more unstable. The physiotherapist needs to be aware of this and be prepared to adjust their treatment accordingly. This is usually a temporary situation from which the patient generally recovers in 24 to 48 hours (Alharbi *et al.*, 2012). There is usually blood on standby for the patient, as often a blood transfusion is necessary. Other complications associated with debridement are pain, infection and risk of removal of healthy tissue (Alharbi *et al.*, 2012). Despite the possibility of complications, early wound closure by skin grafts after debridement has been shown to lead to significantly lower mortality rates (Church *et al.*, 2006; Alharbi *et al.*, 2012).

6.5.3.2.2. Escharotomy

Severely burnt tissue can be tense, firm and leathery in appearance. It is immobile, rigid and constrictive in nature. This type of tissue is called eschar. If eschar is circumferential around a limb or the thorax it can restrict movement, circulation or respiration. In this situation the eschar must be cut to prevent damage. The surgical cutting of eschar is called escharotomy. If escharotomy is necessary, it is usually quite evident soon after admission or within the first few hours. Escharotomy is usually a surgical emergency to prevent death of tissue or limb loss. If eschar is affecting the limbs, longitudinal incisions are generally used, starting, if possible, on unburned tissue, cutting through the eschar to expose the fatty tissue below and ending in unburned tissue. These incisions can be very extensive and in multiple sites simultaneously (Alharbi *et al.*, 2012). Due to the amount of tension in the tissues, this longitudinal incision often widens substantially after the procedure. This is in direct proportion to the amount of pressure the tissues were under prior to the escharotomy being carried out. The site may require grafting at a later stage for skin closure.

Key Message

The physiotherapist should observe for signs such as peripheral cyanosis, reduced capillary refill, reduced limb temperature and weak or non-palpable pulses, which would indicate poor circulation to the extremities. In patients with circumferential thoracic burns, look out for signs of respiratory compromise such as tachypnea, dyspnea, decreased chest wall excursion and deteriorating arterial blood gas values. If any of these signs are present, the surgical team should be alerted.

6.5.3.2.3. Fasciotomy

Fasciotomy is a surgical procedure in which an incision is made in the skin that extends into the fascia to relieve pressure for suspected compartment syndrome, such as in the case of circumferential burns to the wrist (carpal tunnel syndrome), thigh or calf (Fig. 6.4). If necessary, it is usually required in the early stages of wound care. Compartment syndrome can be life or limb threatening.

After fasciotomy, limb movement can continue, with elevation of the part to reduce postoperative swelling. Maintenance of joint range of motion (ROM) and muscle length is crucial after fasciotomy; splinting of the joint is effective to maintain muscle length. The area in which the fasciotomy was performed might need to be grafted once the tissue swelling subsides (Alharbi *et al.*, 2012).

6.5.3.3. *Wound management*

The main aims of burn wound management are to prevent wound infection and facilitate the closure of wounds. This can generally be achieved

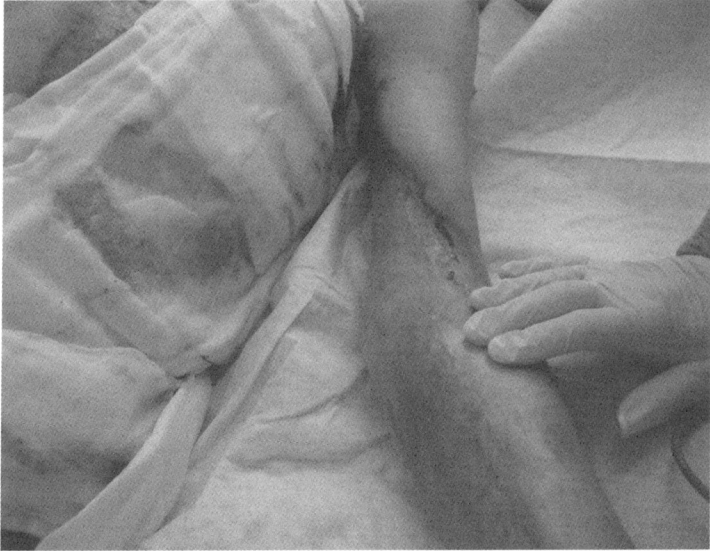

Fig. 6.4: Healed scar following fasciotomy for compartment syndrome in the forearm.

spontaneously in superficial burns. After any of the abovementioned surgical procedures, the open wound will require coverage. The various methods of wound closure are discussed below.

6.5.3.3.1. Autograft

Autograft refers to permanent wound coverage with the patient's own skin (skin grafting). This is ideal as there is less chance of skin graft rejection. Autograft can be in the form of a split (partial) thickness skin graft (SSG) or a full thickness skin graft (FTSG). Healthy skin from another site is used to cover the wound. This is called donor skin and the area it was taken from is referred to as the donor site. Autografting may be limited if the patient has little healthy skin available to use, and other grafting methods may therefore be required.

6.5.3.3.1.1. *Split thickness skin graft.* Split thickness skin graft harvesting is carried out under general anaesthetic as it is a painful procedure. Grafting may take place in several stages that can involve multiple operations (Church *et al.*, 2006; Leung and Fish, 2009). The Dermatome is an instrument with a rapidly oscillating blade and is used to obtain skin from the donor site. It can be set to shave different thicknesses of skin. Donor skin is usually taken from the anterior or lateral aspect of the thigh but can also be taken from the back. The epidermis and part of the dermis is removed. The graft can be passed through a meshing device to maximise the area to be covered and to minimise the amount of donor skin required (Figs 6.5A and B). The graft is then applied to the prepared wound bed and attached with staples or surgical glue (Leung and Fish, 2009).

Particularly where donor sites are limited, expanded skin grafts, using a Meek or modified Meek approach (meshing of graft), may be used. Expanded skin grafts are usually held in place using adhesive glue and are covered with fine gauze (Hsieh *et al.*, 2008).

Split thickness skin grafts applied over the face and arms are not meshed in order for a more desirable cosmetic effect. Meshed grafts are also avoided over joint areas as they are more likely to contract (Leung and Fish, 2009). New blood vessels grow in 36 hours, which is why it is imperative that no movement of the skin graft takes place. After grafting, the

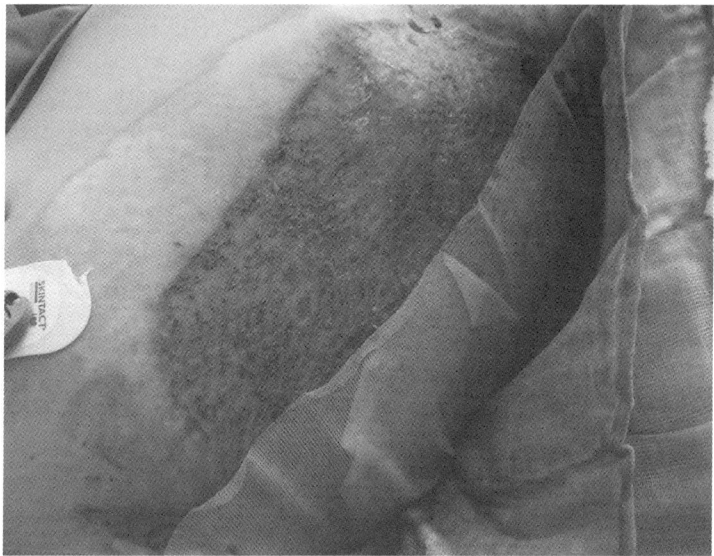

Fig. 6.5A: Healed meshed split skin graft applied over burns to the lateral trunk.

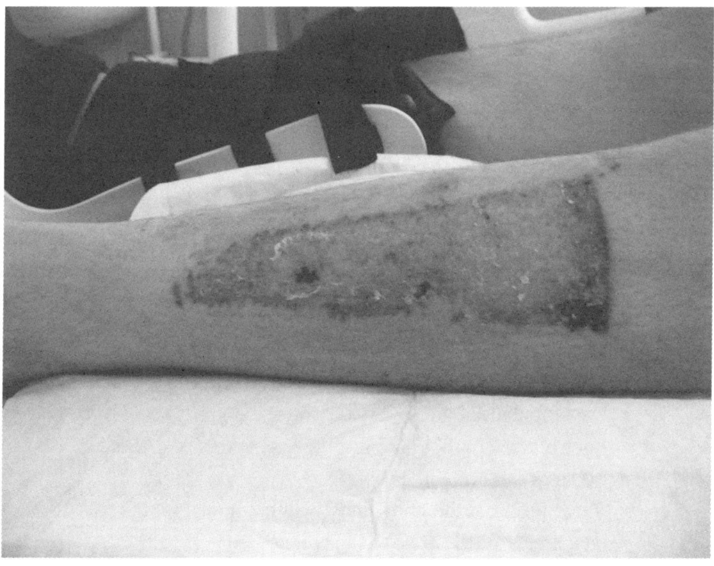

Fig. 6.5B: Healed donor site on the lower leg.

plastic surgeon may apply a splint to the graft area to prevent any incidental movement of the site. During this immobilisation period the patient's own blood vessels start to grow into the graft tissue and it starts to function as healthy tissue. Movement may lead to graft failure. Table 6.7 highlights other factors that may lead to graft failure (Leung and Fish, 2009).

Key Messages

- It is important to closely monitor circulation distal to the splinted area after skin graft to ensure that the bandages are not too restrictive. This is particularly important for sedated patients who are unable to verbalise circulatory compromise.
- Always check with the surgical team prior to mobilising any joint that may be affected by a skin graft.

At the end of the period of immobilisation, the splint is removed, the dressings removed and the 'take' of the graft determined. If there is an odour, excessive pain or discharge, the graft is likely to be exposed earlier to determine the cause. Sensation in a grafted area may never completely return to normal. The grafted skin has no oil glands or sweat glands and becomes dry. The itchiness that arises from dry skin is called pruritis and can be a long-term consequence of skin grafting. The patient is advised to keep the grafted area hydrated with the application of a water based cream like aqueous cream or coconut oil up to five times a day. Patients are also advised to keep the graft site out of the sun for at least 12 months or until the scar reaches maturity after grafting to prevent hyper-pigmentation.

Table 6.7: Reasons for skin graft failure.

• Development of a haematoma under the graft
• Poor blood supply to the graft, e.g. smokers or diabetics
• Local or systemic infections
• Shear forces at the graft site which could disrupt the attachment of the graft to the wound bed
• Rejection

The donor site can be covered with an artificial skin substitute to promote healing and allow early mobility. As it is a surgical wound, there may be a certain degree of reluctance on the part of the patient to move the area. Early mobility of the donor site from the day after grafting is usually commenced by the attending physiotherapist. Split thickness skin grafts have the advantage that, once the donor site has healed after 10 days, it can be used for re-harvesting. This is particularly useful in patients with limited healthy donor sites (Leung and Fish, 2009).

6.5.3.3.1.2. *Full thickness skin grafts.* These grafts involve the use of the epidermis, dermis and hypodermis as donor areas and are used mainly for facial burns to achieve optimal results. The full thickness grafted skin has sweat and oil glands and is elastic so cosmesis is better. This type of graft may also be used on the soles of the feet and on the palms of the hands (see Fig. 6.6) (Landau *et al.*, 2008). The donor area often requires an SSG to cover the deficit left following the FTSG.

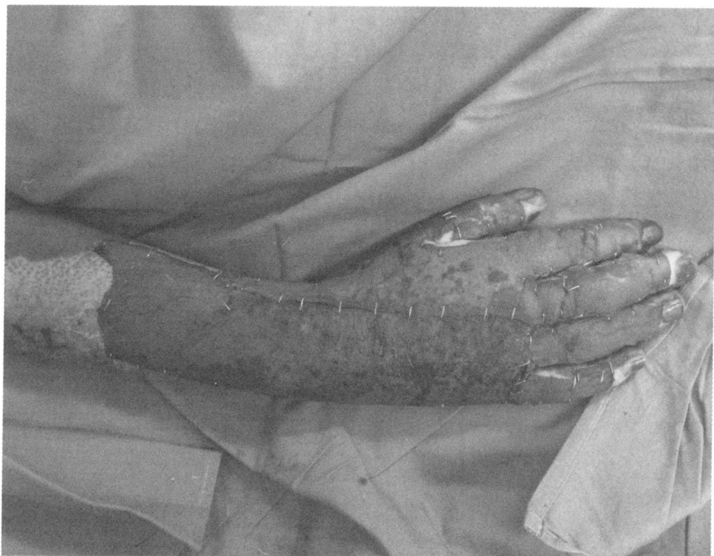

Fig. 6.6: Full thickness skin graft of the forearm and hand.

6.5.3.3.2. Cultured epithelial grafts

Biotechnology has produced a new type of skin graft using living cells from a patient skin biopsy to grow new sheets of cells in the laboratory. The major advantage is that rejection seldom occurs as the graft is grown from the patient's own skin. It is extremely fragile (almost like tissue paper) as it is only 10–15 cells thick so this skin is easily torn (Halim *et al.*, 2010). As it takes time to grow this skin in the laboratory, this makes it costly. This type of graft is useful in patients who have large surface area burns and limited skin that can be harvested for grafting (Lee, 2012; Menon *et al.*, 2013). It takes approximately three weeks from initial biopsy of the skin to readiness for transplantation. Mucosal epithelial cells are reported to have higher proliferation ability than epidermal epithelial cells. Cultured mucosal epithelial cells sprayed onto deep dermal burns after debridement show promising cosmetic outcomes (Ueda, 2010). Cultured epithelial grafts have been used successfully in both the adult and paediatric population (Ueda, 2010; Lee, 2012; Menon *et al.*, 2013).

6.5.3.3.3. Dermal substitutes (prosthetic grafts)

Prosthetic dermal substitutes are used in cases in which donor sites are not available, such as in patients with large TBSA wounds and in cases where allografts or xenografts are not available. There are two categories of dermal substitutes, namely wound dressings and substitutes used for wound closure. These are summarised in Table 6.8 (Leung and Fish, 2009; Alharbi *et al.*, 2012).

More information about dermal substitute therapy is provided in Section 6.5.3.3.6 and Section 6.10.

6.5.3.3.4. Allografts

Allografts consist of cadaveric skin and provide temporary wound cover to burn wounds. Cadaver skin is stored in the skin bank from organ donors. The skin is tested for communicable diseases prior to usage. This type of graft is usually used in cases where there is a large surface area to be covered. An autograft would need to be done after the cadaver skin is rejected but it has the advantage of providing quick temporary coverage of the area, thereby reducing fluid loss and the potential for infection. The

Table 6.8: Categories of dermal substitutes[*].

	Purpose	Examples
Wound dressings	Provides temporary wound cover and prepares the wound bed for a permanent graft	• Biobrane® • Dermagraft® • Allogenic keratinocytes • Amniotic membrane • Suprathel®
Wound closure	These substitutes are integrated into the wound bed and some provide permanent wound cover	• Integra® • Alloderm® • Autologous keratinocytes • Matriderm®

[*]Adapted from Leung and Fish (2009).

cadaver skin promotes vascular growth in preparation for autografting. A major drawback to the use of allografts is that they are not readily available and have a high rate of rejection by the recipient (Leung and Fish, 2009; Alharbi *et al.,* 2012).

6.5.3.3.5. Xenograft

A xenograft is skin taken from animal species (bovine or swine) to provide temporary burn wound cover in patients with a large percentage of TBSA burns. This temporary covering has the advantage of stimulating the formation of granulation tissue in preparation for autografting (Alharbi *et al.*, 2012).

6.5.3.3.6. Wound dressings

There are many different types of wound dressings. The type selected is dependent on depth, site and extent of the burn wound and the required result, e.g. an occlusive dressing versus a dressing needed to treat infection. Wound dressings can be sub-categorised into composites, films, foams, gels and sprays (Wasiak *et al.*, 2009). The ideal wound dressing has most of the features outlined in Table 6.9. Cost, availability and reason for use of dressings may influence the ultimate choice made.

The attending doctor may also have a preference for using a certain type of dressing. Each of these dressings are summarised in Table 6.10.

Table 6.9: Properties of the ideal wound dressing*.

- Protection of the wound from physical damage and contamination with micro-organisms
- Comfortable and durable
- Accommodates movement
- Allows gaseous exchange
- Allows high humidity of the wound
- Is compatible with topical agents
- Is non-toxic, non-adherent and non-irritant

*Wasiak *et al.*, (2009).

6.5.3.3.6.1. *Artificial skin substitutes.* Artificial skin substitutes are made out of molecules and polymers that are not present in normal skin. Animal products containing collagen and chondroitin are used in combination with silicone to form a skin substitute for large area burns. Artificial skin substitutes are biodegradable and provide an adequate environment for tissue regeneration (Halim *et al.*, 2010). These substitutes are fitted very close to the skin, almost like a glove. They are transparent, which makes it easier to assess the underlying tissue. This is a temporary covering and allows for immediate coverage to reduce fluid loss and the likelihood of infection. It starts to loosen around the edges fairly quickly and this can be trimmed off with scissors, but must only be trimmed at the edges as it loosens. It is usually held in place by staples or clips. It is flexible and conforms well to surface irregularities. The artificial skin substitute can also be used on the patient's donor site to encourage faster healing; thus this site could be used for further harvesting, which is useful if there are limited donor areas available (Wasiak *et al.*, 2009; Halim *et al.*, 2010).

Key Message

With artificial skin substitute dressings in place *no* movement of the part, especially over joint areas, is advised, as this may cause shearing of the skin substitute. Therefore *no* limb physiotherapy should be carried out at this time. This is often approximately five days but the plastic surgeon will advise.

Table 6.10: Examples of wounds dressings used for burn injuries*.

Wound dressing	Usage	Brand name
Hydrocolloid dressings	Gel substrate used for autolytic debridement of the wound bed.	• Comfeel® • DuoDerm®
Polyurethane film dressings	Transparent adhesive-coated sheets that are used for absorption of wound exudate.	• OpSite® • Tegaderm®
Hydrogel dressings	High water content gels used for absorption of wound exudate and debridement of the wound.	• Loose hydrogels (IntraSite®, Solugel®) • Hydrogel sheets (Aqua clear®, Nu-gel®)
Silicon coated nylon dressings	Direct wound contact layers which allow drainage of exudates through the mesh structure of the dressing. It reduces potential damage to the wound during dressing changes.	• Mepitel®
Artificial skin substitutes (see information in Section 6.5.3.3.6.1.)	Provides immediate wound cover and assists with tissue regeneration.	• Biobrane® • Dermagraft® • Integra® • Matriderm® • Trans Cyte®
Antimicrobial dressings (see information in Section 6.5.3.3.6.2.)	Silver-containing sustained release dressings used to reduce wound site infection.	• Acticoat® • Contreet® • Avance® • Aquacel Ag®
	Iodine dressings used for wound cleaning.	• Iodosorb® range • Indaine®
Fibre (alginate) dressings	Limit wound secretions and minimise bacterial contamination.	• Algosteril® • Comfeel® • Alginate® • Kaltostat®
Wound dressing pads	Woven cotton pads applied directly over the wound for coverage.	• Medicated pads (with iodine or chlorhexidine) • Non-medicated pads (paraffin-gauze)

*Wasiak *et al.* (2009); Matsumura *et al.* (2013).

6.5.3.3.6.2. *Antimicrobial dressings.* Dressings that contain silver deliver a sustained-release of silver directly onto the wound bed, which contributes to the reduction of wound site infection (Percival *et al.*, 2012). The dressing has a non-adherent contact layer, which permits the passage of wound exudate. These dressings are available in multiple shapes and sizes, and are also available in glove form. This dressing can be left *in situ* for up to seven days. Silver dressings are usually covered with secondary dressings and are used to prepare the wound bed for later grafting.

Iodine-type dressings can also be used for wound cleaning. Large swabs can be soaked in an iodine solution and then applied to the patient, covered with a secondary dressing. These moist impregnated bandages keep the wound bed hydrated and have an anti-bacterial effect. Iodine dressings can be messy to apply but are less costly than other types of dressings. These dressings can be changed daily or even twice a day if the wound is very infected. Iodine dressings can be used to prepare the wound bed for later grafting. Iodine creams are available for smaller-sized wounds (Wasiak *et al.*, 2009).

6.5.3.3.6.3. *Negative pressure wound therapy.* Negative pressure wound therapy can be used in the care of patients with burn wounds that produce large amounts of exudate. A piece of foam is cut to the size of the wound and placed inside the wound. Underneath the foam one end of a perforated tube is placed in the wound and the other end is attached to a vacuum pump. The foam is sealed with a transparent adherent dressing to create a seal. Negative pressure is applied to the sealed wound site through the vacuum pump. This type of therapy keeps the wound clean and stimulates tissue granulation. Negative pressure wound therapy can be used for wound care in a variety of patients (Chapter 5, Fig. 5.9B) and can also be used after debridement of a burn wound before a skin graft is applied (Landau *et al.*, 2008). It can be used after skin graft, providing there is a non-adherent dressing applied on top of the skin graft under the negative pressure wound therapy foam in order to preserve the graft when removing the negative pressure foam and transparent dressing. An advantage of negative pressure wound therapy is that the patient can be mobilised with the foam and dressing *in situ*, as the tubing can be clamped and unclamped when the patient leaves and returns to the bedside, thereby maintaining mobility.

6.6. Physiotherapy Aims of Management

Physiotherapists are regarded as essential members of the interdisciplinary team (Table 6.11) involved in the management of burn survivors (Sheridan *et al.*, 2005; Holavanahalli *et al.*, 2011). It is widely advocated that specialist burn therapists be involved in the physiotherapeutic management of burn survivors (Parry and Esselman, 2011). In the absence of specialisation, an effective standard of physiotherapy care in the burn patient has been described (Simons *et al.*, 2003). The accepted standards of care that form the basis of physiotherapeutic management of the burn patient includes the importance of team work, continued education of patients and caregivers, appreciation for potential complications on the road to recovery, effective pain control measures, evaluation and re-evaluation throughout the continuum of care, the importance of infection control and the use of outcome measures (Simons *et al.*, 2003).

In Chapter 5 (Section 5.4) the importance of individual patient assessment and goal setting, using specific, measureable, attainable, realistic, time-based (SMART) goals, was discussed. The same principles apply to patients with burn injuries, whether these patients are admitted to the ICU or the burn ward. The effects of burn injuries, anaesthesia and immobility

Table 6.11: Interdisciplinary team members involved in the care of the patient with burns in the acute and chronic phases after injury.

- Specialist or generic physiotherapist
- Anaesthetist and pain management specialist
- Medical practitioner, intensivist and plastic surgeon
- Nursing practitioner
- Dietician
- Occupational therapist
- Speech and language therapist
- Pharmacist
- Social worker
- Clergy (pastoral care)
- Interpreter
- Orthotist and prosthetist
- Psychologist
- Play or music therapist

are the same in infants and children as in adults; however, the potential for respiratory complications may be greater in infants and children because of anatomical and physiological differences between them and the adult population (Chapter 2, Section 2.2).

Patients with severe burn injury are often admitted to the ICU, whereas those with less severe injury are admitted to the burns ward. Those in the ICU may be intubated and sedated due to the severity of their injuries and therefore physiotherapy management is aimed at preventing respiratory and musculoskeletal complications, as far as possible. As soon as the patient regains consciousness and becomes cooperative, the focus of physiotherapy management shifts to active rehabilitation in the ICU setting. Important aims of management of patients with burn injury, which need to be considered by the physiotherapist based on individual patient assessment findings in the ICU environment, are listed in Table 6.12.

Important aims of management for patients with burn injuries in the burns ward are listed in Table 6.13. Physiotherapy approaches to patient

Table 6.12: Aims of physiotherapy management for patients with burn injury in the ICU.

- Enhance mucociliary escalator function through adequate humidification of the airways
- Mobilise and remove excessive retained secretions from the airways of patients who are intubated, especially those with inhalation injuries, in order to prevent the development of secondary chest infections
- Enhance the patient's cough effort in order to assist with secretion clearance
- Increase posterior and basal lung volumes of patients who are intubated and sedated in order to prevent the development of atelectasis
- Increase the patient's lung compliance in order to optimise and restore lung function
- Improve the patient's oxygenation
- Improve respiratory muscle strength as soon as the patient becomes conscious and cooperative in order to assist with weaning from mechanical ventilation (MV), especially when weaning has been prolonged
- Maintain or restore passive ROM of all limbs in order to prevent or reduce joint stiffness in patients who are intubated and sedated
- Provide splints to maintain ROM as indicated
- Restore muscle power of the peripheries when the patient regains consciousness and is cooperative
- As the patient regains consciousness and their condition stabilises, aim to restore functionality in order for them to gain independence with activities of daily living (ADL)

Table 6.13: Aims of management for patients with burn injury in the ward setting.

- Improve the patient's self-dependence through encouragement of active and active-resisted ROM exercises of affected extremities and trunk and ensure that end-of-range motion is achieved
- Restore muscle power in affected and unaffected extremities and the trunk
- Restore normal posture
- Restore normal gait pattern for patients with burn injuries to the lower extremities and feet
- Restore independent function in the ward
- Improve and restore cardiorespiratory exercise endurance in order to obtain the health benefits of exercise
- Humidify the airways for as long as the patient receives oxygen therapy
- Enhance the patient's self-dependence by teaching them to mobilise and remove excessive retained secretions independently
- Maintain optimal lung volumes during the patient's stay in the ward
- Maintain optimal lung compliance during the patient's stay in the ward

management should be focussed on early active rehabilitation of awake and cooperative patients. The aims of management listed here are also important for the progression of management of patients that are discharged from the ICU to the ward, based on each individual patient's assessment findings prior to ICU discharge.

6.6.1. *Paediatric considerations*

The aims of physiotherapy intervention are similar between adults and children, but the pre-morbid functional and developmental level of the child must be taken into account when devising short-term and long-term aims of treatment.

6.6.2. *Functional assessment prior to discharge*

Prior to discharge home the adult or paediatric patient with burn injury should undergo a functional assessment similar to that described in Chapter 5 (Section 5.4.2). The impact of the functional assessment outcomes on the patient's ability to perform ADL should be assessed. Based on these findings, the rehabilitation goals for post-discharge care should be discussed with the patient and their family and agreed upon. Post-discharge goals for the continued management of a patient with burn injuries should include the following

- Return to pre-injury functional ability and social integration.
- Empowerment of the patient to take responsibility for skin care, management of scar tissue and prevention of contractures.
- In children especially, long-term follow-up is essential as they grow and therefore may outgrow even the best surgical results. Children also seem to form worse hypertrophic scars that need prolonged scar management (Sheridan, 2002).

For more information about the rehabilitation of burn survivors after hospital discharge, refer to Section 6.10. Guidelines for exercise rehabilitation for trauma survivors can be found in Chapter 10 (Section 10.6).

6.7. Precautions and Contraindications Related to Physiotherapy Management

Recommendations provided here are mostly based on expert opinion derived from clinical practice due to paucity in the literature in certain aspects of patient care in the acute care setting.

6.7.1. *General precautions to physiotherapy in intensive care*

The reader is referred to Chapter 5 (Section 5.5.1) for a list of general precautions that should be adhered to during the treatment of any trauma patient in the acute care setting.

6.7.2. *Specific precautions and contraindications to physiotherapy in patients with burn injuries*

6.7.2.1. *Adult patient with burn injury*

- Due to the vulnerability of burn survivors to infections and the rapid development of severe sepsis, physiotherapists must be vigilant in clinical practice to ensure a safe environment for patients. A vigilant practice is based on a thorough knowledge of universal infection control precautions and the elements responsible for bacterial transfer. This practice includes correct hand washing, wearing of protective clothing (gloves, aprons and goggles) and cleansing of equipment used during patient care (stethoscope, goniometry and other rehabilitation equipment) (Kasten *et al.*, 2011; Rafla and Tredget, 2011).

- After an escharotomy has been performed there are generally no restrictions placed on mobilising the area unless the patient is actively bleeding from the site. If this is the case, postponement of physiotherapy intervention should be discussed with the attending surgeon.
- It is generally accepted that the joints above and below the area which received a skin graft should not be mobilised for a period following the graft. However, the time period necessary is not clear. Suggestions include the immediate active mobilisation (no passive mobilisation) of joints or alternatively three to five days of rest (immobility) after skin graft. The detrimental effects of bed rest must also be considered in the risk–benefit of this decision (Holavanahalli *et al.*, 2011). Physiotherapists should therefore consult with the surgeon to determine the optimal timeframe to initiate joint mobilisation following the placement of grafts. In some centres the skin graft is marked with a pen (usually on a piece of tape stuck on top of the covering bandages) which alerts other health care staff (e.g. radiographers) to the fact that the limb must not be moved. The date of the graft is also written on the tape.
- Danger of damage to new skin must always be considered during passive stretching. Stretches should be gentle, prolonged and gradual. Stretching only to the point of blanching is recommended (Spires *et al.*, 2007).
- It is essential that the physiotherapist liaise with interdisciplinary team members to ensure that there is sufficient pain relief for functional activities. In addition to the pain which results from the injury, this population is also exposed to pain as a result of nursing and physiotherapeutic interventions. The experience of the patient during these therapeutic interventions increases anxiety levels and the patient's compliance with interventions.
- Ambulation must be initiated at the earliest appropriate time. Physiotherapists should be aware that patients with burn wounds to the

legs may suffer from orthostatic intolerance, which could prevent timely ambulation.

- In the burn patient great care should be taken to ensure the security of all lines and tubes before mobilisation is attempted. This population is particularly vulnerable for line displacement and contracting infections due to line replacement.
- The head-down tilt position for postural drainage is contraindicated in patients with inhalation injury due to facial oedema that might worsen in these positions and compromise the integrity of the airways.
- Manual chest therapy techniques should not be administered directly over acute burn wounds on the chest wall or over newly grafted skin on the chest wall. Alternative methods of secretion mobilisation should be considered instead.
- Considering the ciliary damage caused by inhalation injury, special care should be taken not to insert the suction catheter beyond the distal end of the endotracheal tube (ETT) or tracheostomy tube, as deep endotracheal suctioning may lead to further ciliary damage. Suctioning should occur after mobilisation of secretions in the intubated patient or when a specimen is needed for microbiological culture; it should not be routinely performed in patients with inhalation injury.
- Manual hyperinflation should not be used routinely in patients with inhalation injury due to the risk of further cellular airway damage.

6.7.2.2. *Paediatric patient with burn injury*

Similar precautions and contraindications as described above apply to paediatric patients with burn or inhalation injuries.

- Tracheal displacement to facilitate therapeutic coughing should only be used in paediatric patients aged one year or older and as long as there is no upper airway involvement, face or neck burns. It should be noted that this technique is being discouraged in many clinical settings due to the potential danger it poses to airway integrity.
- Tracheal rubs are contraindicated in children less than nine months of age, as the trachea is still very compliant and pressure may result in severe airway obstruction.

- Manual hyperinflation should not be used routinely in the paediatric population due to the increased risks of barotrauma and volutrauma in this population (Bassani *et al.*, 2009).

6.8. Physiotherapy Interventions

Rehabilitation is an essential part of the care that patients with burn injuries can expect to receive and spans from admission to hospital to full integration of the patient into society. However, there is a paucity of research to clarify the optimal therapeutic interventions to be used (Esselman *et al.*, 2006; Esselman, 2007). We will describe the current best evidence available in this section. Where evidence is not available, expert opinion based on clinical experience is shared.

To provide some form of standardisation of physiotherapeutic management of critically ill patients, step-wise intervention protocols were published in recent years by Morris *et al.* (2008) and Hanekom *et al.* (2011b). Although these protocols were written for the general ICU population and not specifically for patients with burn injuries, many of the principles of management remain the same and can be implemented for the patient recovering from burn wounds or inhalation injuries.

Analgesia is the single most important consideration in optimising pulmonary and general function in adults and children following burn injury. In the acute stage early after injury, physiotherapy management for the severely injured patient focuses on support of the respiratory system. As the patient's condition stabilises and they wake up from sedation in the ICU and become more cooperative, rehabilitation is immediately commenced.

6.8.1. *Education*

Continued education of the patient, family members, care givers and staff is an essential component of an effective physiotherapeutic management plan. The continued education of patient and family members needs to ensure a full awareness of the consequences of the choices they make. This includes the benefits and risks of planned therapeutic interventions as well as the consequences of non-compliance. Due to the proximity of care givers and nursing staff to the patients, they are essential partners in promoting independent functional ability of patients and ensuring optimal positioning and splinting interventions. Providing ongoing support and continued education is a strategic priority of the physiotherapeutic management plan.

6.8.2. *Pain*

It is widely accepted that therapy-induced pain cannot be effectively managed by pharmacological interventions alone. There is increasing interest in alternative management for therapy-related pain for patients with burn injuries. This includes the use of relaxation, deep breathing and visualisation in the acute phase after burns and transcutaneous electrical nervous stimulation (TENS) when wound healing has taken place. Promising work is being done using virtual reality in the acute phase management of patients with burn injuries during therapeutic interventions to break the anxiety and pain cycle (Morris *et al.*, 2009, 2010; Hoffman *et al.*, 2011; Kipping *et al.*, 2012).

Physiotherapists must build trusting relationships with their patients to ensure optimal benefits from interventions used. Involving the patient and family in goal setting and establishing ground rules for how far the therapist can push the patient is essential for building these relationships. The timing of physiotherapeutic interventions to coincide with maximum benefits from pharmacological relief and application of interventions when bandages are removed while the patient is in the bath are examples of strategies which can be employed to maximise therapeutic benefit without increased pain. Physiotherapists also need to be aware and consider the impact of pain medication on the patient's performance. This includes drowsiness, nausea, impaired memory, an inability to communicate effectively, postural hypotension, which could result in fainting, and lastly constipation.

6.8.3. *Respiratory system management*

6.8.3.1. *Oxygenation*

6.8.3.1.1. Intubated patient

Oxygenation may be improved for intubated and ventilated patients with burn injuries by utilising regular body position changes to enhance V/Q matching. A certain degree of V/Q mismatch is created by MV as air flows to areas of least resistance in the lungs; these are often the anterior and apical lung segments in a supported sitting position. Ventilation is optimal in gravity-dependent areas of the lungs, which are the basal and posterior lung segments. As a result V/Q matching cannot be optimal while the patient is receiving MV. Body positioning such as 45–60º head-up high supported sitting is used to prevent aspiration and may provide better V/Q matching than side-lying positions (when assumed for extended time periods). In side-lying the ventilated patient experiences more V/Q mismatch due to preferential ventilation of the upper-most lung versus preferential perfusion of the bottom lung.

6.8.3.1.2. Spontaneously breathing patient

Body position changes may also be used for spontaneously breathing patients to improve V/Q matching and therefore oxygenation. The reader is referred to Chapter 4 (Section 4.2.3) for more information.

6.8.3.2. *Humidification*

6.8.3.2.1. Intubated patient

The reader is referred to Chapter 5 (Section 5.6.1.2) for more information. Patients with burn injuries and a history of chronic lung disease should always be treated with heated water humidification applied through the ventilator circuit (AARC, 2003).

6.8.3.2.2. Spontaneously breathing patient

Humidification of the airways of a spontaneously breathing patient can be achieved through a heated water humidifier using an oxygen mask. Alternatively, intermittent nebulisation with 0.9% sodium chloride (NaCl) solution can also be used. This solution can be administered through a small volume (jet) nebuliser attached to a face mask or a mouth piece. The reader is referred to Section 6.5.3.1.5 for information about additional medication that can be administered via nebulisation for patients with inhalation injury.

6.8.3.3. *Management of pulmonary secretions*

Clearance of airway debris is primarily dependent on the effective functioning of the mucociliary clearance system and secondarily on an effective cough mechanism. Coughs can be reflexive or voluntary. The increased expiratory flow rate, which results from a cough, causes a sheering force which dislodges secretions from the airway walls (Fink, 2007). It is one of the strongest physiological reflexes and is responsible for maintaining an open airway. Due to destruction of cilia as a result of inhalation burn, therapeutic coughing is essential to remove debris from the airways.

6.8.3.3.1. Intubated patient

For an intubated and mechanically ventilated patient, pulmonary secretion mobilisation and removal can be achieved through the use of modified postural drainage positions, manual chest clearance techniques (within the limitation of precautions and contraindications described in Section 6.7), suction and manual hyperinflation (MHI). The reader is referred to Chapter 4 (Section 4.2) for information on safe and effective applications of these techniques. Recent studies indicate that ventilator hyperinflation (VHI) (Chapter 4, Section 4.2) results in similar volumes of secretions cleared as MHI. When ventilated with positive end-expiratory pressure (PEEP) above eight cmH_2O it has been recommended that VHI is used (Berney and Denehy, 2002; Hanekom *et al.*, 2011a). The head-down position combined with MHI increases the volume of secretions cleared and expiratory flow rates in intubated adult patients (Berney *et al.*, 2004). The techniques outlined here may be used in intubated and ventilated patients who have suffered burn or inhalation injuries, but head-down tilt should only be used after oedema of the face, neck and airways has subsided. In some clinical settings mechanical insufflation-exsufflation (Chapter 4, Section 4.2.2.3) is used for secretion clearance and is reported to be effective together with negating the need for hands-on chest wall manual therapy. Currently no research evidence is available on the use of mechanical insufflation-exsufflation in the respiratory management of patients with burn injuries.

The reader is referred to Chapter 4 (Section 4.2.7.1) for information on the safe and effective performance of suctioning through artificial airways.

During airway suction normal saline (0.9% NaCl) may be instilled in small amounts down the endotracheal or tracheostomy tube in an attempt to stimulate a cough to enhance secretion clearance; however, close monitoring of the patient's peripheral oxygen saturation during saline instillation is advised. Saline instillation should not be a routine procedure during suction but should only be done in the presence of viscous, difficult to clear secretions (Roberts, 2009). It is important to note that normal saline does not mix with mucus and therefore does not thin mucus but merely serves to stimulate a cough to assist with clearance of secretions (Halm and Hagel, 2008).

The reader is referred to Chapter 5 (Section 5.6.1.3.1) for information about open suction and closed suction systems.

6.8.3.3.2. Spontaneously breathing patient

Physiotherapists must use a variety of techniques to stimulate an effective cough in spontaneously breathing patients (Hanekom *et al.*, 2012). The spontaneously breathing patient with burn injuries may be shown how to perform the active cycle of breathing technique (ACBT) (Chapter 4, Section 4.2.1.2) in order to assist with secretion mobilisation and clearance. Encouragement to huff (forced expiratory technique), cough and expectorate retained secretions is vitally important. It has been recommended that deep breathing exercises and coughing be implemented every two hours to reduce the risk of secretion retention in patients with inhalation burns (Mlcak *et al.*, 2007). This has not been confirmed in clinical trials. Some patients who breath spontaneously may be too weak or in too much pain to clear secretions effectively with ACBT alone. These types of patients will benefit from the addition of modified postural drainage positions and manual chest therapy techniques (applied within the limitations of precautions and contraindications discussed in Section 6.7), as well as suction with a Yankauer at the back of the throat to facilitate secretion clearance. Manual chest therapy techniques may be performed over the chest wall when wound healing has taken place. Mobilisation around the ward and active exercises are alternative and effective methods to facilitate secretion mobilisation.

6.8.3.4. *Lung capacity and volumes*

6.8.3.4.1. Intubated patients

Patients with severe burn and inhalation injuries are at risk of developing partial or complete atelectasis as a result of immobility in the ICU and cast formation in the airways (after inhalation injury) that may lead to airway obstruction. Prolonged bed rest results in a loss of lung capacity, especially functional residual capacity (FRC), as airways close prematurely. Reduction in FRC leads to decreased surface area for gas exchange and results in poor oxygenation. The application of positive expiratory pressure (PEP) to the airways of intubated and spontaneously breathing patients assists with the restoration of FRC. Patients on MV receive PEP in the form of PEEP. Soon after initiation of MV, PEEP levels might be set at a high level to recruit partially collapsed alveoli, increase FRC and improve the patient's oxygenation. As the patient's condition stabilises, PEEP is weaned to the lowest possible level while optimal oxygenation is maintained. The advantage of PEEP is that the alveoli remain distended for prolonged periods, stimulating surfactant production in those alveoli that were previously collapsed.

Body position changes that involve moving from side to side, supine to sitting and upright standing (for alert and cooperative patients in the ICU) lead to improvements in FRC and lung volumes (as discussed in Chapter 4, Section 4.2.3.1). Techniques such as MHI can be used to improve inspiratory lung volumes in patients who are intubated and mechanically ventilated. Manual hyperinflation reduces airway resistance and assists with improvement of lung compliance, thereby increasing lung volumes (Paratz *et al.*, 2002; Choi and Jones, 2005).

As soon as the intubated patient regains consciousness, ACBT can be initiated, with emphasis on the thoracic expansion exercises component, to encourage collateral ventilation through the peripheral airways and thereby improve lung volumes. The patient should be encouraged to observe their tidal volume on the ventilator screen (biofeedback) and to increase the volume with every breath during the thoracic expansion exercises component of ACBT to further encourage lung expansion.

6.8.3.4.2. Spontaneously breathing patient

Spontaneously breathing patients may improve lung volumes by performing active exercises, mobilisation out of bed, ACBT or incentive spirometry. Care should be taken during the use of incentive spirometry to encourage lateral costal deep breathing in order to correct the patient's breathing pattern from apical to diaphragmatic breathing (Chapter 4, Section 4.2.2.1). The American Association for Respiratory Care (AARC) recommends that incentive spirometry be used in combination with deep breathing, directed coughing and early mobilisation in order to have a beneficial effect on lung volume (AARC, 2011).

Oscillating PEP may be administered to the patient through the use of a bubble PEP bottle or a flutter device. The reader is referred to Chapter 4 (Section 4.2.2.4.1.2) for a description on the safe and effective application of oscillatory PEP devices in patient care. Continuous PEP may be administered through the use of a PEP mask if no facial burns are present (Chapter 4, Section 4.2.2.4.1.1). Currently no research evidence is available to support the effectiveness of PEP mask, bubble PEP bottle or flutter devices in the management of patients with inhalation injuries.

6.8.3.5. *Respiratory muscle training*

The reader is referred to the discussion in Chapter 5, Section 5.6.1.5, as the same principles apply for patients with burn injuries who undergo prolonged MV.

6.8.3.6. *Paediatric considerations*

Generally, similar techniques can be used for the young and old, but these need to be adapted and tailored according to the patient's age, developmental level and acuity of presentation. The reader is referred to Chapter 4 for more information about the respiratory system management of patients with traumatic injury, as these principles can be applied for those who have suffered burn injury.

6.8.4. *Neuromusculoskeletal system*

6.8.4.1. *Joint range of motion*

Patients with extensive burns (greater than 20% TBSA), deep partial thickness and full thickness burns, inhalation burns and amputations have a high risk of developing contractures (Schneider *et al.*, 2006; Tan *et al.*, 2012). Intensive physiotherapy and positioning regimes should be implemented from day one to limit the development of contractures. Patients will adopt flexion positions for comfort. Unfortunately these are also the positions that facilitate contracture development. The development and implementation of anti-contracture positions should be spearheaded by the physiotherapist (Table 6.14) (Spires *et al.*, 2007). The success of this strategy is dependent on the support of the interdisciplinary team members, including the patient and family members (Holavanahalli *et al.*, 2011).

When the patient is exposed, either during bathing activities or whilst dressings are being done, it is very useful for the physiotherapist to assess the burn wounds, taking note of the distribution and depth for planning purposes and to ascertain how much healing has occurred. Physiotherapy to the limbs can also be carried out when the patient's wounds are exposed. This can be very effective in gauging joint range and muscle extensibility in the absence of restrictions posed by wound dressings and bandages. Often with patchy burns the tendency is to wrap the entire arm in bandages, so if the physiotherapist can assess the burns visually, then they can make a decision on the amount of mobility and stretching that can be safely carried out. The physiotherapist is also able to see potential joint restrictions and can adjust patient positioning and treatment accordingly. It is then possible for the physiotherapist to advise the nurse on the most beneficial positions for the patient to be nursed in. Hand and finger mobilisation and web space stretching is most effective when the patient's wounds are exposed, as there are no dressings to restrict ROM.

6.8.4.1.1. Intubated patients

It is essential to reach full passive ROM of all affected joints (neck, trunk and extremities) once daily through gentle passive stretching to end of

Table 6.14: Anti-contracture body positions to avoid shortening of flexor muscles affected by burn injury.

Body position	Description
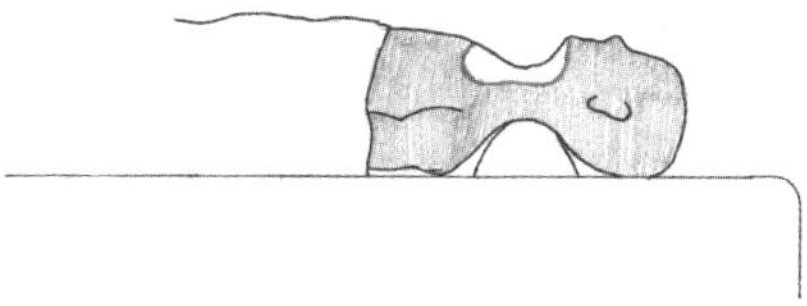	Positioning a patient with anterior neck burns in supine with a pillow under the neck facilitates lengthening of the neck flexors to ensure neck extension ROM is maintained.
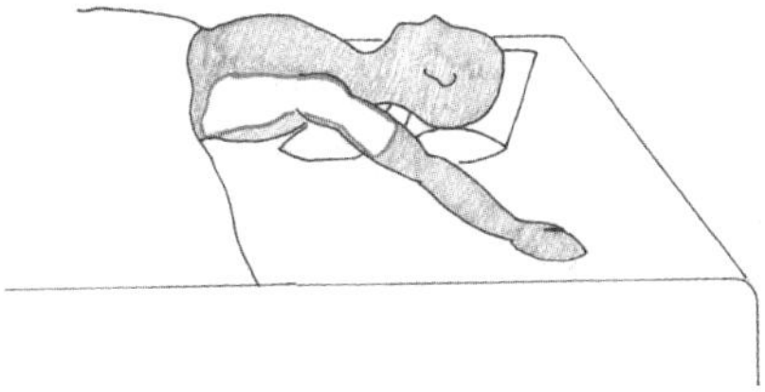	A patient with burns over the axilla, anterior aspect of the shoulder girdle and lateral trunk should be positioned with their arm in abduction to facilitate the lengthening of the pectoralis major and anterior deltoid muscles. A shoulder abduction splint (Fig. 6.8) is beneficial to meet these treatment goals.
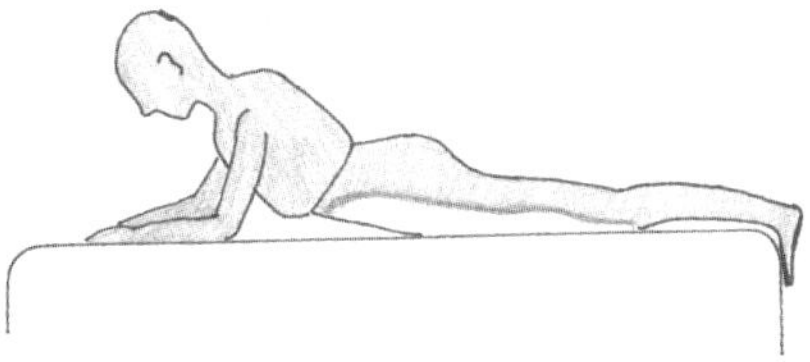	Positioning a patient with burns over the anterior aspect of the hip and upper part of the leg in prone facilitates lengthening of the hip flexors to ensure hip extension ROM is maintained.
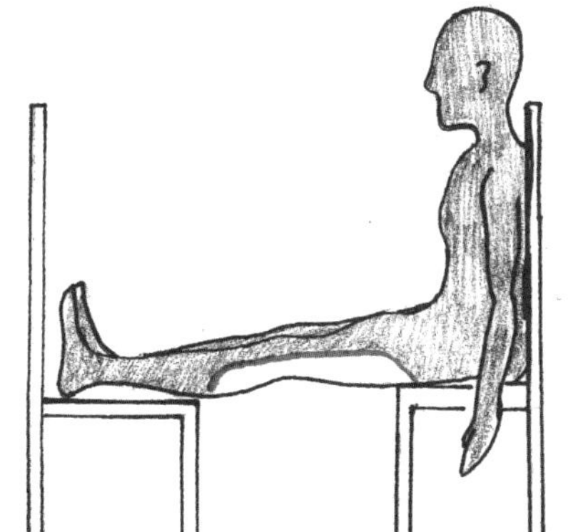	A patient with burns to the posterior aspect of the knee should be positioned in upright sitting in a chair with the lower part of the leg resting on another chair. This position allows gravity to facilitate lengthening of the knee flexors to obtain a neutral knee position.

joint range. Passive stretching is reported to decrease joint stiffness and increase muscle extensibility in healthy subjects (Gosselink *et al.*, 2011). In the ventilated and sedated patient with a burn injury it is important to maintain ROM and muscle extensibility, paying special attention to the shoulder on the side of the ventilator (this side often doesn't get put through as complete a range as the non-ventilated side due to the obstruction posed by the ventilator circuit). Hand and finger mobility and full forearm supination are important to maintain during the sedation phase.

Passive cycling in bed to maintain or improve ROM of the lower extremities may also be used for the sedated patient with burn injuries if the equipment is available locally. The benefits of a 20-minute daily passive cycling programme in addition to usual respiratory care in critically ill, non-burn injured patients on prolonged MV were shown in terms of improvement in functional status, exercise endurance and duration of hospital stay (Burtin *et al.*, 2009). These benefits may translate to the burn injured critical care population, although there is paucity in the literature regarding its effectiveness on the outcomes of these patients.

6.8.4.1.2. Spontaneously breathing patients

It is important that therapists make patients aware of the value of optimal positions for the prevention of contractures during the day (Table 6.14) and encourage them to use these positions during ADL. An example would be to encourage patients with burns of the hips and knees to watch television while in prone in order to stretch the hip flexors and knee extensors. By placing a television screen at the head of the bed, children with burns of the neck can be encouraged to lie supine while playing video games overhead in order to stretch the neck flexors.

Proprioceptive neuro-facilitation techniques or muscle energy techniques such as hold-relax, contract-relax and rhythmic stabilisation can also be used when the patient is able to participate in treatment to ensure that active ROM equal to passive ROM is achieved. When there is limitation in passive ROM, decisions related to the choice of technique to be used should be based on the end-feel of the joint.

Patients with burns to the upper limb should be taught simple stretch exercises to maintain the length of two-joint muscles. Table 6.15 shows

Table 6.15: Simple upper limb stretch exercises.

Stretch	Description
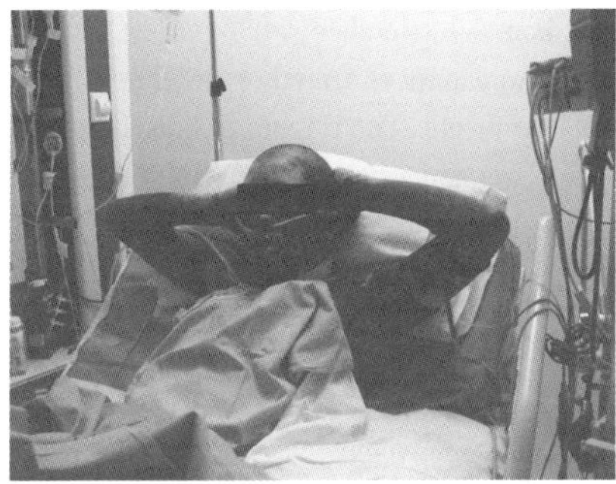	On the beach stretch. The patient is placed in supported sitting in bed with shoulders in abduction and hands meeting behind the head. The aim is to push the elbows backwards onto the bed to stretch the anterior aspects of the shoulders.
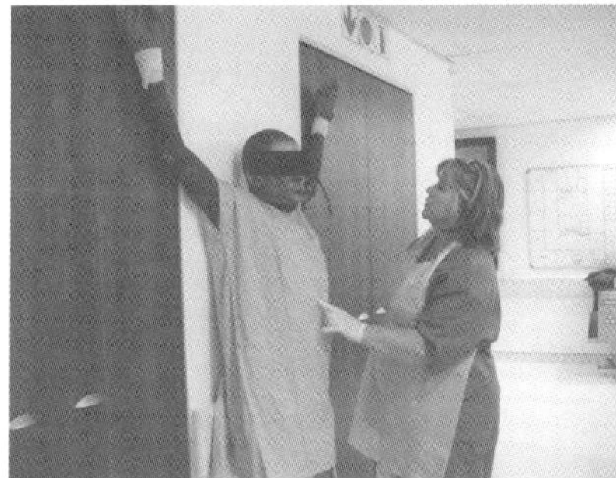	Hallelujah stretch. Once the patient is mobile this stretch can be carried out with the patient standing facing a wall. The arms are lifted upwards with elbows extended as if in praise, with the wall offering support to the patient. Mark the wall with the date and the level of stretch achieved to give the patient visual input and encouragement. Progression of this stretch would be for the patient to place their back against the wall while performing the stretch to ensure end of range shoulder elevation is achieved.
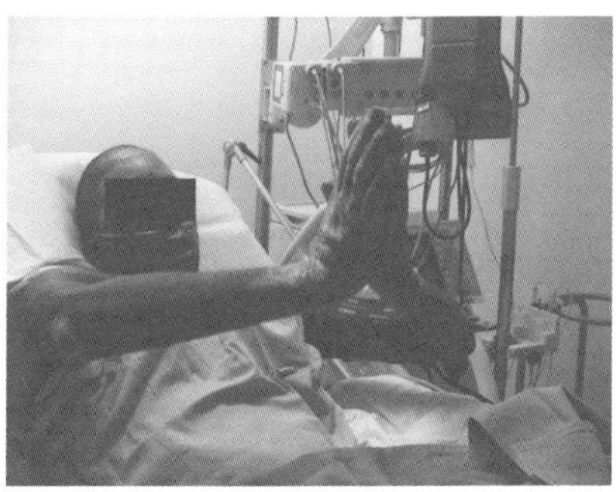	Prayer position stretch. The patient is seated or standing upright. Hands are placed together in front of the body with fingers pressed against each other and elbows elevated to 90°. Wrist extension and flexion is then carried out to improve wrist mobility.

(*Continued*)

Table 6.15. (*Continued*)

Stretch	Description
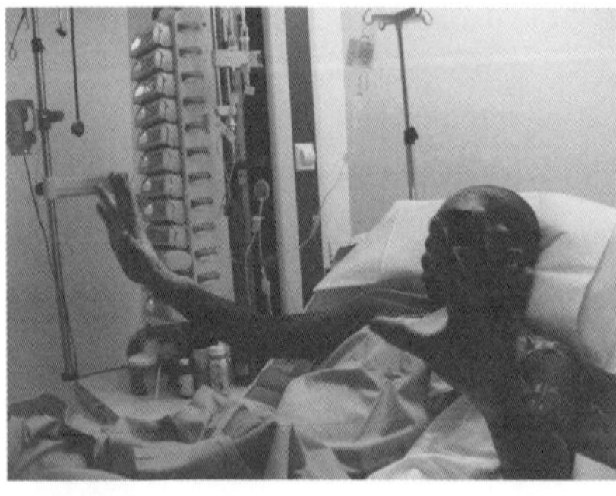	Big five stretch. The patient is seated or standing upright. The fingers of both hands are actively stretched as wide as possible. Alternatively, the physiotherapist can apply stretch to the patient's fingers with emphasis on prolonged stretch of the first web space.
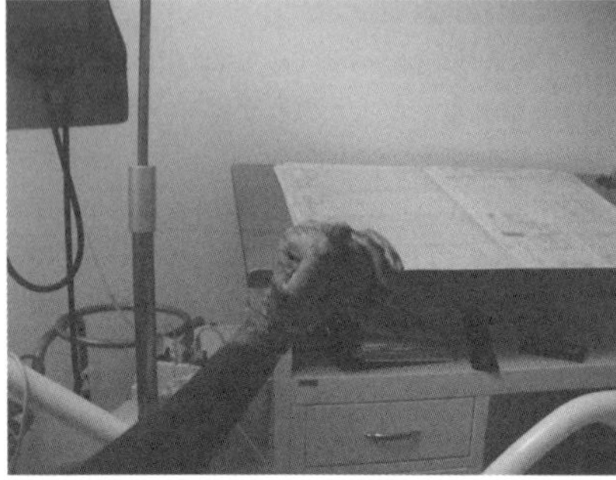	Pull down stretch. The patient is seated or standing upright. Using the thumb of the same hand they are encouraged to pull the index finger into full metacarpo-phalangeal joint flexion while maintaining interphalangeal joint extension. Repeat this with the other fingers of the same hand.

examples of simple stretch exercises that the patient can perform several times a day to maintain ROM of the upper limbs.

Key Message

When a patient with burn injury starts losing ROM, the physiotherapist should reconsider their approach to care and revert to methods that will assist in gaining the lost ROM as quickly as possible.

6.8.4.2. *Splinting*

There are two schools of thought about the use of splinting in the burn injured population. Splinting has been recommended for prophylactic use to prevent the development of contractures or, alternatively, as a therapeutic intervention to correct areas of decreased motion. The depth of the burn and the area of the burn are most often cited as a motivation for prophylactic splinting, especially in patients who are unable to move actively (Gosselink *et al.*, 2011). Prophylactic splinting should be considered for partial thickness and full thickness burns of the axilla, elbow, ankle and hand.

The joints that are most often reported to be splinted therapeutically are the neck, elbow, hands and the knees. Generally it is accepted that splinting should be considered when full passive ROM cannot be maintained (Holavanahalli *et al.*, 2011). Ankle foot orthoses (AFO or foot drop) splints may be used on the ventilated patient with burn injury, even if the legs are spared, due to the natural tendency for the resting position of the feet to be slightly plantar-flexed, thereby allowing the Achilles tendon to shorten (Fig. 6.7). This is especially important in the severely injured patient who may be on bed rest for a prolonged period of time.

Shoulder-abduction elbow-extension splints are frequently used in the clinical setting for patients with burn injuries. The splint is applied to the

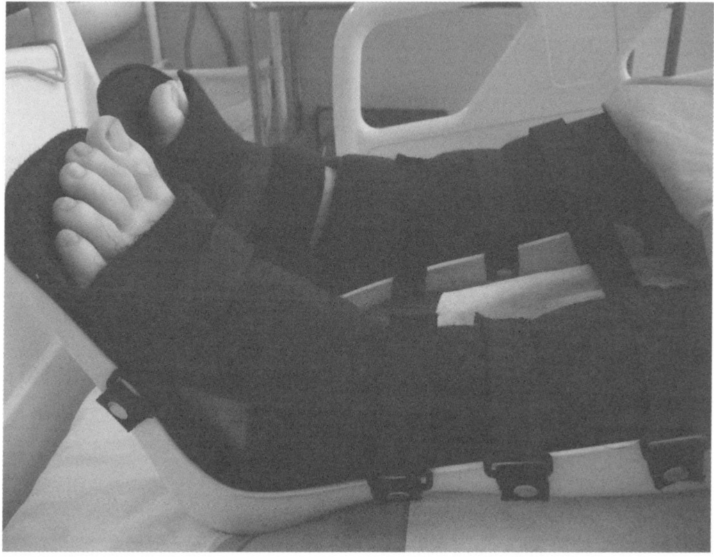

Fig. 6.7: Ankle foot orthoses to maintain the length of Achilles tendons in a ventilated patient in the ICU.

lateral aspect of the trunk and anterior or posterior aspects of the shoulders and arms to prevent contracture formation (Fig. 6.8).

Resting hand splints are used to maintain ROM in patients with hand burn injuries during the sedation phase of their management in the ICU (Fig. 6.9). As soon as the patient's condition is stabilised and they are able to cooperate with treatment, dynamic hand splints may be used to encourage end-of-range metacarpo-phalangeal flexion (Fig. 6.10).

6.8.4.3. *Muscle strength*

As soon as consciousness is regained, active-assisted, active and active-resisted exercises should be initiated (within the limits of the precautions and contraindications listed in Section 6.7) to improve muscle strength in affected and non-affected areas. The types of exercises that can be used to improve muscle strength for patients with burn injuries are displayed in Fig. 6.11. The reader is referred to Chapter 4 (Section 4.1) for information on exercise prescription guidelines for resistance exercise training.

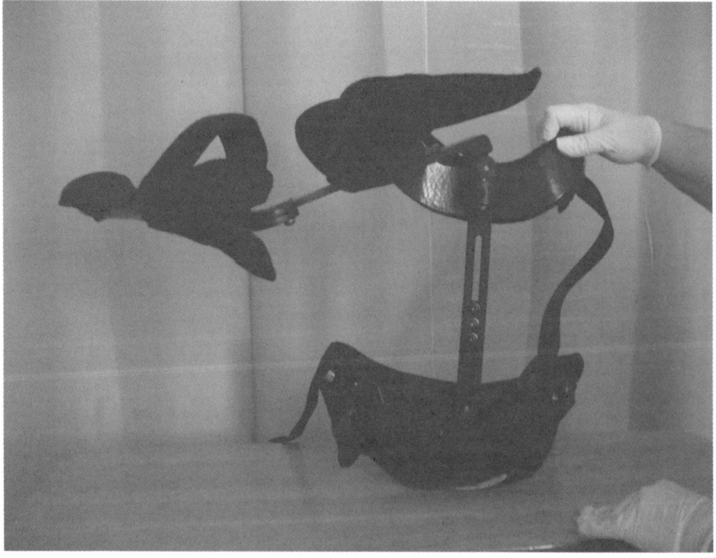

Fig. 6.8: Posterior view of shoulder-abduction elbow-extension splint. The splint is secured around the trunk and arm with Velcro straps.

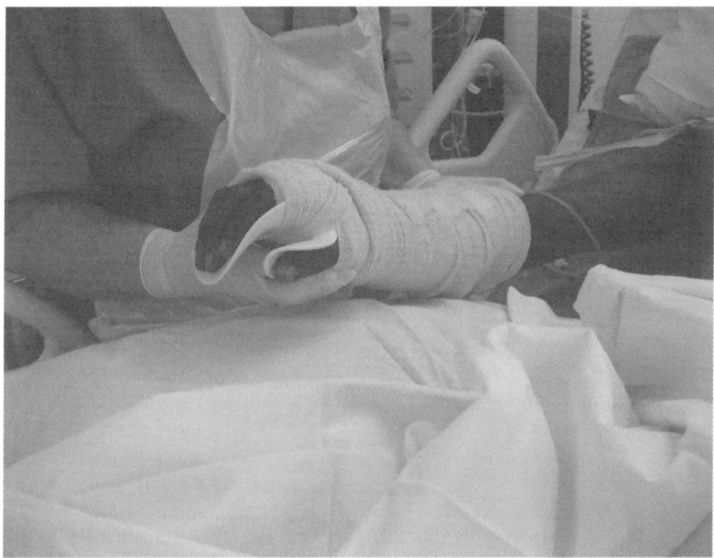

Fig. 6.9: Resting splint for a patient with burn injury to the hands.

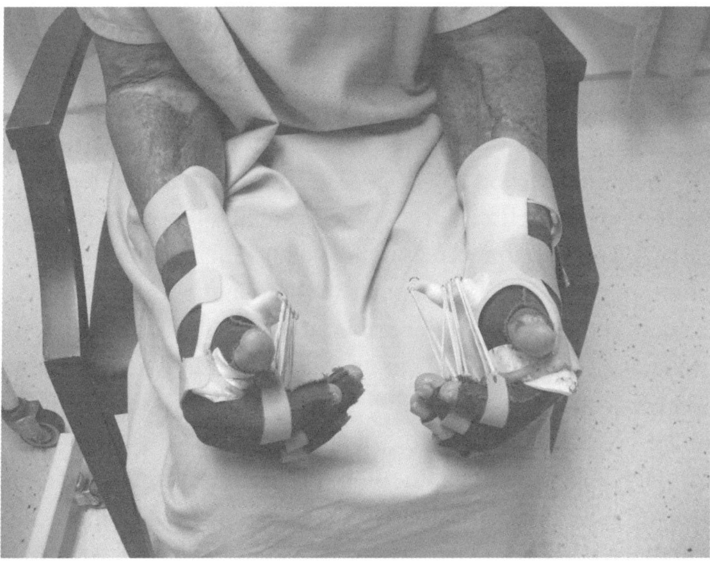

Fig. 6.10: A patient wearing pressure garments and using dynamic hand splints to improve metacarpo-phalangeal joint flexion.

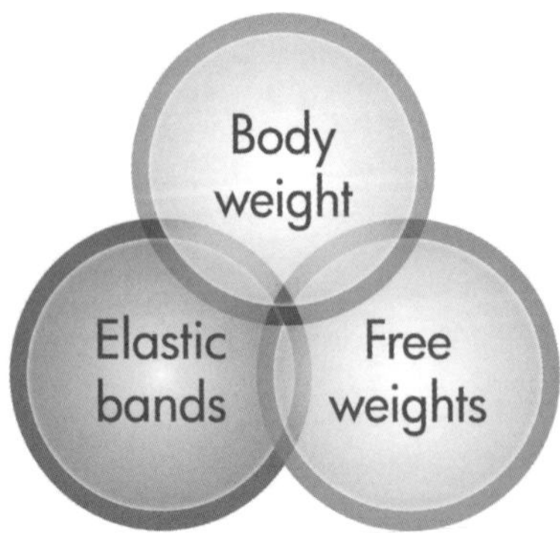

Fig. 6.11: Types of exercises that may be used to improve muscle strength for patients with burn injuries.

The patient's response to resistance exercise training should be assessed regularly using muscle charting as an objective marker of treatment outcome.

6.8.4.4. *Functional activities and mobilisation*

6.8.4.4.1. Intubated patient

There is increasing evidence that stable critically ill patients can be mobilised safely out of bed, resulting in improved functional ability at discharge from the unit, a decrease in ventilation days and a decrease in delirium (Schweickert and Kress, 2011). This therapeutic intervention has not been evaluated in clinical trials with critically ill burn injured patients; however, early ambulation is recommended for this population to optimise ventilation, improve muscle tone and strength and prevent contractures.

As soon as the patient with burn injuries regains consciousness in the ICU, is haemodynamically stable and able to follow verbal commands, functional activities such as rolling in bed, bridging, sitting up over the edge of the bed, standing upright, stepping and walking should form part of their physiotherapy rehabilitation programme. Team work among members of the ICU interdisciplinary team is important to safely mobilise such patients out of bed. Devices such as electronic hoists, standing hoists or walking frames can be used to assist with transferring the patient out of bed into a chair by the bedside. In addition to monitoring physiological variables during mobilisation, sufficient pain management strategies need to be in place to ensure optimal benefits derived from this therapeutic intervention (Hanekom *et al.*, 2011b).

Standing balance should be assessed prior to mobilisation. Mobilisation of the patient should take the form of walking short distances away from the bedside regularly during the day. Walking aids and assistance from the physiotherapist and nursing staff should be provided as needed. The physiotherapist should aim to increase the walking distance away from the bedside daily as a progression of mobilisation (Fig. 6.12). The physiotherapist should make the patient with burn injuries to the trunk and lower limbs aware of attention to posture correction as well as restoration of normal heel-toe gait pattern during ambulation.

As mentioned previously, patients with burn injuries to the legs may suffer from orthostatic intolerance during ambulation. Gradually increasing the time spent in the upright position through the use of a tilt table could prepare such patients for standing.

6.8.4.4.2. Spontaneously breathing patients

Similar activities to those described above should be encouraged in this group of patients to improve functional ability in the ICU and on the ward. Static and dynamic standing balance exercises should form part of patient rehabilitation, especially for those with burns to the legs and feet (Fig. 6.12A, B and C).

If the patient mobilises well with a walking aid (Fig. 6.13), gradual weaning of the patient off the walking aid to achieve independent mobilisation should be encouraged (Fig. 6.14).

6.8.4.5. *Exercise endurance*

As the patient's condition improves and wound healing takes place, activities to improve exercise tolerance should be added to the patient's rehabilitation programme. These activities should be graded and progressive. The reader is referred to Chapter 4 (Section 4.1) for exercise prescription guidelines for aerobic exercise training. Figure 6.15 displays examples of activities that may be used to improve exercise endurance.

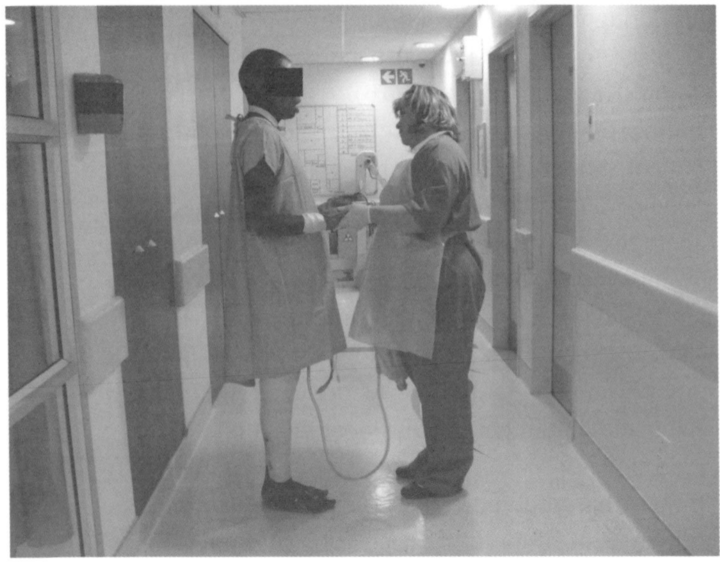

(A)

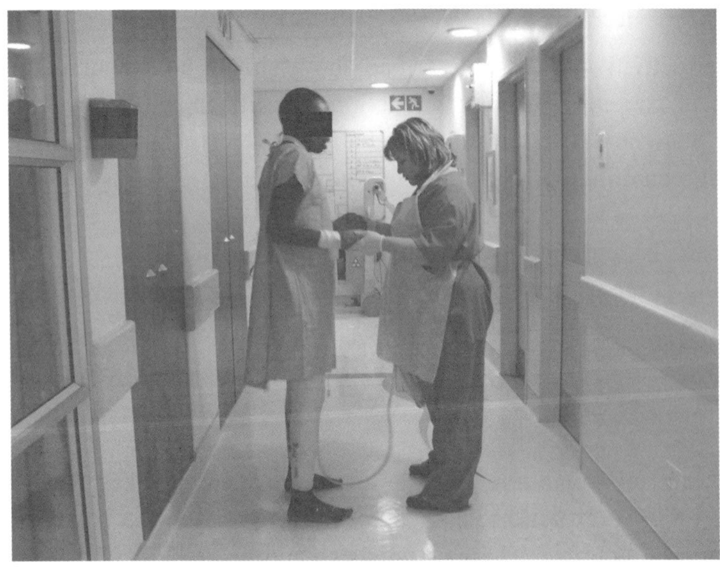

(B)

Fig. 6.12: (A) and (B) Stepping sideways to improve dynamic standing balance.

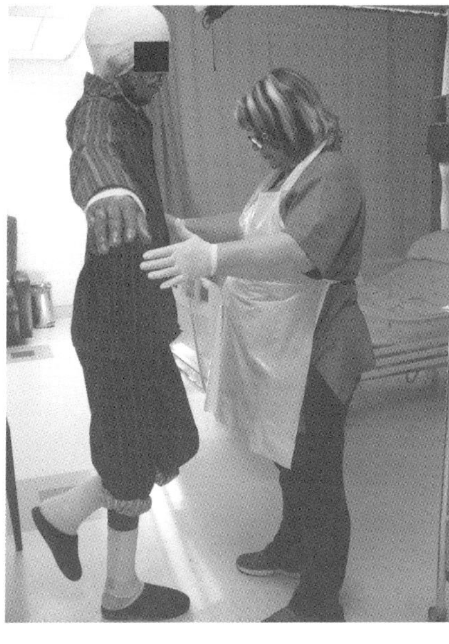

(C)

Fig. 6.12: (C) One-legged standing to improve static standing balance.

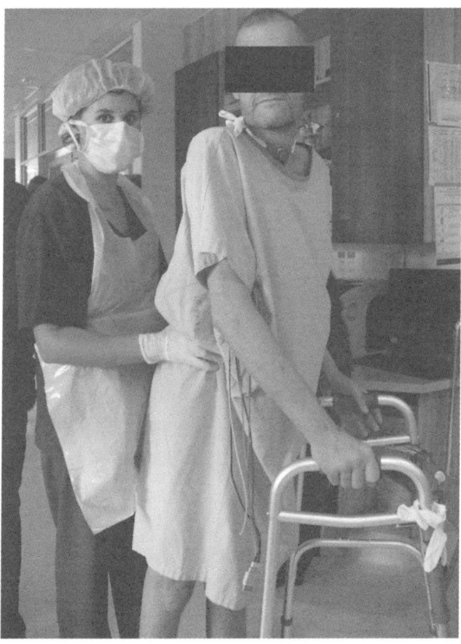

Fig. 6.13: Mobilisation of a patient with trunk and thigh burns away from the bedside in the ICU using a walking frame with supervision of the physiotherapist to ensure patient stability.

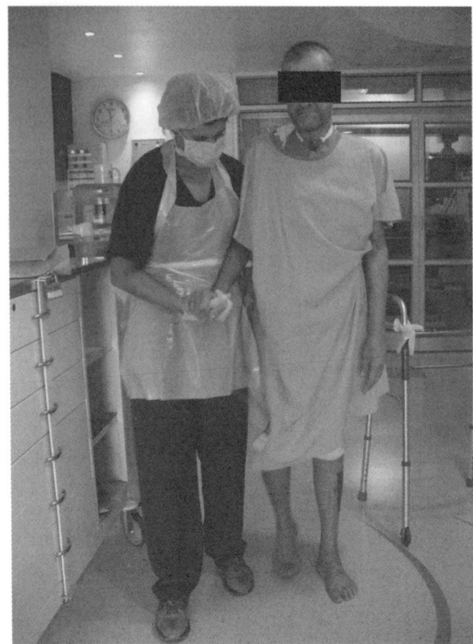

Fig. 6.14: Progression of mobilisation to walking without a frame.

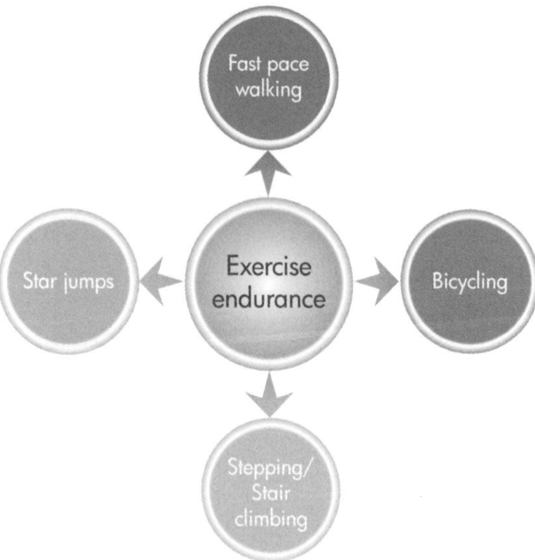

Fig. 6.15: Examples of aerobic-type exercises that may be used for patients with burn injuries to improve exercise endurance.

Step climbing by the bedside can be used in appropriately selected intubated and cooperative patients who are weaning from MV. Spontaneously breathing patients should perform step climbing on a staircase as progression of treatment (Fig. 6.16).

The duration of aerobic exercise activities as well as the frequency of exercise training per day should be increased according to each patient's ability in order to improve endurance prior to discharge from the hospital. As exercise endurance improves, the patient should be able to perform more ADL independently and with less effort.

6.8.4.6. *Paediatric considerations*

The neuromusculoskeletal management of children with burn injuries is similar to that for adults, as described above. Emphasis should be placed

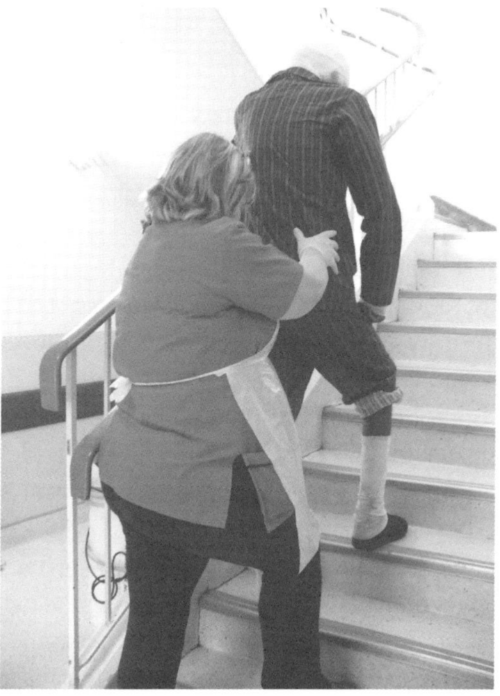

Fig. 6.16: A patient with burn injuries to the legs is performing step climbing with minimal support provided by the physiotherapist to improve his exercise endurance.

on early mobilisation when possible in order to optimise V/Q matching and to prevent the numerous complications of immobility. Mobilisation occurs on a continuum from turning in bed to sitting, standing and walking; a similar approach as that described for the adult patient. The developmental level of the child as well as any associated injuries must be taken into account with appropriate precautions when moving children who have sustained burn trauma.

Most young children do not require specific ROM exercises; however, the size and site of the burn injury may dictate such exercises. Bedridden children and infants will benefit from simple rolling games to reach toys, for example, or, if they are able to sit independently or with support, trunk rotational or side-flexion exercises using play will improve chest expansion and thoracic mobility for those with chest wall burns.

Upper extremity exercises are also essential, especially following burns to the shoulder and trunk areas, to prevent loss of ROM at the shoulder and postural deformities. This can again be accomplished through play in children (e.g. throwing or hitting a balloon or ball).

6.8.5. *Rehabilitation strategies for the management of complications associated with burn injuries*

6.8.5.1. *Exposed tendons*

Burn wounds to the hand and ankle easily result in full thickness burns due to the lack of skin thickness around these areas. The development of boutonnière deformity has been documented in up to 22% of patients presenting with burns to the hand (Feldmann *et al.*, 2008; Omar and Hassan, 2011). Boutonnière deformity is characterised by the joint closest to the knuckle displacing towards the palm and the farthest joint displacing upwards away from the palm. Optimal management of hand injuries is important, as they are predictive of a patient's health-related quality of life (QOL). Splinting of the hand with the extensor tendons in a slack position has been recommended to prevent boutonnière deformity. Tendon glide has been recommended to maintain the anatomical ROM of the proximal inter-phalangeal joint without placing tension on the tendons. Pinning of the joints has also been recommended when it is not possible to complete early grafting of the hand (Feldmann *et al.*, 2008; Omar and Hassan, 2011).

The management of an exposed Achilles tendon is dependent on the extent of the exposure. Splinting in a neutral or slight plantar flexion position has been recommended. The use of early active ankle exercise has also been described. There is no consensus on the ambulation of patients with exposed Achilles tendons. Weight bearing with a splint, non-weight bearing walking or no ambulation has all been documented as management options. Individual assessment of the patient, the clinical judgment of the physiotherapist and consultation with the rest of the interdisciplinary team members should inform decision making.

6.8.5.2. *Heterotopic ossification*

Heterotopic ossification refers to the formation of bone tissue outside of the skeleton. The mechanism for this bone formation is unknown. It can develop in patients who have sustained severe burn injury, especially around the elbow joint. Gentle passive terminal stretch, strengthening in terminal range and active assisted ROM exercises of the elbow has been recommended to minimise the development of heterotopic ossification. However, once it is suspected, active movement that is limited to a pain-free range is recommended.

6.8.5.3. *Hypertrophic scars*

Following severe burn injuries patients are at risk of developing hypertrophic scarring. Hypertrophic scars are red, elevated and rigid and can result in contractures and deformity, especially when they cross over joints. As with many of the techniques used in the rehabilitation of burn injured patients, the use of pressure garments is widely advocated, even though there are few controlled studies to confirm its use (Schneider *et al.*, 2006) (Fig. 6.17). Issues related to the timing of the intervention are also inconclusive. The use of pressure garments is recommended when it takes 10–14 days for wounds to close spontaneously or when skin grafting is required. Current practice is that custom-made pressure garments are worn 23 hours per day from the time of wound healing onwards to prevent

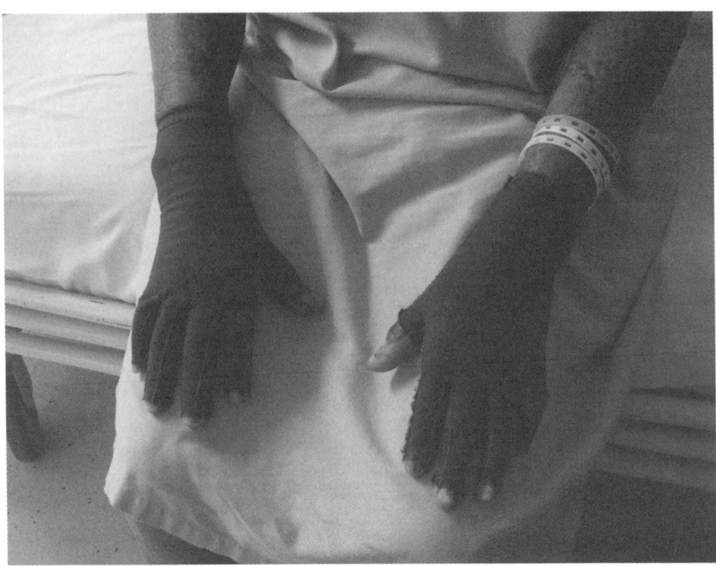

Fig. 6.17: A patient with hand burn injury wearing pressure garments.

the development of hypertrophic scarring. It is also suggested that the garments be re-fitted at two-to-three month intervals to ensure consistent pressure. Patient compliance (especially when presenting with injuries to the face) remains a concern (Esselman *et al.*, 2006).

Scar massage can be used to decrease the sensitivity of the skin and increase the pliability of the scar tissue. Scar massage should be used in combination with the wearing of pressure garments for optimal effect (Gabriel, 2011).

6.8.6. *Patient response to treatment*

The use of objective measures to monitor the patient's recovery process from ICU admission to full social integration after discharge is essential to ensure optimal patient outcome. These outcomes must be specified and the results reported in patient documentation. Outcomes include the appropriate evaluation of physical, psychological and functional dimensions (Oster *et al.*, 2009; Tan *et al.*, 2012). The reader is referred to Chapter 4 (Section 4.3) for a list of subjective and objective markers, as well as outcome measurement tools to use for the evaluation of the effectiveness of treatment interventions used during the rehabilitation of patients with burn injury.

6.9. Clinical Case Scenarios

6.9.1. *Case scenario of an adult patient*

A light aircraft crashed into the house of a 31-year-old woman. As a result she sustained severe full thickness burns to the right side of her face and right ear, neck, chest, abdomen, arms, hands, upper thighs and back with inhalation injury (42% TBSA). This accident took place in a neighbouring country to South Africa, and the patient was airlifted to a level one trauma centre in Johannesburg for specialised burns care.

On admission she received a CT scan to establish the presence of other traumatic injuries. The only orthopaedic injuries that she sustained were fractures of the bones in her right hand. Her past medical history was unknown. She spoke French and also presented with obesity. Her Glasgow coma score (GCS) on admission was 14/15, temperature 38°C and lactate was 4.9. Arterial blood gas analysis (on supplemental oxygen) on admission:

pH	7.25
PaO_2	142 mmHg (18.9 kPa)
$PaCO_2$	37.8 mmHg (5 kPa)
HCO_3	16 mmol/L
BE	–9.5
SaO_2	98.3%

The extent of her burn wounds and the inhalation injury led to admission to the ICU, where she was sedated, intubated and mechanically ventilated on biphasic positive airway pressure ventilation (FiO_2 of 0.5; PEEP of 10 cmH_2O). Her blood pressure was 91/71 mmHg and therefore she was placed on inotropic support. Later that day she was taken to theatre for extensive debridement involving her right arm, upper thigh and abdomen. Amputation of the fingers of her left hand at the metacarpo-phalangeal joints was undertaken due to severe tissue necrosis; the thumb was spared. A partial right breast mastectomy was done for the same reason.

Following surgery she required three units of blood, as her haemoglobin levels had dropped to 8.2 and the dosage of inotropic support was increased. Iodine wound dressings were applied to all burn wounds. On auscultation her breath sounds were equal throughout all lung fields but with marked high-pitched wheezing in most of the airways due to bronchoconstriction. The nursing staff reported that they suctioned thick, carbonaceous secretions from her ETT on return to the ICU.

On day two of her admission a tracheostomy was performed as it was expected that she would have a prolonged stay in the ICU. She was taken back to theatre for debridement of her left arm. On day four she was taken back to theatre for amputation of her right thumb tip and index finger due to the development of deep tissue necrosis. K-wires were inserted into her right hand to stabilise the fractures and a resting splint was applied to maintain metacarpo-phalangeal joint flexion and interphalangeal joint extension. The dosage of analgesia administered in the ICU was frequently assessed and adjusted according to her needs. During her stay in the ICU the wound dressings were changed to silver-containing dressings and a number of SSG were done to achieve wound closure. She eventually developed sepsis, which was successfully managed with antibiotics during her stay in the ICU.

- What precautions and contraindications would you assess prior to the treatment of this patient?
- How would you manage this patient during her stay in ICU?

6.9.1.1. *Discussion*

6.9.1.1.1. Precautions and contraindications

Regarding her pulmonary system, it would be important to ensure that bronchodilator therapy was administered to address her bronchospasm prior to the use of manual chest clearance techniques. Manual chest percussion and shaking should not be used over acute burn wounds on the chest wall; gentle manual vibrations may be used but ensure firm pressure of the physiotherapist's hands against the chest wall to avoid any sliding friction on the open wounds, which may increase bleeding. In the case of a skin graft on the chest wall, no manual chest therapy techniques may be used until the skin graft has taken; in this instance MHI or VHI to mobilise and clear excessive retained secretions might be a better option. Ensure that a pressure manometer is placed in the MHI circuit to monitor the amount of pressure administered to the airways, especially in the case of inhalation injury. Ensure that the patient is pre-oxygenated at 100% prior to suction and that a sterile suction procedure is used.

In relation to her neuromusculoskeletal system, it is important to assess the amount of bleeding that occurs after debridement; if bleeding is excessive, physiotherapy rehabilitation should be postponed until bleeding is under control. In the case of skin grafting, the graft area should be immobilised to allow the graft time to take. The duration of immobilisation should be discussed with the plastic surgeon to guide rehabilitation intervention.

It is also important to communicate regularly with the nursing staff to ensure optimal analgesia during physiotherapy treatment sessions. The patient's response to physiotherapy interventions should be monitored closely during each treatment session, and adverse responses should be addressed rapidly with the assistance of the nursing and medical personnel.

6.9.1.1.2. Physiotherapy interventions in the ICU

During the sedation phase of her ICU stay, frequent body position changes (two to four hourly) should be used to enhance lung ventilation and the drainage of secretions and to prevent the development of pressure sores. When turning her onto her right side there should be a towel placed supporting the side of her forehead so that no pressure is placed on her burned ear or on the lower right side of her face. Body positioning is also important to prevent contracture formation. She should be nursed with her head lying on a towel, not a pillow, to reduce the risk of neck flexor contracture development.

Modified postural drainage positions (no head-down tilt) using side-lying with the bed in a neutral position can be utilised during chest physiotherapy sessions to assist with secretion clearance if indicated. Gentle manual chest vibrations may be used together with careful suctioning of the ETT and later the tracheostomy tube. Manual hyperinflation or VHI may be added to her treatment as her condition stabilises and the inhalation injuries heal. It is important to obtain a sputum sample for microbiology, culture and sensitivity analysis as early as possible during her stay in the ICU. Chest physiotherapy should be performed twice daily or daily, according to the patient's needs.

Passive ROM exercises with end-of-range stretch should be carried out daily for all joints affected by burn wounds. Important areas to focus on are her peri-oral area, neck, shoulders, elbows, forearms, wrists, fingers, hips and knees. It is particularly important to stretch the web spaces between the fingers with attention to the first web space. The physiotherapist can use two wooden tongue depressors to stretch the peri-oral area diagonally and vertically. All joints not covered by burns should also be stretched through full passive ROM until the patient is able to perform active exercises. Splinting should be used to prevent the shortening of two-joint muscles. Ankle-foot orthoses should be made to maintain a neutral ankle position and prevent a shortening of the Achilles tendon due to inactivity. The right-hand splint should be removed during physiotherapy treatment sessions to allow for ROM exercises to be done within the precautions posed by the patient's surgery. Outside of physiotherapy treatment sessions, splinting is done for two hours at a time and then removed for two hours. This sequence is continued during the course of the day. Splints are left *in situ* during the night.

As she regains consciousness and the ability to participate in treatment sessions, techniques such as ACBT and biofeedback through the ventilator may be added to her management to increase lung volumes, strengthen her respiratory muscles and assist with weaning from ventilation. Directed coughing should be encouraged to enable her to practise protecting her airways effectively prior to extubation. If she is stable enough, she can be assisted to sit up over the edge of the bed. In this position, active or active-assisted ROM exercises of her neck, trunk, upper and lower limbs can be performed. Gentle stretching of the joints to end-of-range is important until full active ROM is achieved. The height of the ICU bed should be adjusted to ensure that her feet are well supported on the floor during active exercises. The physiotherapist should show her various types of active peri-oral exercises that she can continue with on her own (a mirror can be incorporated). Self-stretches of the web spaces of her remaining fingers should be emphasised, as her grip is dependent on the functionality of the first web space of both hands. Sit-to-stand exercises can be performed from the edge of the bed and the patient can be assisted to transfer from the bed to the chair. If the patient is not able to stand on her own or with assistance, a tilt table or a standing frame can be used instead.

Muscle strengthening exercises may also be initiated at this stage to address muscle weakness resulting from the injuries, as well as her critical illness using her own body weight and manual resistance from the physiotherapist and later elastic bands and free weights if the patient is able to use these devices. The intensity and frequency of exercise should be graded according to the patient's ability and should be progressed when applicable.

After successful extubation, early mobilisation away from the bedside, incentive spirometry and oscillating PEP may be added to her bronchial hygiene regimen. The physiotherapist should assess whether the patient would benefit from a walking aid at this stage due to her deconditioned status and burn injuries to her upper thighs to allow for more independence in mobilising to and from the bathrooms in the ICU. If she presents with a shortening of the Achilles tendon (which in our experience occurs often in patients with burn injuries, despite judicious stretching and splint application), lunge-type movements can be encouraged while she walks to increase the dorsiflexion range. This allows the tibia to translate anteriorly over the talus and achieve better locomotion.

Progression of this rehabilitation programme should continue as she is transferred from the ICU to the burns ward.

6.9.2. *Case scenario of a paediatric patient*

A three-year-old girl sustained a fire burn when a candle tipped over and set her bedding alight. She sustained 15% TBSA burns to her face, axillae and hands (a combination of full thickness and partial thickness burns) with inhalation injury. She required intubation and MV, for which she was admitted to the paediatric ICU.

She was ventilated for two weeks, during which time she underwent numerous dressing changes under anaesthesia and skin grafts to the axillae and hands. She developed ventilator-associated pneumonia, culturing

Acinetobacter baumannii, for which she received appropriate antibiotics. As a complication of the pneumonia, she developed right middle and upper lobe atelectasis.

During this time she was nursed with the head of bed raised and regular changes of position. She was sat out of bed when haemodynamically stable. Analgesia was ensured with continuous morphine infusions as well as regular additional analgesia and boluses of morphine prior to stretching of the burned areas.

- What would your treatment approach be towards this patient?

6.9.2.1. *Discussion*

Rehabilitation should include daily passive and active ROM exercises and stretches to all major joints and muscles, according to her levels of sedation and cooperation. Emphasis should be placed on the hands and axillae, and these burned areas should be stretched under general anaesthesia by the physiotherapist. After grafting, the axillae and hands should be splinted to maintain ROM whilst they cannot be moved.

Chest physiotherapy consisting of chest wall shaking and vibrations in side-lying and half-sitting positions can be performed to mobilise tenacious secretions and endotracheal suctioning used to remove the secretions. The lobar atelectasis should be resolved radiographically and clinically within two sessions of chest physiotherapy.

After resolution of the atelectasis and pneumonia, the patient should be weaned and extubated. After extubation, nasal prong oxygen therapy may be used to support oxygenation, which should later be weaned to room air. During this time the patient should be mobilised and encouraged to move independently by means of play activities like throwing and catching balloons and bubbles. She should be encouraged to perform breathing exercises using bubbles and whistles (fun forms of PEP) and coughing, using mimicry if necessary.

It is essential to maintain ROM in all affected joints, as well as full facial movement, and to improve muscle strength following ICU deconditioning. To this end, active and active assisted exercises should be encouraged, using full ROM. Examples include drawing on large sheets of paper;

playing 'Simon says'; reaching and hitting balloons with open hands and full shoulder elevation; pushing balls up the wall and bouncing big balls; crawling with flat hands; climbing up frames or ladders; and later using play dough and playing with shaving cream on a mirror once all wounds are healed. Passive stretching should be continued as needed. Active exercises of the facial muscles should be done regularly by pulling faces and giving different sizes and textures of food to eat.

In the later stages of recovery, scar massage should be conducted daily and pressure garments made, if indicated. Interdisciplinary team members such as occupational and speech and language therapists should be involved with this child's rehabilitation. The patient may also be referred to a psychologist and play therapist to work with her on issues relating to body image and reintegration into home and playschool.

6.10. Suggested Reading Material for Further Study

Baux score for assessment of mortality risk (Osler *et al.*, 2010); burn wound infections (Church *et al.*, 2006); skin grafts (Leung and Fish, 2009); burn survivor rehabilitation (ANZBA, 2007).

6.11. Conclusion

Rehabilitation of patients with burn injuries starts on admission to the hospital and each member of the interdisciplinary team plays an important role to effect the best possible outcome for the patient. The information provided here should equip the physiotherapist with basic knowledge of the interdisciplinary team management of patients with burn trauma and should enable them to provide high-quality evidence-based rehabilitative care to patients with such injuries in the acute care setting in which they work.

Acknowledgement

We would like to thank Shahieda Khan for providing input on the paediatric component of this chapter.

Bibliography

Alharbi, Z., Piatkowski, A., Dembinski, R., *et al.* (2012). Treatment of burns in the first 24 hours: simple and practical guide by answering 10 questions in a step-by-step form, *World J. Emerg. Surg.,* **7**, 13. [Online] Available at: http://www.wjes.org/content/7/1/13 [Accessed 15 November 2014].

Australian and New Zealand Burn Association (ANZBA). (2007). *Burn Survivor Rehabilitation: Principles and Guidelines for the Allied Health Professional.* Allied Health Forum. [Online] Available at: http://www.aci.health.nsw.gov.au/__data/assets/pdf_file/0008/162629/anzba_ahp_guidelines_october_2007.pdf [Accessed 24 July 2014].

American Association of Respiratory Care (AARC) Evidence-Based Clinical Practice Guidelines. (2003). Care of the ventilator circuit and its relation to ventilator-associated pneumonia, *Respir. Care,* **48**, 869–879.

American Association of Respiratory Care (AARC) Clinical Practice Guideline. (2011). Incentive spirometry, *Respir. Care,* **56**, 1600–1604.

Arnoldo, B.D., Purdue, G.F., Kowalske, K., *et al.* (2004). Electrical injuries: a 20-year review, *J. Burn Care Rehabil.,* **25**, 479–484.

Atiyeh, B., Masellis, A., and Conte, C. (2009a). Optimizing burn treatment in developing low- and middle-income countries with limited health care resources (part 1), *Ann. Burns Fire Disasters,* **22**, 121–125.

Atiyeh, B., Costagliola, M., and Hayek, S. (2009b). Burn prevention mechanisms and outcomes: pitfalls, failures and successes, *Burns,* **35**, 181–193.

Balan, B., and Lingam, L. (2012). Unintentional injuries among children in resource poor settings: where do the fingers point? *Arch. Disabil. Child.,* **97**, 35–38.

Bassani, M., Filho, F., Coppo, M., *et al.* (2009). Peak pressure and tidal volume are affected by how the neonatal self-inflating bag is handled, *J. Pediatr. (Rio J.),* **85**, 217–222.

Berney, S., and Denehy, L. (2002). A comparison of the effects of manual and ventilator hyperinflation on static lung compliance and sputum production in intubated and ventilated intensive care patients, *Physiother. Res. Int.,* **7**, 100–108.

Berney, S., Denehy, L., and Pretto, J. (2004). Head-down tilt and manual hyperinflation enhance sputum clearance in patients who are intubated and ventilated, *Aust. J. Physiother.,* **50**, 9–14.

Birchenough, S., Gampper, T., and Morgan, R. (2008). Special considerations in the management of pediatric upper extremity and hand burns, *J. Craniofac. Surg.,* **19**, 933–941.

Blumetti, J., Hunt, J., Arnoldo, B., *et al.* (2008). The parkland formula under fire: is the criticism justified? *J. Burn Care Res.,* **29**, 180–186.

Burtin, C., Clerckx, B., Robbeets, C., *et al.* (2009). Early exercise in critically ill patients enhances short-term functional recovery, *Crit. Care Med.,* **37**, 2499–2505.

Cassell, O., Hubble, M., Milling, M., *et al.* (1997). Baby walkers--still a major cause of infant burns, *Burns,* **23**, 451–453.

Chan, M., and Chan, G. (2009). Nutritional therapy for burns in children and adults, *Nutrition,* **25**, 261–269.

Choi, J.S.P., and Jones, A.Y.M. (2005). Effects of manual hyperinflation and suctioning on respiratory mechanics in mechanically ventilated patients with ventilator-associated pneumonia, *Aust. J. Physiother.,* **51**, 25–30.

Church, D., Elsayed, S., Reid, O., *et al.* (2006). Burn wound infections, *Clin. Microbiol. Rev.,* **19**, 403–434.

De Castro, R.J.A., Leal, P.C., and Sakata, R.K. (2013). Pain management in burn patients, *Rev. Bras. Anestesiol.,* **63**, 148–158.

Demling, R.H. (2008). Smoke inhalation injury: an update, *Eplasty,* **8**, 254–282.

Dissanaike, S., and Rahimi, M. (2009). Epidemiology of burn injuries: highlighting cultural and socio-demographic aspects, *Int. Rev. Psychiatry,* **21**, 505–511.

Dissanaike, S., Boshart, K., Coleman, A., *et al.* (2009). Cooking-related pediatric burns: risk factors and the role of differential cooling rates among commonly implicated substances, *J. Burn Care Res.,* **30**, 593–598.

Dorafshar, A.H., Gitman, M., Henry, G., *et al.* (2010). Guided surgical debridement: staining tissues with methylene blue, *J. Burn Care Res.,* **31**, 791–794.

Dries, D.J., and Endorf, F.W. (2013). Inhalation injury: epidemiology, pathology, treatment strategies, *Scand. J. Trauma Resus. Emerg.,* **21**, 31. [Online] Available at: http://www.sjtrem.com/content/21/1/31 [Accessed 15 November 2014].

Edwards, J. (2010). Hydrogels and their potential uses in burn wound management, *Brit. J. Nurs.,* **19** [Suppl], S12–S16.

Esselman, P.C. (2007). Burn rehabilitation: an overview, *Arch. Phys. Med. Rehabil.,* **88** [Suppl], S3–S6.

Esselman, P.C., Thombs, B.D., Magyar-Russell, G., *et al.* (2006). Burn rehabilitation: state of the science, *Am. J. Phys. Med. Rehabil.,* **85**, 383–413.

Fink, J.B. (2007). Forced expiratory technique, directed cough and autogenic drainage, *Respir. Care,* **52**, 1210–1221.

Feldmann, M.E., Evans, J., and O, S.J. (2008). Early management of the burned pediatric hand, *J. Craniofac. Surg.,* **19**, 942–950.

Forjuoh, S.N. (2006). Burns in low-and middle-income countries: a review of available literature on descriptive epidemiology, risk factors, treatment and prevention, *Burns,* **32**, 529–537.

Freiburg, C., Igneri, P., Sartorelli, K., *et al.* (2007). Effects of differences in percent total body surface area estimation on fluid resuscitation of transferred burns patients, *J. Burn Care Res.,* **28**, 42–48.

Gabriel, V. (2011). Hypertrophic scar, *Phys. Med. Rehabil. Clin. N. Am.,* **22**, 301–310.

Gosselink, R., Clerckx, B., Robbeets, C., *et al.* (2011). Physiotherapy in the intensive care unit, *Neth. J. Crit. Care,* **15**, 66–75.

Hall, K.L., Shahrokhi, S., and Jeschke, M.G. (2012). Enteral nutrition support in burn care: a review of current recommendations as instituted in the Ross Tilley burn centre, *Nutrients,* **4**, 1554–1565.

Halm, M.A., and Hagel, K.K. (2008). Instilling normal saline with suctioning: beneficial technique or potentially harmful sacred cow? *Am. J. Crit. Care,* **17**, 469–472.

Halim, A.S., Khoo, T.L., and Yussof, S.J.M. (2010). Biologic and synthetic skin substitutes: an overview, *Indian J. Plast. Surg.,* **43** [Suppl], S23–S28.

Hanekom, S., Berney, S., Morrow, B., *et al.* (2011a). The validation of a clinical algorithm for the prevention and management of pulmonary dysfunction in intubated adults — a synthesis of evidence and expert opinion, *J. Eval. Clin. Pract.,* **17**, 801–810.

Hanekom, S.D., Brooks, D., Denehy, L., *et al.* (2012). Reaching consensus on the physiotherapeutic management of patients following upper abdominal surgery: a pragmatic approach to interpret equivocal evidence, *BMC Med. Inform. Decis. Mak.,* **12**, 5. [Online] Available at: http://www.biomedcentral.com/1472-6947/12/5 [Accessed 15 November 2014].

Hanekom, S.D., Gosselink, R., Dean, E., *et al.* (2011b). The development of a clinical management algorithm for early physical activity and mobilisation of critically ill patients: synthesis of evidence and expert opinion and its translation into clinical practice, *Clin. Rehabil.,* **25**, 771–787.

Herrera, F.A., Hassanein, A.H., Potenza, B., *et al.* (2010). Bilateral upper extremity vascular injury as a result of a high-voltage electrical burn, *Ann. Vasc. Surg.,* **24**, 825.e1–825.e5.

Hoffman, H.G., Chambers, G.T., Meyer, W.J. III, *et al.* (2011). Virtual reality as an adjunctive non-pharmacologic analgesic for acute burn pain during medical procedures, *Ann. Behav. Med.,* **41**, 183–191.

Holavanahalli, R.K., Helm, P.A., Parry, I.S., *et al.* (2011). Select practices in management and rehabilitation of burns: a survey report, *J. Burn Care Res.,* **32**, 210–223.

Hsieh, C.S., Schuong, J.Y., Huang, W.S., *et al.* (2008). Five years' experience of the modified meek technique in the management of extensive burns, *Burns,* **34**, 350–354.

Huzar, T.F., George, T., and Cross, J.M. (2013). Carbon monoxide and cyanide toxicity: etiology, pathophysiology and treatment in inhalation injury, *Expert Rev. Respir. Med.,* **7**, 159–170.

Johnson, C.F., Ericson, A.K., and Caniano, D. (1990). Walker-related burns in infants and toddlers, *Pediatr. Emerg. Care,* **6**, 58–61.

Kasten, K.R., Makley, A.T., and Kagan, R.J. (2011). Update on the critical care management of severe burns, *J. Intensive Care Med.,* **26**, 223–236.

Kipping, B., Rodger, S., Miller, K., *et al.* (2012). Virtual reality for acute pain reduction in adolescents undergoing burn wound care: a prospective randomised controlled trial, *Burns,* **38**, 650–657.

Krieger, Y., Bogdanov-Berezovsky, A., Gurfinkel, R., *et al.* (2012). Efficacy of enzymatic debridement of deeply burned hands, *Burns,* **38**, 108–112.

Kumar, S., Verma, A.K., Ali, W., *et al.* (2013). A study of unnatural female death profile in Lucknow, India, *Am. J. Forensic Med. Pathol.,* **34**, 352–356.

Landau, A.G., Hudson, D.A., Adams, K., *et al.* (2008). Full-thickness skin grafts: maximizing graft take using negative pressure dressings to prepare the graft bed, *Ann. Plast. Surg.,* **60**, 661–666.

Latenser, B.A. (2009). Critical care of the burn patient: the first 48 hours, *Crit. Care Med.,* **37**, 2819–2826.

Lee, H. (2012). Outcomes of sprayed cultured epithelial autografts for full-thickness wounds: a single centre experience, *Burns,* **38**, 931–936.

Leung, J.J., and Fish, J. (2009). Skin grafts, *Univ. Toronto Med. J.,* **86**, 61–64.

Li, W., Wu, X., and Gao, C. (2013). Ten-year epidemiological study of chemical burns in Jinshan, Shanghai, PR China, *Burns,* **39**, 1468–1473.

Lowell, G., Quinlan, K., and Gottlieb, L.J. (2008). Preventing unintentional scald burns: moving beyond tap water, *Pediatrics,* **122**, 799–804.

Matsumura, H., Ahmatjan, N., Ida, Y., *et al.* (2013). A model for quantitative evaluation of skin damage at adhesive wound dressing removal, *Int. Wound J.,* **10**, 291–294.

Mayes, T., Gottschlich, M., Scanlon, J., *et al.* (2003). Four-year review of burns as an etiologic factor in the development of long bone fractures in pediatric patients, *J. Burn Care Rehabil.,* **24**, 279–284.

Menon, S., Li, Z., Harvey, J.G., *et al.* (2013). The use of the meek technique in conjunction with cultured epithelial autograft in the management of major paediatric burns, *Burns,* **39**, 674–679.

Mlcak, R.P., Suman, O.E., and Hemdon, D.N. (2007). Respiratory management of inhalation injury, *Burns,* **33**, 2–13.

Morris, P.E., Goad, A., Thompson, C., *et al.* (2008). Early intensive care unit mobility therapy in the treatment of acute respiratory failure, *Crit. Care Med.,* **36**, 2238–2243.

Morris, L.D., Louw, Q.A., and Crous, L.C. (2010). Feasibility and potential effect of a low-cost virtual reality system on reducing pain and anxiety in adult burn injury patients during physiotherapy in a developing country, *Burns,* **36**, 659–664.

Morris, L.D., Louw, Q.A., and Grimmer-Somers, K. (2009). The effectiveness of virtual reality on reducing pain and anxiety in burn injury patients: a systematic review, *Clin. J. Pain,* **25**, 815–826.

Mosier, M.J., Dechristopher, P.J., and Gamelli, R.L. (2013). Use of therapeutic plasma exchange in the burn unit: a review of the literature, *J. Burn Care Res.,* **34**, 289–298.

Nachiappan, M., Gurusinghe, D., and Bhandari, S. (2012). Hypothermia in burns intensive care: use of the intravenous temperature management system Thermogard XP®, *Crit. Care,* **16**, A15. [Online] Available at: http://ccforum.com/content/16/S2/A15 [Accessed 15 November 2014].

Olaitan, P.B., and Jiburum, B.C. (2008). Chemical injuries from assaults: an increasing trend in a developing country, *Indian J. Plast. Surg.,* **41**, 20–23.

Omar, M.T., and Hassan, A.A. (2011). Evaluation of hand function after early excision and skin grafting of burns versus delayed skin grafting: a randomised clinical trial, *Burns,* **37**, 707–713.

Osler, T., Glance, L.G., and Hosmer, D.W. (2010). Simplified estimates of the probability of death after burn injuries: extending and updating the baux score, *J. Trauma,* **68**, 690–697.

Oster, C., Willebrand, M., Dyster-Aas, J., *et al.* (2009). Validation of the EQ-5D questionnaire in burn injured adults, *Burns,* **35**, 723–732.

Palao, R., Monge, I., Ruiz, M., *et al.* (2010). Chemical burns: pathophysiology and treatment, *Burns,* **36**, 295–304.

Panté, M.D., Andrew, N., and Pollak, M.D. (2010). 'Burn Trauma', in American Academy of Orthopaedic Surgeons (eds), *Advanced Assessment and Treatment of Trauma*, Jones and Bartlett Learning, Sudbury, pp. 188–216.

Paratz, J., Lipman, J., and McAuliffe, M. (2002). Effect of manual hyperinflation on hemodynamics, gas exchange and respiratory mechanics in ventilated patients, *J. Intensive Care Med.,* **17**, 317–324.

Parbhoo, A., Louw, Q.A., and Grimmer-Somers, K. (2010). Burn prevention programs for children in developing countries require urgent attention: a targeted literature review, *Burns,* **36**, 164–175.

Parry, I., and Esselman, P.C. (2011). Rehabilitation Committee of the American Burn Association: clinical competencies for burn rehabilitation therapists, *J. Burn Care Res.,* **32**, 458–467.

Peck, M.D. (2011). Epidemiology of burns throughout the world. Part I: distribution and risk factors, *Burns,* **37**, 1087–1100.

Peck, M.D. (2012). Epidemiology of burns throughout the world. Part II: intentional burns in adults, *Burns,* **38**, 630–637.

Percival, S.L., Thomas, J., Linton, S., *et al.* (2012). The antimicrobial efficacy of silver on antibiotic-resistant bacteria isolated from burn wounds, *Int. Wound J.,* **9**, 488–493.

Rafla, K., and Tredget, E.E. (2011). Infection control in the burn unit, *Burns,* **37**, 5–15.

Rennekampff, H.O., Schaller, H.E., Wisser, D., *et al.* (2006). Debridement of burn wounds with a water jet surgical tool, *Burns,* **32**, 64–69.

Rice, P.L., and Orgill, D.P. (2012). *Classification of Burns*. [Online] Available at: http://www.uptodate.com/contents/classification-of-burns#H10 [Accessed 10 May 2013].

Roberts, F.E. (2009). Consensus among physiotherapists in the United Kingdom on the use of normal saline instillation prior to endotracheal suction: a Delphi study, *Physiother. Can.,* **61**, 107–115.

Russell, K.W., Cochran, A.L., Mehta, S.T., *et al.* (2014). Lightning burns, *J. Burn Care Res.,* **35**, e436–e438.

Salehi, S.H., Fatemi, M.J., Aśadi, K., *et al.* (2014). Electrical injury in construction workers: a special focus on injury with electrical power, *Burns,* **40**, 300–304.

Saracoglu, A., Kuzucuoglu, T., Yakupoglu, S., *et al.* (2014). Prognostic factors in electrical burns: a review of 101 patients, *Burns,* **40**, 702–707.

Schneider, J.C., Holavanahalli, R., Helm, P., *et al.* (2006). Contractures in burn injury: defining the problem, *J. Burn Care Res.,* **27**, 508–514.

Schweickert, W.D., and Kress, J.P. (2011). Implementing early mobilisation interventions in mechanically ventilated patients in the ICU, *Chest,* **140**, 1612–1617.

Shaha, K.K., and Mohanthy, S. (2006). Alleged dowry death: a study of homicidal burns, *Med. Sci. Law,* **46**, 105–110.

Sharma, R.K., and Parashar, A. (2010). Special considerations in paediatric burn patients, *Indian J. Plast. Surg.,* **43**, 43–50.

Sheridan, R.L. (2002). Burns, *Crit. Care Med.,* **30** [Suppl], S500–S514.

Sheridan, R., Barillo, D., Hemdon, D., *et al.* (2005). Burn specialty teams, *J. Burn Care Rehabil.,* **26**, 170–173.

Sheridan, R.L., Baryza, M.J., Pessina, M.A., *et al.* (1999). Acute hand burn in children: management and long-term outcome based on a 10- year experience with 698 injured hands, *Ann. Surg.,* **229**, 558–564.

Simons, M., King, S., and Edgar, D. (2003). ANZBA: occupational therapy and physiotherapy for the patient with burns: principles and management guidelines, *J. Burn Care Rehabil.,* **24**, 323–335.

Smith, G.A., Bowman, M.J., Luria, J.W., *et al.* (1997). Babywalker-related injuries continue despite warning labels and public education, *Pediatrics,* **100**, e1–e5.

Spires, M.C., Kelly, B.M., and Pangilinan, P.H., Jr. (2007). Rehabilitation methods for the burn injured individual, *Phys. Med. Rehabil. Clin. N. Am.,* **18**, 925–948.

Tahir, C., Ibrahim, B.M., and Terna-Yawe, E.H. (2012). Chemical burns from assault: a review of seven cases seen in a Nigerian tertiary institution, *Ann. Burns Fire Disasters,* **25**, 126–130.

Tan, W.H., Goldstein, R., Gerrard, P., *et al.* (2012). Outcomes and predictors in burn rehabilitation, *J. Burn Care Res.,* **33**, 110–117.

Teo, A.I., Van As, A.B., and Cooper, J. (2012). A comparison of the epidemiology of paediatric burns in Scotland and South Africa, *Burns,* **38**, 802–806.

Ueda, M. (2010). Sprayed cultured mucosal epithelial cell for deep dermal burns, *J. Craniofac. Surg.,* **21**, 1729–1732.

Van Niekerk, A., Rode, H., and Laflamme, L. (2004). Incidence and patterns of childhood burn injuries in the western Cape, South Africa, *Burns,* **30**, 341–347.

Wasiak, J., Cleland, H., and Campbell, F. (2009). Dressings for superficial and partial thickness burns (review), *Cochrane Database Syst. Rev.,* **4**, CD002106.

Whitcomb, D., Martinez, J.A., and Daberkow, D. (2002). Lightning injuries, *South. Med. J.,* **95**, 1331–1334.

Chapter 7

Multiple Orthopaedic Injuries

Written by N. Plani, H. van Aswegen and B.M. Morrow

An increase in death rate due to traumatic injury is projected by the World Health Organisation by 2030, with road traffic accident mortality figures rising from 1.3 million in 2004 to 2.4 million in 2030. Patients who suffer high-energy traumatic injuries frequently have orthopaedic involvement and those who present with extremity fractures may also suffer from abdominal, chest, spinal cord or traumatic brain injuries.

This chapter discusses the following topics related to the management of traumatic orthopaedic injuries:

- The causes and mechanisms of fractures.
- Types of fractures.
- The orthopaedic injuries commonly encountered in the polytrauma patient.
- Classification of fractures.
- The complications associated with fractures.
- The medical and surgical management of a patient who sustained multiple orthopaedic injuries.
- Mechanism of bone healing.
- The physiotherapy aims of management of a patient in the intensive care unit and trauma ward who sustained orthopaedic injuries.
- The contraindications and precautions related to the physiotherapy management of a patient with orthopaedic injuries.
- The physiotherapy interventions for patients who have suffered fractures.
- Adult and paediatric clinical case scenarios.

The reader is referred to the chapters in this book that discuss trauma-related injuries other than orthopaedic injuries for additional information on the management of the polytrauma patient.

7.1. Causes and Mechanisms of Injury

7.1.1. *Causes of injury in adults*

In countries such as South Africa, trauma-related injuries are common occurrences. There are approximately 20 non-fatal incidents that result in disability for each violent fatality (Groenewald *et al.*, 2008; South African Medical Research Council, 2008). Motor cycle, motor vehicle and pedestrian vehicle accidents, as well as assault, are listed as the main causes of injury in adults. Many of these patients are critically injured and require extensive treatment in an intensive care unit (ICU).

The American College of Surgeons' national trauma data bank indicated that, in 2013, motor vehicle-related injuries accounted for 27% of cases in the data bank, especially in persons aged 19. Across the data bank, the leading two causes of death were fall-related injury followed by motor vehicle-related injury. Case fatality rates were reported to increase with the severity of injury sustained (National Trauma Data Bank Report, 2013). Multiple orthopaedic injuries account for approximately 10% of inpatient rehabilitation admissions in the USA (Uniform Data System for Medical Rehabilitation, 2004; Dubov *et al.*, 2008).

High-energy injuries, such as road traffic accidents or a fall from a height, may result in traumatic brain injury or spinal cord injury together with pelvic, femoral shaft or tibial plateau fractures, as well as hip or knee dislocations in young adults. Elderly patients may sustain pelvic, femur or tibial plateau fractures from low energy injuries, such as a simple fall (Ip, 2008).

7.1.2. *Causes of injury in paediatrics*

Common sites of injury in children with polytrauma are the head, chest, abdomen, genitourinary and musculoskeletal systems. Mortality in these children is usually associated with traumatic brain, abdominal or chest injuries (Kay and Skaggs, 2006; Abdelgawad and Kanlic, 2011).

Orthopaedic injuries constitute a high proportion of injury in paediatric polytrauma cases, with fractures accounting for up to 25% of childhood injuries (Rennie *et al.*, 2007). Although these injuries are rarely life-threatening in themselves, they can cause long-term morbidity and disability (Kay and Skaggs, 2006; Abdelgawad and Kanlic, 2011). Children have a greater potential for recovery from polytrauma than adults, both in terms of musculoskeletal and other system injuries (Kay and Skaggs, 2006); the reason being that many of the processes that encourage healing are already in motion in children at the time of the fracture (Gaston and Simpson, 2007).

The most common orthopaedic injuries in children with polytrauma are open fractures (about 10% of fractures in children with multiple injuries), compartment syndrome, pelvic injuries, multiple bone fracture, fracture-associated vascular injuries and spinal injuries (Abdelgawad and Kanlic, 2011). In the setting of high-energy or multiple traumas, children should always be assumed to have a spinal injury unless proven otherwise (Skaggs and Flynn, 2006). The presence of a pelvic fracture indicates that the child has been exposed to high-energy trauma and careful exclusion of other injuries is essential (Abdelgawad and Kanlic, 2011).

Most fractures are sustained during falls, motor vehicle accidents and other accidental injuries, including crush injuries (Rennie *et al.*, 2007). However, non-accidental injury (NAI) should always be suspected in children presenting with multiple injuries, unless a clear and validated history to the contrary is obtained (Kemp *et al.*, 2008; Abdelgawad and Kanlic, 2011). Warning signs of NAI include humeral fractures in children under three years and femur or tibia and fibula fractures in children less than 18 months of age (Pandya *et al.*, 2009; Abdelgawad and Kanlic, 2011). Other fracture locations with a high specificity for NAI include the ribs, scapula, lateral end of the clavicle and vertebrae. In addition, the presence of fractures in different stages of healing, digital fractures in non-mobile children and bilateral fractures should raise a high index of suspicion for NAI (Jayakumar *et al.*, 2010).

7.1.3. *Mechanism of injury in adults*

Bone has complex mechanical properties, combining strength, elasticity and adaptability. It has a unique ability to repair itself, but fails when overloaded. The rate at which a bone is loaded, and the orientation of the bone microstructure in relation to the direction of the applied force, influences the amount of load it can withstand. Direct injury to the bone may result in a fracture. With indirect traumatic loading, bone might be subjected to a combination of axial, bending and torsional loads that can lead to fractures (McRae, 2006). Fractures occur when the local stress or strain exceeds the strength of the bone in that area. Fracture patterns will depend on the type and direction of load applied and may be complex. In addition, high loads might cause comminution of the fracture (Hipp and Hayes, 2009).

The mechanical properties of bone slowly degrade with age. There is net bone mass loss and increased brittleness with decreased ability to absorb energy, leading to an increased fracture risk. The most significant change in ageing bone is the ease with which a fracture progresses through the bone (Hipp and Hayes, 2009). Fragility fractures, such as neck of femur fractures, become more common as age progresses. Increasing age has been shown to play a role in the inhibition of fracture healing (Gaston and Simpson, 2007).

7.1.4. *Mechanism of injury in paediatrics*

There are a number of differences between paediatric and adult bone structure that influence the injuries incurred during trauma. Children have a thicker periosteum, which commonly results in an intact periosteum on one side of the bone following a fracture, making closed reduction easier. The intact periosteum decreases the amount of fracture displacement, even in response to high-energy trauma. However, the limited bulk in children (fat and muscle mass) means that the bone is often more vulnerable to injury, as it is less protected than in adults (Musgrave and Mendelson, 2002). In children, a larger sub-periostial haematoma forms, which, together with the thicker periosteum, enhances the rapid formation of callus and hence bone healing (Gaston and Simpson, 2007).

In flat bones, bone formation occurs by either membranous, appositional bone formation or by endochondral ossification. Endochondral ossification in long bones occurs at the growth plates (physes), which allows longitudinal bone growth until skeletal maturity (about 14 years in girls and 16 years in boys) (Musgrave and Mendelson, 2002). Injury to the growth plates is common in children (about 25% of all paediatric fractures), whereas in adults the ligaments and insertions are the weakest periarticular structures. In children the growth plates are significantly weaker than the ligaments; therefore therapists should be aware that 'sprains' in children might be unrecognised fractures (Musgrave and Mendelson, 2002). Physeal injuries in skeletally immature bone may lead to the formation of physeal bridges, a well-recognised complication of physeal fractures (Khoshhal and Kiefer, 2005). Physeal bridge formation leads to growth plate arrest (closure), especially in early adolescence when the physis is at its thickest and the cartilage at its weakest (Khoshhal and Kiefer, 2005). Some physeal bridges resolve spontaneously but others may result in the shortening of the affected limb (leg length discrepancy) if the growth plate closure is complete, or angular limb deformity if the closure is incomplete (Khoshhal and Kiefer, 2005; Abdelgawad and Kanlic, 2011). Some physeal bridges lengthen spontaneously with growth (Khoshhal and Kiefer, 2005). Physeal fractures tend to heal faster than metaphyseal or diaphyseal fractures, so the window for remanipulation of a physeal fracture is short: generally no more than five days after injury (Skaggs and Flynn, 2006).

7.2. Types of Fractures

Table 7.1 outlines the types of fractures commonly seen in patients who have suffered traumatic injury, as well as a description of each fracture type (McRae, 2006; Staheli, 2006; Ratini, 2014).

7.3. Orthopaedic Injuries Commonly Encountered in the Polytrauma Patient

7.3.1. *Shoulder girdle*

A variety of shoulder injuries can result from high- or low-energy trauma. Table 7.2 provides a summary of the structures of the shoulder girdle that may be injured, the mechanism of injury and associated injuries.

Rotator cuff tears are surgically repaired only after the patient's life-threatening injuries are stabilised. This might be after discharge from the

Table 7.1: Description of fracture types.

Type of fracture	Description
Simple transverse	These fractures run at a 90° angle to the long axis of a bone. There is minimal displacement of bony ends at the fracture site and shortening of the bone is not a concern.
Simple oblique	These fractures run at an oblique angle (30° or more) along the long bone.
Simple spiral	These fractures result from indirect torsional forces to a long bone. The fracture line runs around the bone and displacement is minimal because large areas of bone remain in contact.
Greenstick	This is an incomplete fracture of the bone in which the bone is bent. It is a common type of fracture in children.
Buckle	The ends of the bones in the fractured site are driven into each other with this type of fracture. It is often called an impacted fracture and is commonly seen in children.
Compression (crush)	These occur when cancellous (spongy) bone is compressed beyond its tolerance limit. Crush fractures of the vertebral bodies are associated with spinal flexion injuries. Crush fractures of the ankle are encountered when a person falls from a height.
Comminuted	This type of fracture has more than two fragments. Examples of comminuted fractures are: • Spiral wedge fracture caused by torsion forces (Fig. 7.1) • Bending wedge fracture caused by direct or indirect violence After reduction, the main fragments will still have bony contact. Comminuted fractures are rare in children due to higher proportions of cellular and porous bone, which reduce tensile strength and the tendency to propagate.
Compound	Compound fractures are fractures with an associated open wound of the skin. They are classified as Grade I, II or III depending on the size of the open wound. Compound fractures are more prone to infection, and open reduction and internal fixation (ORIF) of these fractures may be associated with chronic sepsis.
Multifragmentary complex	These types of injuries are caused by significant violence and are difficult to manage. Three types of complex fractures are identified: • Complex spiral fractures (more than two spiral fragments) • Complex segmental fractures (minimum of one separate complete bone segment) (Fig. 7.2) • Complex irregular fractures (the fractured segment is split into many irregular fragments) After reduction there is no contact between the main bone fragments, and delayed union and joint stiffness are common complications.

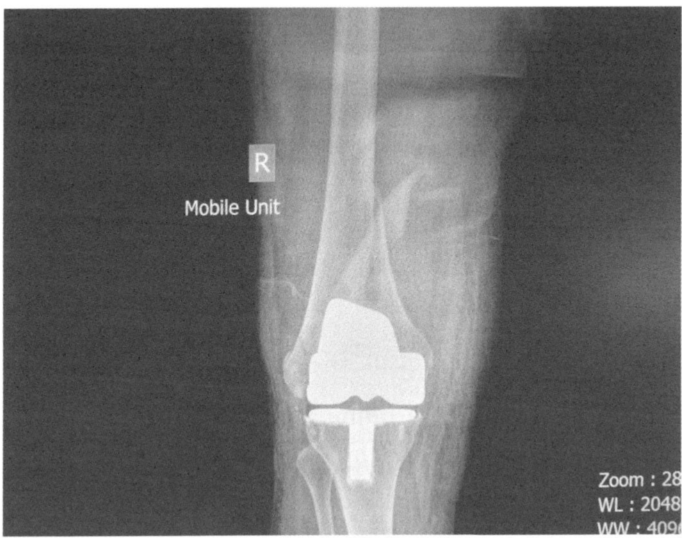

Fig. 7.1: A patient with a comminuted spiral wedge femur fracture and previous total knee replacement.

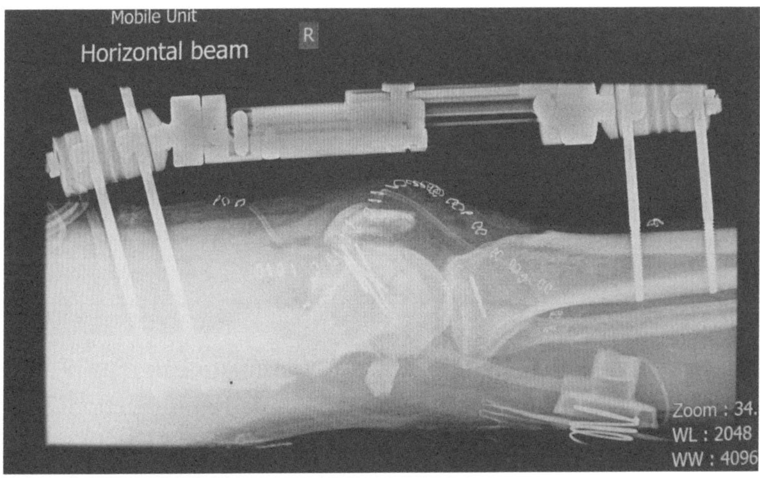

Fig. 7.2: A patient with multifragmentary complex fractures of the distal femur managed with an external fixator.

Table 7.2: Commonly encountered injuries to the shoulder girdle.

Structure	Mechanism of injury	Associated injuries
Clavicle	Injury may result from a fall on the side of the shoulder or from a heavy blow to the front of the shoulder.	• Assessment for acromioclavicular joint involvement is important, especially if the lateral end of the clavicle is fractured (McRae, 2006). • Clavicle fractures may result in injury to the brachial plexus and careful assessment for decreased usage of the affected upper limb is essential for diagnosis (Dandy and Edwards, 2009).
Scapula	Injury may result from a direct blow to the scapula. Scapula blade and scapula spine fractures heal quickly without complications.	If the scapula neck is injured, the integrity of the glenohumeral joint should be assessed closely. The glenoid can be fractured from a direct blow on the lateral side of the shoulder (McRae, 2006; Dandy and Edwards, 2009).
Rotator cuff tear	May be present in a patient with upper limb trauma (McRae, 2006).	Not applicable.
Anterior shoulder dislocation	It is the most common form of shoulder dislocation. It often occurs due to a fall that leads to external rotation and abduction of the shoulder and is also seen with motorcycle accidents.	Axillary nerve palsy may occur with anterior shoulder dislocation (McRae, 2006).

acute care setting. Rehabilitation protocols for rotator cuff repairs are well described in the literature and the reader is referred to Section 7.12 for further information.

7.3.2. *Humerus*

Table 7.3 outlines typical humerus fractures seen in patients who suffered traumatic injury.

Table 7.3: Commonly encountered injuries of the humerus.

Structure	Mechanism of injury	Associated injuries
Fracture of the surgical neck of the humerus or greater tuberosity	A fall onto an outstretched arm.	The axillary nerve and the posterior circumflex artery may be damaged.
Fracture of the humerus shaft	Direct or indirect blows to the arm.	Radial nerve palsy is commonly associated with fractures of the middle third of the humerus (McRae, 2006; Dandy and Edwards, 2009; Carroll *et al.*, 2012).
Supracondylar fractures (most common humeral fractures seen in children)	Hyperextension of the elbow when a child tries to catch themselves during a fall.	Radial or ulnar nerve injury (15%), vascular compromise (20%) and compartment syndrome (infrequent) are reported as associated injuries (Skaggs and Flynn, 2006). Injury to the median nerve may also occur.
Lateral condyle fractures of the distal humerus (second most common humeral fractures in children)	Fall onto an extended elbow leads to the impaction of the head of the radius into the distal humerus.	Fewer complications and less associated soft tissue injury are reported (Skaggs and Flynn, 2006).

7.3.3. *Radius and ulna*

Incidents such as a fall or direct blow to the elbow often result in a fracture of the radial head, the radial neck or both. Direct violence to the forearm, such as when warding off a blow during assault, results in shaft fractures of the radius or ulna. Commonly, fracture of one leads to dislocation of the other. A Monteggia fracture is a fracture of the ulna with dislocation of the radial head and is the most common fracture-dislocation injury in the forearm. Conversely, a Galeazzi fracture is a fracture of the radial shaft accompanied by a dislocation of the distal radio-ulna joint (McRae, 2006; Dandy and Edwards, 2009).

Distal radial or ulna fractures are the most common forearm fractures seen in children. Where these fractures involve the metaphysis, they usually involve both bones. Diaphyseal fractures are commonly seen in girls between 10 and 12 years and in boys between 12 and 14 years of age. Monteggia fractures may occur in children under 10 years of age, with 20% presenting with nerve palsy. Fractures of the proximal radius in children usually involve the metaphyseal neck or the physis and not the head, as seen in adults. In children, a loss of supination and pronation is common, despite optimal management (Skaggs and Flynn, 2006). The childhood equivalent of a Galeazzi fracture is the distal radial and ulnar Salter-Harris type-2 epiphyseal fracture (Staheli, 2006).

7.3.4. *Hand and wrist*

Hand and wrist injuries are complex due to the number of articular joints, innervation and blood supply. Even minimal injury may lead to large dysfunction. If immobilisation is required, this may severely impact on function and recovery time may be extended (Adams and Hamblen, 2005). Hand and wrist injuries commonly occur in children. Growth plate injuries are commonly seen in hand fractures, but growth problems are rare. The reader should refer to Section 7.12 for more information on various types of hand and wrist injuries.

7.3.5. *Pelvis*

Fractures of the pelvis are often associated with significant haemorrhage due to the rich blood supply to the pelvis. Internal haemorrhage may be severe and pelvic fractures carry a mortality rate of up to 40% if the haemorrhage is not timely managed (Mejaddam and Velmahos, 2012). Unstable pelvic fractures are those in which the pelvic ring is broken at two levels and free to open out ('open book'). An 'open book' pelvic fracture leads to significant blood loss due to damage to vascular structures and is associated with a high mortality rate. Stable pelvic fractures involve isolated injuries to the pelvic ring, e.g. superior or inferior pubic rami fractures, and do not include displacement (McRae, 2006). Figure 7.3 shows an example of a left superior pubic ramus fracture.

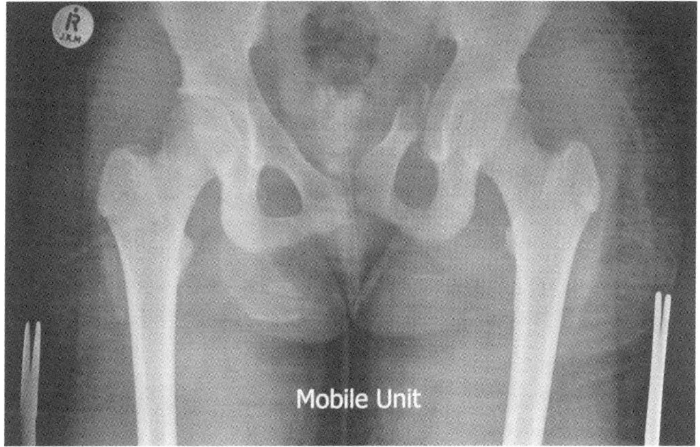

Fig. 7.3: Left superior pubic ramus fracture.

In the long term following complex pelvic fractures, patients may experience lingering pain, pelvic instability, leg length discrepancies, nerve and soft tissue damage and difficulty in sitting or, for females, giving birth (Adams and Hamblen, 2005; Hall and Brody, 2005).

Because the pelvis in children is more elastic than adults (requiring higher force to fracture), pelvic fractures in young children are rare (Musgrave and Mendelson, 2002). Most pelvic fractures that do occur in children are stable, with no widening of the symphysis pubis or sacroiliac joints (Abdelgawad and Kanlic, 2011). The vast majority of pelvic fractures in children can be managed without surgical intervention, but associated serious injury may cause significant morbidity and mortality, with the mortality rate for children with closed pelvic fractures being as high as 9% and up to 50% in children with 'open book' pelvic fractures (Musgrave and Mendelson, 2002; Skaggs and Flynn, 2006).

7.3.6. *Acetabulum*

A direct blow to the side of the hip joint or to the front of the knee in a seated position (dashboard injury) may drive the femur head into the pelvis and result in an acetabulum fracture. In the elderly, low-energy injury such as a simple fall may lead to acetabulum fracture due to osteoporotic bone. Table 7.4 lists the most common types of acetabular fractures

Table 7.4: Acetabular fractures and their associated complications.

Most common types of acetabular fractures	Injuries associated with acetabular fractures	Long-term complications
Posterior acetabulum wall fracture	Soft tissue detachment at the time of injury	Avascular necrosis of the femur head
Both anterior and posterior column fractures	Gynaecological, urinary or rectal injury	Heterotopic ossification of the acetabulum
Transverse acetabulum fracture with posterior wall fracture	Sciatic nerve injury (30% of cases)	Traumatic osteoarthritis of the hip
Transverse fracture only	Vascular injury	
Transverse fracture with medial acetabular wall fracture (also called T-shaped fracture)		

encountered, as well as associated complications (Kim *et al.*, 2011; Wheeless, 2012; Weatherford, 2014).

7.3.7. *Hip dislocation*

Hip dislocation may result from dashboard injuries during motor vehicle accidents, with energy transmitted up the femoral shaft into the hip joint. It may also occur with falls from a height or assault to the back of someone who is kneeling (McRae, 2006). Posterior dislocation of the hip (adduction and internal rotation abnormality) is most commonly seen with high-energy injury. Central hip dislocation may occur with acetabular fractures (Ip, 2008).

Traumatic hip dislocations are generally uncommon in children and fracture dislocations are seen in adolescents (Staheli, 2006). Hip dislocation in children may be from trivial trauma (in toddlers and young children), or from significant trauma in older children and teenagers. In young children without associated injury, closed reduction is usually performed and avascular necrosis is rare. In older children, however, avascular necrosis is more common and related to the severity of injury. If spontaneous reduction has occurred, the injury may be missed and tissue may be interposed within the joint. Adolescents with hip dislocation

Table 7.5: Femoral injuries and associated complications in adults and children.

Type of fracture	Complications
Femur neck	• Neurovascular injury • Avascular necrosis (a third to half of hip fractures) • Growth disturbance with physeal damage • Coxa vara (not with internal fixation)
Femur shaft	• Closed femur fractures are associated with blood loss into the surrounding tissue of up to two litres in adults; greater blood loss is seen with open (compound) femur fractures • Femoral shaft fractures in children seldom lead to levels of blood loss requiring replacement, although signs of shock in children may still indicate occult bleeding

may have the additional problem of an unstable femoral epiphysis (Skaggs and Flynn, 2006).

7.3.8. *Femur*

Femoral injury is often the result of high-energy activity in younger adults or children (road traffic accidents, falls from a height, crushing injury), or low-energy activity such as a simple fall or trip in the elderly. Table 7.5 summarises the types of fractures and associated complications related to femur fractures (McRae, 2006; Staheli, 2006; Ip, 2008; Dandy and Edwards, 2009).

Always consider the possibility of NAI in a child presenting with a femur fracture if the history is not clear, particularly in non-ambulatory infants. About 70% of paediatric femur fractures are shaft (diaphyseal) fractures (Musgrave and Mendelson, 2002). Femur fractures in children are often not as problematic as their adult counterparts, owing to the thick periosteum and good remodelling potential, which usually leads to good long-term outcomes.

7.3.9. *Knee dislocation*

Knee (tibio-femoral) dislocation can be classified according to type, e.g. anterior, posterior, medial or lateral, and rotary dislocation, e.g. anteromedial, anterolateral, posteromedial and posterolateral. High-velocity knee

Table 7.6: Mechanisms of injury associated with knee dislocation.

Type of dislocation	Mechanism of injury
Anterior	Characterised by forced hyperextension of the knee caused by motor vehicle or pedestrian vehicle accidents, unexpectedly stepping into a hole in the ground or sporting activities such as rugby or football
Posterior	Characterised by a direct force applied to the tibia while the knee is in a flexed position, such as when an athlete falls or when the knee strikes the dashboard in a motor vehicle accident
Medial or lateral	Characterised by varus or valgus forces applied to the knee
Rotary	Characterised by rotary forces applied to the knee

dislocations are very likely to involve extensive neurovascular and soft tissue injury. Lower rates of injury and better functional recovery are associated with low-velocity knee dislocations (Henrichs, 2004). Table 7.6 lists the mechanism of injury for each type of knee dislocation (Henrichs, 2004).

Anterior knee dislocation commonly occurs and is associated with significant knee ligament damage, vascular injury (especially the popliteal artery), common peroneal nerve palsy, displacement of menisci and fractures of the tibial spine (McRae, 2006; Ip, 2008).

Knee dislocations are rarely seen in children. They usually follow high-energy injuries and are more prevalent in older children and adolescents. There is a high risk of associated neurovascular injury, compartment syndrome and multiple ligamentous injury (Musgrave and Mendelson, 2002).

7.3.10. *Patella injury*

Any direct blow to the patella may result in joint cartilage damage, with or without fracture or dislocation. In the long term, patients may develop cartilage breakdown. Some may even develop erosion of the joint cartilage, with the associated development of degenerative joint disease.

Patellar sleeve injuries, characterised by avulsion of the patellar ligament from the distal pole of the patella, are unique to children and should be considered in any trauma patient who does not have full active knee extension (assuming the child is generally able to move actively) (Skaggs and Flynn, 2006; Staheli, 2006).

7.3.11. *Floating knee injury*

Ipsilateral fractures of the femur and tibia (combinations of diaphyseal, metaphyseal and intra-articular fractures) are called floating knee injuries. Floating knee injuries are generally the result of high-energy impact in the polytrauma patient. Concomitant knee ligament injury is often identified (Lundy and Johnson, 2001; Ip, 2008).

7.3.12. *Tibial plateau*

The tibial plateau is injured with violent blows (inwardly or outwardly) to the lateral side of the knee during weight bearing (also known as axial loading). This type of injury may occur as the result of a pedestrian vehicle or motor vehicle accident or with a fall from a height. Injuries that accompany tibial plateau fractures include meniscus, ligament and patella injuries (Ip, 2008).

7.3.13. *Tibia and fibula*

Direct trauma to the lateral side of the lower leg can result in fracture of the fibula alone. Dislocation of the fibula head may lead to peroneal nerve injury (Wheeles, 2012). Direct trauma to the lower leg (e.g. fall from a height) may result in a fracture of the tibia alone. Open fractures are common with tibial fractures in which the subcutaneous section of the tibia is injured. The popliteal artery may be damaged with fractures of the upper tibia. Commonly, both the tibia and fibula are fractured with road traffic accidents (McRae, 2006; Dandy and Edwards, 2009).

7.3.14. *Foot*

Traumatic injury to the foot can be categorised as forefoot, midfoot and calcaneal injury. Metatarsal bone fractures make up 80% of all fractures of the foot and ankle and extensive soft tissue injury is commonly seen (Clements and Schopf, 2013). Fractures to the first metatarsal bone and first metatarso-phalangeal joint are associated with significant functional impairment due to the limitation imposed on the amount of anatomical movement that usually takes place around these structures. Recovery from forefoot trauma can therefore be prolonged (Clements and Schopf, 2013). Calcaneus fractures are caused by high-energy impact injury such as fall from a height or motor vehicle accident. A twisting action often causes a crack in the calcaneus, whereas head-on collision (in the case of a motor vehicle) leads to shattering of the bone. The subtalar joint may be damaged with calcaneus injury and results in balance impairment when a patient walks on an uneven or slanted surface. Short-term outcomes after traumatic foot injury are influenced by the extent of the soft tissue damage, whereas long-term outcomes are affected by the extent of the bone injury (AAOS, 2010; Kinner *et al.*, 2011).

Foot injuries account for up to 6% of all children's fractures, with about half involving the metatarsal bones. Soft tissue injuries are relatively common, owing to the vulnerability of the paediatric foot (Musgrave and Mendelson, 2002).

7.4. Classification of Fractures

In many hospitals a fracture is described by site of anatomical injury, e.g. undisplaced fractured head of humerus; however, various classification systems for fractures can be used in orthopaedic practice to describe injury severity and the need for surgical intervention. Some of the most commonly used classification systems in clinical practice are discussed in this section.

7.4.1. *Long bones*

The most commonly used classification system is the Arbeitsgemeinschaft für Osteosynthesefragen/Orthopaedic Trauma Association (AO/OTA) classification of fractures of long bones. This complex system describes fractures of the humerus, radius and ulna, femur, tibia and fibula. Fracture types are described as least severe (Type A), intermediate (Type B) or most severe (Type C). This classification is used for each fracture that the patient suffers from. Comminuted fractures are generally described as Type B and complex fractures as Type C (McRae, 2006).

7.4.2. *Pelvis*

The Tile classification is used for pelvic fractures. Three categories with sub-categories are described (McRae, 2006) (Table 7.7).

7.4.3. *Acetabulum*

The AO classification system, which incorporates components of the Judet and Letournel classification, is used to determine the severity of acetabulum fractures (Table 7.8).

Table 7.7: Tile classification for pelvic fractures.

Type A (stable)	Type B (rotationally unstable fractures of the pelvic ring that are vertically stable)	Type C (rotationally and vertically unstable)
A1: Pelvic fractures that do not involve the pelvic ring	B1: Open book fractures (antero-posterior compression fractures)	C1: Unilateral fractures
A2: Minimally displaced stable fractures of the pelvic ring	B2: Ipsilateral compression fractures	C2: Bilateral fractures
	B3: Contralateral compression fractures	C3: Associated with acetabular fractures

Table 7.8: AO classification of acetabulum fractures.

Type	Description
Type A	Partial articular fracture, involving only one of the two columns of the acetabulum A1: Posterior wall fracture A2: Posterior column fracture A3: Anterior wall or column fracture
Type B	Partial articular fracture involving a transverse component B1: Pure transverse fracture B2: T-shaped fracture B3: Anterior column and posterior hemi-transverse fractures
Type C	Complete articular fractures involving both columns C1: High variety extending to the iliac crest C2: Low variety extending to the anterior border of the ilium C3: Extension into the sacroiliac joint

7.4.4. *Floating knee*

The Waddell-Fraser classification system is used to determine the severity of floating knee injuries. Two types of injuries are identified with subcategories (Ip, 2008):

- Type I: extra-articular injury;
- Type IIA: femoral shaft fracture with intra-articular tibial fracture;
- Type IIB: Intra-articular distal femur fracture with tibial shaft fracture; and
- Type IIC: Ipsilateral intra-articular fractures of both the distal femur and tibial plateau.

7.4.5. *Tibial plateau*

The Schatzker classification is the most popular system used to describe tibial plateau fractures. Types IV–VI are related to high-energy impact injuries (Ip, 2008).

- Type I: lateral tibial plateau fracture without depression.
- Type II: lateral tibial plateau fracture with depression.
- Type III: focal depression of articular surface with no associated split.
- Type IV: medial plateau and tibial spine injury with associated ligament injury.
- Type V: bicondylar fracture with split fractures of both the lateral and medial plateaus.
- Type VI: meta-diaphyseal dissociation with associated proximal tibial shaft fracture.

7.4.6. *Physeal fractures in children*

Physeal fractures are commonly classified using the Salter-Harris system (Musgrave and Mendelson, 2002) (Fig. 7.4).

- Type I: complete fracture through the hypertrophic zone of the physis (complete separation of the epiphysis and metaphysis). May be displaced or non-displaced.

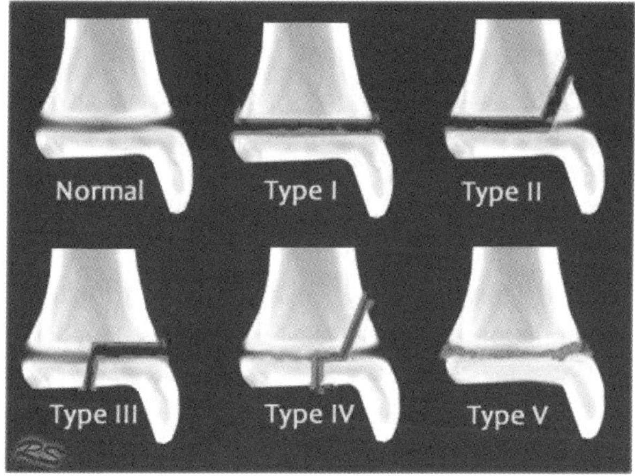

Fig. 7.4: Salter-Harris classification of physeal fractures (printed with permission from the Radiological Society of the Netherlands).

- Type II: type I plus a metaphyseal spike attached to the epiphyseal fragment on the compression side of the fracture (Thurston-Holland sign).
- Type III: fracture through the physis that extends through the epiphysis, disrupting the articular surface.
- Type IV: fracture traversing the metaphysis, physis and epiphysis.
- Type V: compression fracture involving the physis (has the highest rate of growth plate disturbance).

The aim is to achieve anatomic reduction of the physis without further injury that could affect growth.

7.4.7. *Open fractures*

Open fractures are graded according to the Gustilo-Anderson classification system, which takes into account the amount of energy, extent of soft tissue injury and contamination in order to grade fracture severity (Gustilo *et al.*, 1984). This classification system is still widely utilised and is described below.

- Type I: open fracture associated with skin laceration less than 1 cm, minimal periosteal stripping and muscle contamination and a relatively clean wound.

- Type II: open fracture associated with skin laceration less than 10 cm, with significant soft tissue damage.
- Type IIIA: open fracture associated with skin laceration greater than 10 cm, with severe soft tissue damage, underlying segmental fracture, or high-energy injury; soft tissue coverage is adequate for delayed primary closure.
- Type IIIB: open fracture associated with skin laceration greater than 10 cm, with extensive soft tissue damage, periosteal stripping and gross contamination. A soft-tissue flap is needed to achieve delayed soft-tissue coverage.
- Type IIIC: open fracture associated with a vascular injury requiring repair.

7.5. Complications Associated with Orthopaedic Injuries

Patients with orthopaedic injuries are at risk of developing various complications associated with soft tissue damage, fractured bones, anaesthesia or prolonged immobility. Table 7.9 lists the complications associated with soft tissue damage and fractured bones (McRae, 2006; Brautigam *et al.*, 2009; Dandy and Edwards, 2009).

Table 7.9: Complications associated with bony fractures and soft tissue injury.

Fractures	Soft tissue injury
Malunion, delayed union or non-union	Internal or external bleeding
Joint stiffness	Vascular injury and haemarthrosis
Avascular necrosis	Neural injury
Myositis ossificans	Ligamentous injury
Osteitis (inflammation of bone)	Muscle and skin injury
Muscle tendon complications	Infection
Fat embolism	Metabolic responses to trauma such as electrolyte shifts and protein breakdown
Compartment syndrome	
Implant complications	

7.5.1. *Avascular necrosis*

Avascular necrosis refers to the death of bone cells due to a lack of blood supply. This complication occurs more frequently in younger adults (aged 45 or less) and typically affects the femoral head, knee, talus, humeral head and scaphoid (Gao *et al.*, 2013). Avascular necrosis results mostly from glucocorticoid therapy, alcohol abuse, long smoking history and blood clotting disorders.

7.5.2. *Myositis ossificans*

Bone formation in the surrounding tissue outside the bony skeleton is referred to as myositis ossificans or heterotopic ossification. It is occasionally seen in patients with long bone fractures and causes severe pain and limited joint range of motion (ROM). Factors that predispose a patient to the development of myositis ossificans are still unclear. Precautions for the physiotherapy management of patients with this complication are discussed in Section 7.9.

7.5.3. *Fat embolism*

Fat embolism syndrome develops when fat molecules accumulate in the lung parenchyma and peripheral circulation. The syndrome develops within 72 hours of fractures of the long bones and pelvis or major trauma. It is more frequent in closed than open fractures (Gupta and Reilly, 2007). Patients with fat embolism syndrome develop distinct changes related to the respiratory system, neurological changes and petechial skin rash. Respiratory system changes include dyspnoea, tachypnoea and hypoxaemia, and some patients may require mechanical ventilation (MV) (Gupta and Reilly, 2007). Neurological changes develop after the onset of respiratory distress and may range from mild confusion to severe seizures (Gupta and Reilly, 2007). Petechial rash typically develops in the conjunctiva, oral mucus membranes, neck, axilla and skin folds of the upper body (Gupta and Reilly, 2007).

Key Message

A patient with bilateral closed femur fractures and no chest-related trauma that suddenly develops breathlessness may have a pulmonary embolism. The physiotherapist should immediately inform the orthopaedic or critical care team of the change in symptoms so that a ventilation-perfusion scan of the lungs can be performed to confirm or refute the presence of an embolism.

Table 7.10: Complications associated with prolonged immobility.

Atelectasis and pneumonia
Pressure sores
Deep venous thrombosis
Muscle wasting
Decalcification of bone
Calcium deposits in the urinary tract
Urinary tract infections

Patients who undergo surgical repair of fractures may develop complications associated with general anaesthesia and surgery, e.g. sore throat, nausea and vomiting, hypothermia, nerve injury, atelectasis, pneumonia, anaemia, shock from blood loss or wound infection. Those who are placed on a period of bed rest due to the severity of their injuries or after surgery are at risk of developing a number of additional complications, as listed in Table 7.10 (McRae, 2006; Dandy and Edwards, 2009).

Physiotherapists generally spend more time with patients during the day than the medical and surgical teams and therefore physiotherapists are often the first members of the interdisciplinary team to note the development of complications after injury. It is thus important that physiotherapists take cognisance of the complications that may arise after orthopaedic injury and act as advocate for the patient in immediately informing the patient's doctor or surgeon if these complications are suspected or identified.

Key Message

A patient with a pelvic fracture that suddenly develops a hot swollen calf may have a deep venous thrombosis. The physiotherapist should immediately inform the orthopaedic or critical care team of the change in condition so that a duplex ultrasound can be performed to confirm or refute the diagnosis.

7.6. Mechanism of Bone Healing

Fractured bone heals mainly through physiological processes. The stability of the fracture site will determine the rate at which repair takes place and load-bearing capacity is restored. A degree of micro movement between bone fragments facilitates healing (Hipp and Hayes, 2009).

7.6.1. *Phases of bone repair*

Bone repair takes place through three distinctive phases that are summarised below (McRae, 2006; Gaston and Simpson, 2007; Dandy and Edwards, 2009; Hipp and Hayes, 2009).

7.6.1.1. *Reactive phase*

The reactive phase involves the inflammatory process that follows fracture of the bone. A haematoma forms around the bone ends and as it coagulates blood clots are formed. Fibroblast activity increases, the clots are broken down and granulation tissue is formed.

7.6.1.2. *Reparative phase*

This phase involves the formation of soft and then hard callus. Periostial cells above the fracture gap form into chondroblasts, responsible for the formation of hyaline cartilage. Periostial cells below the fracture gap form into osteoblasts that produce woven bone. As these tissues are formed they grow towards each other until the fracture gap is bridged. This is called callus formation, but the strength of the bone remains weak for a period of four to six weeks after the fracture occurred. In children, the greater subperiostial haematoma and stronger periosteum result in more rapid callus formation than in adults. This rapidly formed callus is strong enough to render the fracture healed (Lindaman, 2001).

Whilst some micro movement is essential for callus formation, shear motion at a fracture gap can significantly impair fracture healing. Shear motion results in less bone bridging across the fracture gap, and reduces the amount of callus formation and therefore the rigidity at the fracture site (Augat *et al.*, 2003).

Following callus formation, endochondral ossification takes place. During this ossification process the hyaline cartilage and woven bone are replaced with laminar bone. Eventually the laminar bone is replaced with trabecular bone, which restores most of the bone's original strength.

7.6.1.3. *Remodelling phase*

In this last phase of healing, trabecular bone is replaced with compact bone through finely balanced osteoblast and osteoclast activity. Remodelling occurs slowly over months and even years and is facilitated by the loading of the bone through mechanical forces such as walking.

In children remodelling is affected by years of remaining growth (with increasing age the potential for remodelling decreases), the position of the fracture in relation to the joint (greater remodelling for mid-shaft fractures), the growth potential of adjacent physis (upper humeral fractures show much better remodelling than distal humeral fractures), the orientation of the fracture to joint axis (remodelling is greatest for sagittal plane, then frontal plane and least for transverse plane malunions), and physeal status (damage to the physis reduces growth and the potential for remodelling) (Wilkins, 2005; Staheli, 2006). Children generally have greater potential for remodelling than adults.

There is evidence to suggest that innervation of the fracture site is a requirement for timely and good fracture repair (Li *et al.*, 2001; Hipp and Hayes, 2009). Several factors affect the rate at which bone heals (McRae, 2006), and are summarised in Table 7.11.

Table 7.11: Factors that affect the rate of bone healing.

Type of bone: cancellous bone heals within six weeks; cortical bone within nine to 18 weeks
Patient age: the union of fractures is more rapid in children than in adults
Mobility at fracture site: excessive mobility disrupts new bone growth
Separation of bone ends
Infection at the fracture site
Poor blood supply to fracture site, e.g. scaphoid fracture
Joint involvement

7.6.2. *Abnormal bone healing*

7.6.2.1. *Malunion*

Malunion of a fracture site is where bony union has occurred in an abnormal position, which may result in dysfunction or may be cosmetically unattractive. This may occur as a result of inadequate initial reduction or if reduction has been displaced (McRae, 2006; Dandy and Edwards, 2009). The mal-alignment is usually corrected surgically through osteotomy. This involves cutting the bone at the site of or near the fracture and re-aligning the fracture ends through secure fixation using plates, screws or an external frame with pins.

7.6.2.2. *Delayed union*

When a fracture heals at a slower rate than anticipated, it is referred to as delayed union. This may be a result of infection, poor blood supply, inadequate stabilisation, open fractures and severe soft tissue damage and smoking (McRae, 2006; Dandy and Edwards, 2009; Lee *et al.*, 2013). Delayed union is managed in several ways, including replacement of the patient's existing cast, reduction of traction forces, functional bracing, internal fixation or bone grafting.

7.6.2.3. *Non-union*

Non-union of a fracture is where all bone healing has ceased without fracture healing being achieved. This may be due to poor blood supply, infection, inadequate stabilisation of the fracture, poor alignment, open fractures, soft tissue interposed between fracture ends and smoking (McRae, 2006; Dandy and Edwards, 2009; Ebraheim *et al.*, 2013; Lee *et al.*, 2013). Non-union is managed surgically through the removal of all scar tissue from the fracture site followed by bone graft and fixation using plates, screws or external frames with pins.

Patient-related factors such as diabetes (types I and II) and the use of non-steroidal anti-inflammatory drugs within 12 months prior to the fracture injury are associated with malunion, delayed union or non-union of fractures (Hernandez *et al.*, 2012).

7.7. Medical and Surgical Management

7.7.1. *Primary survey and resuscitation of vital functions*

On admission to the emergency department the patient with multiple orthopaedic injuries will be assessed through the internationally accepted 'airways, breathing, circulation, disability, exposure' (ABCDE) approach to advanced trauma life support, as described in Chapter 5. As mentioned previously, this approach is used for all adult and paediatric patients with trauma-related injuries (Musgrave and Mendelson, 2002; Thim *et al.*, 2012). A patient with pelvic injuries may present with excessive haemorrhage; an attempt is made firstly to control the bleeding and thereafter to correct hypotension (Mejaddam and Velmahos, 2012).

X-rays of the chest, cervical spine and pelvis, whole-body x-ray imaging (if available locally) or ultrasound technology form part of the primary survey in order to identify life-threatening injuries that are not visible (Kool and Blickman, 2007) (Figs 7.5A and B).

If the patient sustained thoracic trauma in addition to extremity or pelvic injuries, the patient will be screened for the presence of the 'lethal six injuries' related to thoracic trauma, as discussed in Chapter 5, Section 5.3.1.1.

Care provided to the patient with multiple orthopaedic injuries in the emergency department during the primary survey may include oxygen therapy, placement of an endotracheal tube (ETT) if indicated, nasogastric

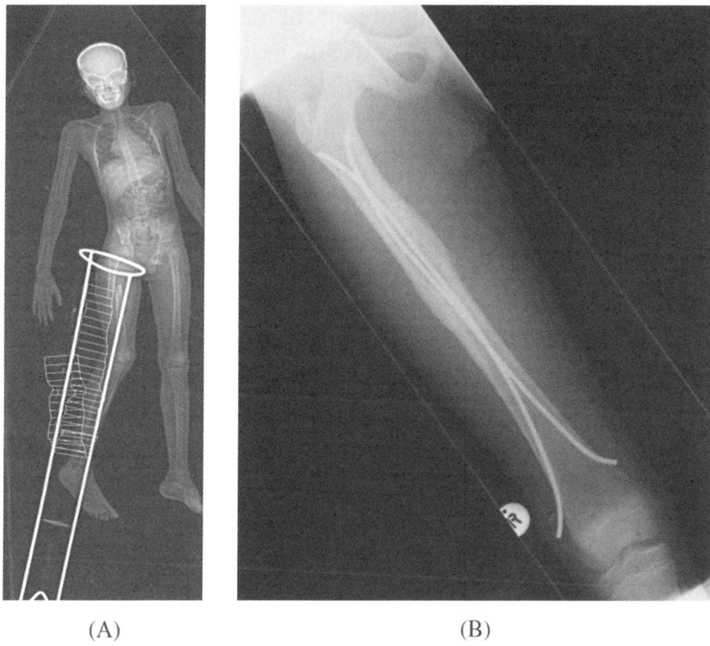

(A) (B)

Fig. 7.5: Whole body x-ray of a 10-year-old child with a right femur fracture. (A) Before fracture reduction; (B) After internal fixation.

tube placement, placement of peripheral intravenous (IV) lines for medication (especially analgesia) administration and fluid replacement therapy and, lastly, insertion of a urinary catheter.

7.7.2. *Secondary survey as adjunct to primary survey*

The secondary survey is a 'head-to-toe' evaluation of the patient (see Chapter 5, Section 5.3.2), which includes taking a detailed history of the patient as well as a complete neurological and physical examination.

X-rays of the thoracic and lumbar spine, as well as the extremities, are performed during the secondary survey. If the mechanism of injury suggests possible pelvic injury, an x-ray of the pelvis is done. In addition, computed tomography (CT) scanning and contrast studies may be requested (Kool and Blickman, 2007).

Care provided to the patient during the primary survey continues in the secondary survey. If patient admission to intensive care is anticipated due to the severity of the patient's injuries, placement of arterial and central venous pressure (CVP) lines are performed. If the patient has sustained thoracic trauma in addition to extremity or pelvic injuries, the patient will be screened for the presence of the 'hidden six injuries' related to thoracic trauma (Chapter 5, Section 5.3.2.1).

7.7.3. *Definitive care*

Orthopaedic injuries can be classified as emergent (life- or limb-threatening), urgent (open fractures, femur fractures, joint dislocations, significant soft tissue injuries) or semi-elective (most other fractures). Treatment is based on the presence and severity of other injuries, physiological stability and the need for orthopaedic intervention. Timing of orthopaedic surgical intervention remains controversial. It is now well recognised that the aggressive orthopaedic approach that was advocated in earlier years may be counterproductive to the other overall goals of successful resuscitation (Deitch and Dayal, 2006). Assessment of the patient's physiological and neurological status and consideration of the impact of anaesthesia and surgery on patient outcome is vital. Patients should be in a physiologically stable condition prior to surgical intervention (Mejaddam and Velmahos, 2012).

The above approach has led to the development of damage control orthopaedics (DCO), in which the minimum is done and external fixators are temporarily placed until optimisation of the patient's condition is achieved. Damage control orthopaedics refers particularly to the care of femur and pelvic fractures and significant soft tissue injuries. It can be defined as the use of treatment techniques that enhance immediate survival with the least stress to the patient's physiological condition and may include (Roberts *et al.*, 2005; Dubov *et al.*, 2008; Bosse and Kellam, 2009; Mooney, 2012):

- splinting for extremity fractures;
- traction for long bone fractures;
- pelvic compression for pelvic fractures; and
- placement of external fixators in stable but critically ill patients.

This approach may be used until the patient is stable enough for delayed definitive surgery, such as in the case of closed head injuries, haemodynamic instability and thoracoabdominal injuries which may delay femur nailing (Bosse and Kellam, 2009). Delay in fracture fixation does not contribute to the development of pulmonary complications such as pneumonia or acute respiratory distress syndrome (ARDS). Pulmonary complications are more likely related to the underlying condition that motivated surgical delay in the first place (Bosse and Kellam, 2009). The patient with unstable pelvic fractures and excessive haemorrhage will be taken to theatre immediately for operative pelvic packing to control the bleeding. Angiography may also be performed if indicated (Mejaddam and Velmahos, 2012). These patients are admitted to the ICU after surgery for monitoring and care. Although there is little evidence regarding the use of DCO for children, it is suggested that these methods are useful as a temporary measure in the management of severe, open (compound) fractures complicated by severe soft tissue injury and bone loss, until the paediatric patient is sufficiently stabilised to allow definitive fracture fixation (Mooney, 2012).

In children, the goals of management are to provide fracture stabilisation, facilitate bone healing, achieve adequate reduction to ensure physiologic alignment by skeletal maturity, permit early ROM to minimise joint stiffness and allow early mobilisation and facilitate rehabilitation so the child can return to functional activities as soon as possible (Musgrave and Mendelson, 2002).

7.7.3.1. *Care provided in the ICU*

Preventable causes of death following multiple traumatic injuries most often include haemorrhage, multiple organ dysfunction syndrome and cardiac arrest (Deitch and Dayal, 2006; Mejaddam and Velmahos, 2012). The care provided to the patient in the ICU aims to optimise the patient's condition in order to avoid the development of these complications. A fine balance between operative and non-operative therapy is of utmost importance (Deitch and Dayal, 2006).

- Pain control must be achieved and optimised early. Pain relief assists and benefits mobilisation.
- Fracture alignment may decrease ongoing muscle damage and stimulation of the inflammatory response. It may decrease the risk of

vascular and neurological injuries (Dubov *et al.*, 2008; Bosse and Kellam, 2009).

- Extremity fractures carry a high risk for the development of deep venous thrombosis, and therefore low molecular weight heparin is prescribed to prevent this (Mejaddam and Velmahos, 2012).
- Patients who are in need of MV are managed according to the ARDS network trial guidelines of low tidal volume ventilation in order to minimise ventilator-induced lung injury (Mejaddam and Velmahos, 2012). The reader is referred to Section 7.12 for sources of additional reading material on ventilator-induced lung injury.
- Some patients with multiple orthopaedic injuries who developed respiratory complications may need a longer period of support from MV. Tracheostomy is performed in such cases to reduce the patient's work of breathing and to facilitate weaning from MV. Care of the tracheostomy is of utmost importance as it will directly influence the patient's outcome. The reader is referred to Chapter 5 (Section 5.3.4.1) for more information about tracheostomy care.
- The formation of stress ulcers is avoided with the administration of proton pump inhibitors or histamine-2-receptor antagonist medication. A bleeding stress ulcer increases the risk for mortality five-fold (Mejaddam and Velmahos, 2012).

7.7.3.2. *Non-surgical interventions*

7.7.3.2.1. Splints, braces or casts

In undisplaced fractures, splints, braces or casts may be used to immobilise the fracture site effectively. Casts are easy to apply and modern material such as fibreglass is lightweight. Most children under six years of age with femur fractures are managed with closed reduction and early spica casting or skin traction. Spica casts are usually kept on for six weeks in children under five years and for eight weeks in children between five and 10 years of age.

If a cast is circumferential, excessive swelling may cause compartment syndrome or muscle ischaemia; therefore the limb should be monitored closely after application. Another disadvantage of casts is that they are often applied over joints adjacent to the fracture, immobilising them. This could lead to joint stiffness, muscle weakness and shortening and prolonged swelling (Boyd *et al.*, 2009).

Key Message

Signs of vascular compromise in a patient wearing a cast include severe swelling, coldness and pain, delayed capillary refill and a dusky appearance of the exposed extremities.

7.7.3.2.2. Traction

Traction can reduce a fracture and maintain good alignment. It is most frequently used for femur, tibial and cervical spine fractures (McRae, 2006).

- Skin traction is used for limb fractures and is usually a temporary measure. Weight of approximately four to five kilograms is applied to achieve alignment of the fractured bone.
- Skeletal traction, such as halo traction or Thomas splint, is applied through pins that are inserted into the bone and heavier loads can be applied. The reader is referred to Chapter 8 (Section 8.6) for information about cervical traction.

Traction must be applied in the correct direction, parallel to the shaft of the fractured bone, and weights must be free hanging (McRae, 2006). Skin traction is commonly used in young children with lower limb fractures (Fig. 7.6). Children may be in skin traction for the full six weeks of healing.

Skeletal traction with a weight greater than five kg has the potential to pull the child off the bed and often needs to be counteracted by tilting the bed so that the child lies in a head down position. Another concern regarding skeletal traction in children is the risk of pins going through the growth plate. Traction and casting are often not considered as management options in children following multiple injuries or a significant head

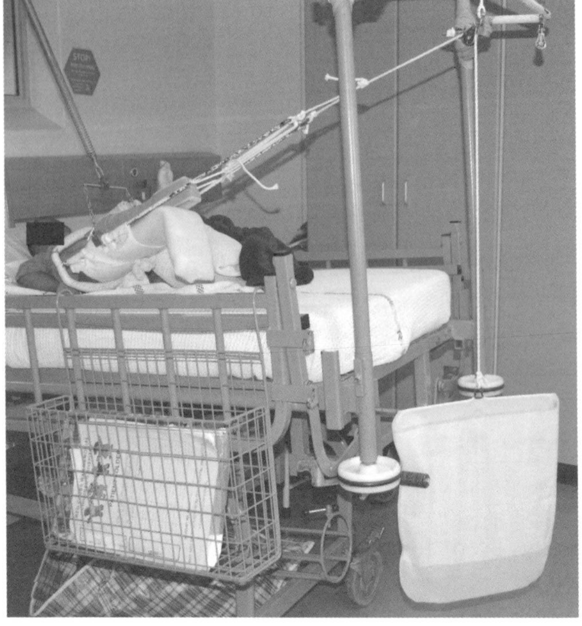

Fig. 7.6: A 3-year-old boy on skin traction for fractured femur.

Table 7.12: Complications associated with the use of traction.

Type of traction	Complications
Skin traction	• Distal oedema • Vascular obstruction • Peroneal nerve palsy • Skin necrosis
Skeletal traction	• Physeal injury to the distal femur or proximal tibia or tibial tubercle in children • Peroneal nerve injury with placement of a pin in the proximal tibia • Popliteal artery injury with placement of a pin in the distal femur

injury, as an operative approach in these circumstances is associated with less complications and shorter hospital stay (Skaggs and Flynn, 2006; Green and Swiontkowski, 2009). Complications encountered with the use of traction for fracture management are listed in Table 7.12 (Green and Swiontkowski, 2009).

Physiotherapists should regularly assess their patients for the development of these complications and notify the orthopaedic surgeon in a timely manner if they suspect the development of complications.

7.7.3.3. Surgical interventions

The main aim of all orthopaedic treatment is to restore function and minimise deformity. Management therefore consists of good reduction of the fracture and maintenance of such reduction in a manner that promotes bone healing. In addition, other concomitant injuries need to be managed. This might include microsurgery to repair damaged nerves and ruptured blood vessels. Fasciotomy may be indicated in the presence of severe soft tissue swelling if compartment syndrome develops (Adams and Hamblen, 2005).

There are a variety of techniques available to treat fractures. The choice of technique may be dependent on the type and site of fracture, the stability of the patient, associated vascular or nerve injuries and surgeon preference. There is, however, one general principle: to obtain sufficient stability to ensure fracture healing. Different fixation methods offer different levels of stability and bones may be subjected to varying types of loads (axial, torsional or bending) of varying magnitude. This is considered when the surgeon chooses fixation devices (Hipp and Hayes, 2009).

7.7.3.3.1. External fixation

External fixation can be applied quickly and therefore it is useful in patients who have suffered multiple injuries and skin loss (Dandy and Edwards, 2009; Carroll *et al*., 2012). There is minimal interference with adjacent joints and during surgery soft tissue damage is limited. External fixation may be used where contact can be achieved between bone segments, but also where there is a gap between bone fragments. Current devices offer many different frame configurations and stability options, such as a pin-to-bar fixator (unilateral frame, Fig. 7.7) or Ilizarov fixator (ring frame with K-wires).

External fixation also provides a means to change the rigidity of the fixation over time. Stability depends on the frame configuration and the

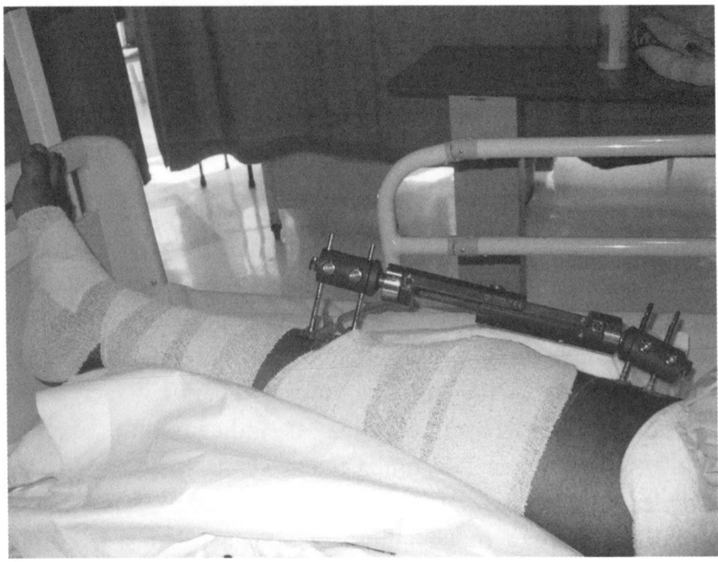

Fig. 7.7: External fixation for distal femur fracture.

interaction between bone fragments and the frame. The direction of applied load, number of pins used and number of sidebars on the frame are all factors that influence rigidity (Fragomen and Rozbruch, 2007).

Pin loosening is a common problem with external fixators, and if the clamps or pins come loose the stability of the fixator is severely compromised. Pin loosening may develop due to pin design and placement, pin site infection and bone necrosis. One must be aware that these connections may fail under relatively low load. The percutaneous pins are typically the weakest part of the system, especially in very unstable fractures. The pin diameter and number of pins determines fixator stiffness, as does bar-to-bone spacing. Care must be taken not to place pins through or very close to open growth plates in children.

Bone contact between fragments will allow load sharing between the fixator and bone, but if there is no contact between the bone fragments, the fixator bears the entire load. This can significantly affect bone healing (Dandy and Edwards, 2009). Pins may also need to pass through muscle, which may become tethered, leading to pain and reluctance to move.

It appears that a more rigid fixation may lead to earlier stiffness at the fracture site, but this does not necessarily coincide with the restoration of bone strength. However, the strength of the bone will return later, irrespective of the level of fixator rigidity. One might want to achieve firm rigidity early during healing to encourage osseous union, but in the latter stages of healing more load transfer across the fracture site might be beneficial to promote bone remodelling (Fragomen and Rozbruch, 2007; Hipp and Hayes, 2009).

Complications associated with external fixation include neurovascular injuries due to percutaneous placement of the pins and infection at the pin sites (Carroll *et al.*, 2012).

In children, external fixators are limited to the stabilisation of open fractures, multiple fractures and polytrauma patients. The advantages of external fixation in paediatric and adult trauma patients include (Fragomen and Rozbruch, 2007):

- reduced infection risk in open fractures;
- observation of the skin and wounds;
- no additional treatment is needed for the fracture; and
- movement and early mobilisation.

In children, complications include neurovascular injuries due to pin insertion, infection at pin sites, the weakening of bones by pin insertion, which can lead to iatrogenic fractures, and the heavy weight of fixators, which may limit movement in small children. Modern fixators, however, lead to fewer complications (Hayek *et al.*, 2004).

7.7.3.3.2. Internal fixation

Internal fixation is generally used when it is not possible to reduce a fracture with closed manipulation, or when it is unlikely that reduction will be maintained. Patients with multiple fractures or associated nerve or vascular injuries appear to do better with internal fixation. It is the technique of choice when early mobilisation is desired. Particularly for the fractured femur and humerus, internal fixation has gained ground in recent years (Hipp and Hayes, 2009; Carroll *et al.*, 2012). In children with open (compound) tibia fractures, operative fixation with flexible nailing is indicated, having better results than external fixation (Kay and Skaggs, 2006).

Internal fixation can cause iatrogenic physeal injury in children, which may limit options for paediatric fracture stabilisation (Musgrave and Mendelson, 2002).

Types of internal fixation devices include intramedullary nails or bone plates and screws.

7.7.3.3.2.1. *Intramedullary nails.* An intramedullary (IM) nail (also referred to as intramedullary rod) is made of metal and is forced into the medullary cavity of a bone through the proximal or distal femur. It is locked in place with bolts on each end of the nail to prevent rotation of the bony fragments. By locking the nail on one end, the forces transmitted through fracture segments increase during weight-bearing. Locking both ends prevents axial displacement of the bone and increases rigidity (Hipp and Hayes, 2009). Intramedullary nails are inserted into the medullary bone cavity through a process called reaming. A bone reamer is used to clear out the bone cavity and widen it to allow the IM nail to be placed in position. Reaming with the insertion of IM nails is associated with high bone union rates and low complication rates (Ricci *et al.*, 2009). Femur and humerus fractures are often managed surgically with IM nailing (Fig. 7.8). The nail acts as an internal splint and the nail and bone both contribute to fracture stability. Complications such as infection, nail deformation and fatigue fractures are rare (Ricci *et al.*, 2009; Carroll *et al.*, 2012).

In the polytrauma patient early IM nailing for femur fractures has been associated with negative patient outcome, due to the strain that reaming places on the patient's immune system. The release of inflammatory mediators, blood loss in theatre and hypothermia are among the factors ascribed to IM nail insertion through reaming that lead to decompensation in these patients. The principle of DCO (initial external fixation followed by IM nailing when the patient is stable) is vital to optimise patient outcome (Ricci *et al.*, 2009).

7.7.3.3.2.2. *Bone plates and screws.* This fixation method is often referred to as ORIF. The bone and plate work together when this type of fixation is used, as some load is supported by the plate and some passes between the bone fragments. The interaction between the plate and bone

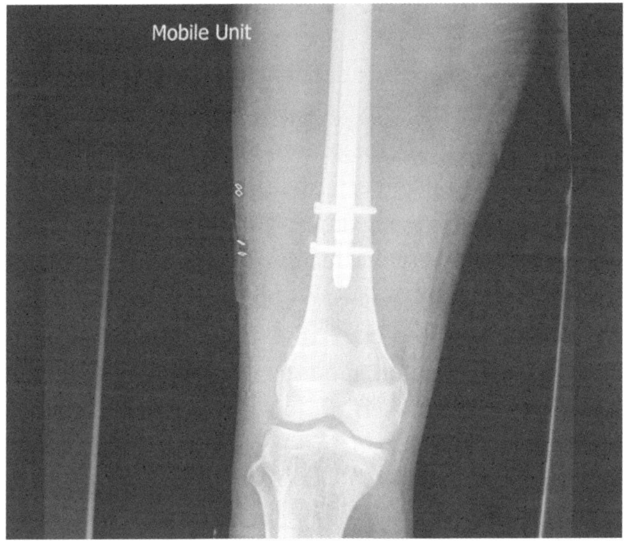

Fig. 7.8: The distal section of an IM nail used to stabilise a proximal femur fracture.

is load dependant, so the plate may provide more stability for one type and direction of load than for others.

The thickness of the plate and the type and integrity of the bone influences the behaviour of the plate–bone system. With comminuted fractures there may not be much load sharing between bone fragments and thus the plate will bear greater loads. This may increase the risk of the plate fatiguing and breaking. Loads may also be transmitted at the site of the bone screws. The amount of load transferred depends on the stage of remodelling, the quality of the bone and how rigidly the plate is applied (Cordey *et al.*, 2000).

Plates and compression plates are applied on the tensile aspect of the fracture, as the bone is particularly weak under loads that bend open a fracture. Similarly, the use of inner screws together with outer screws on a plate system increases rigidity (Cordey *et al.*, 2000).

It appears that there may be an inverse relationship between plate stiffness (how rigidly it is applied and how much micro movement it allows) and callus formation and bone strength (Hipp and Hayes, 2009).

7.7.3.3.3. Amputation

Amputation of a joint or limb is dependent on the severity of soft tissue injury sustained and the viability of salvaging the limb. A patient's functional ability is dependent on the preservation of as much limb length as possible when amputation is performed. A recent meta-analysis on the outcomes of patients following lower limb amputation after traumatic injury showed that patients who received through-knee amputation had better quality of life (QOL) related to physical function than those with above-knee amputation (Penn-Barwell, 2011). Amputation of the forefoot or at calcaneal level is often required following severe foot injuries (Kinner *et al.*, 2011). The reader is referred to Section 7.12 for sources of information on pre-prosthetic and post-prosthetic complications following amputation.

7.8. Physiotherapy Aims of Management

The main aim of physiotherapy treatment is to safely rehabilitate a patient back to previous full function, or to optimise their function as far as their injuries permit, in the shortest possible time. However, the extent and nature of the injury must be taken into consideration and goals set for the patient and by the patient must be realistic. All rehabilitation is performed within the limits set down by the orthopaedic surgeon and their guidance should be sought on limitations in ROM and weight-bearing status for each individual patient. If multiple injuries were sustained, the critically injured patient may spend an extended time on MV with sedation. Muscle mass deteriorates by 1.5–2% per day with strict bed rest and by as much as 5–6% per day with immobilisation in the first three weeks of ICU stay (De Jonghe *et al.*, 2009). If immobilisation is achieved by casting, patients may lose 25% muscle mass in the first week (De Jonghe *et al.*, 2009).

Assessment of the patient with multiple orthopaedic injuries for their risk of developing physical and non-physical morbidity should be performed early during ICU stay. It is important that the patient and their family are involved with short- and medium-term goal setting for rehabilitation. Rehabilitation for 'at risk' patients in the ICU should start as soon as clinically possible (NICE, 2009). An interdisciplinary team approach to the rehabilitation of patients with multiple orthopaedic injuries in the ICU is important. Regular communication should take place between the physiotherapist and dietician regarding nutritional support supplied to the patient to ensure effective rehabilitation can be performed.

For the purposes of this book, physiotherapy-specific aims of intervention for patients with orthopaedic injuries are provided in Table 7.13. These suggested aims of management should be tailored to the needs of each individual patient in the acute care setting.

Before discharge from the ICU, patients should be re-assessed and ward-based care should include a rehabilitation approach that incorporates

Table 7.13: Aims of physiotherapy management for patients with orthopaedic injuries who are in the ICU.

- Enhance mucociliary escalator function through adequate humidification of the airways
- Mobilise and remove excessive retained secretions from the airways of patients who are intubated or spontaneously breathing in order to prevent the development of secondary chest infections
- Once extubated, enhance the patient's self-dependence by encouraging spontaneous coughing and expectoration of retained secretions
- Increase posterior and basal lung volumes of patients who are intubated and sedated in order to prevent the development of atelectasis
- Increase compliance of the chest wall and lung tissue in order to optimise and restore lung function
- Improve the patient's oxygenation
- Soft tissue injuries that result in swelling or tightness must be managed with elevation above the level of the heart
- Maintain passive joint ROM of all joints and muscle length of all two-joint muscles to prevent joint stiffness and contracture formation. This should be done within the limitations posed by the orthopaedic injuries that the patient has sustained
- As the patient wakes up from sedation and is able to cooperate with rehabilitation, encourage active muscle strengthening exercises within the limitations posed by the orthopaedic injuries
- Encourage patients who are awake and responsive to become functionally independent in activities of daily life (ADL)
- Early mobilisation, as soon as the patient is physiologically stable and bearing all contraindications in mind, forms an important component of treatment of the polytrauma patient

Table 7.14: Aims for progression of management for patients with orthopaedic injuries in the ward setting.

- Humidification of the patient's airways for as long as they receive oxygen therapy
- Encouragement of spontaneous cough and expectoration of retained secretions to prevent the development of a secondary chest infection
- Maximisation of lung compliance and lung volumes during the patient's stay in the ward to prevent the onset of secondary chest infections
- Progression of rehabilitation from active exercises to resisted exercises to optimise muscle strength in all affected areas
- Optimisation of muscle strength of all unaffected muscles so that the patient can become independent with transfers and mobilisation (especially if walking aids are used)
- Education of the patient on the safe use of walking aids (walking frames, gutter or elbow crutches) if appropriate
- Re-education of the patient's gait pattern with a walking aid according to the amount of weight-bearing allowed in light of the patient's injuries
- Re-education of stair climbing with the walking aid if appropriate
- Optimisation of the patient's exercise endurance through progressively increasing the frequency of exercise and the distance mobilised in the ward and on the hospital premises
- Any paresis or paralysis due to nerve damage may require intensive physiotherapy

the assessment findings of the 'prior to ICU discharge' assessment, is individualised, structured and progressive. If care is provided by a different team in the ward, a comprehensive handover of the patient's rehabilitation needs and care provided by the ICU team should be performed at the time of patient transfer (NICE, 2009). This is particularly important for physiotherapists, to ensure continuity and progression of care.

Important aims for the progression of the patient's physiotherapy management on the ward are listed in Table 7.14. The aims should be tailored to each individual patient's needs.

7.8.1. *Paediatric considerations*

Rehabilitation is an essential component of paediatric trauma care. The aims of treatment are to return the child to full age-appropriate levels of function and enable the child to reach their maximum potential. Early rehabilitation is especially critical in children who have sustained concomitant neurological injuries (American Academy of Pediatrics and Pediatric Orthopaedic Society of North America, 2008). The same principles and aims of management in the trauma ward apply to children as in adults, but execution differs. This should be appropriate to the child's stage of development, and the therapist needs to be cognisant of the differences in physiology, anatomy and increased vulnerability of the child. Analgesia remains the mainstay of treatment, as a child in pain will not cough or move.

7.8.2. *Functional assessment prior to discharge*

The reader is referred to Chapter 5 (Section 5.4.2) for information on functional assessment. Exercise rehabilitation guidelines for survivors of trauma can be found in Chapter 10 (Section 10.6).

7.9. Precautions and Contraindications Related to Physiotherapy Management

The type and stability of a fracture or joint determines the type of exercises that may be performed, which muscles may be used actively and what ROM may be achieved. It is good practice to discuss these issues with the attending orthopaedic or trauma surgeon prior to the initiation of rehabilitation.

7.9.1. *General precautions related to physiotherapy in intensive care*

The reader is referred to Chapter 5 (Section 5.5.1) for a list of general precautions that should be adhered to during the treatment of any patient with traumatic injury in the acute care setting.

7.9.2. *Specific precautions related to physiotherapy in patients with multiple orthopaedic injuries*

7.9.2.1. *Adult patients*

- In general, fracture sites must be supported during therapy to avoid excessive movement. Rotation and undue pain at the fracture site should be avoided.

- Resistance distal to the fracture site should be avoided.
- The available ROM at a joint should correlate with the pathology and permissible movement. If ROM is initially limited as part of the management of the injury, it should be gradually increased as allowed.
- Stability of the fracture will determine the amount of weight-bearing that may occur, and this must be established prior to mobilisation. Unstable fractures will generally not allow any degree of weight-bearing.
- If a patient has sustained multiple fractures, especially when they are of different limbs (such as bilateral lower extremity fractures or an upper and lower extremity fracture), mobilisation may be difficult. More staff may be required to assist when the patient has limited ability to participate. Care must be taken to ensure that patients do not bear excessive weight on any limb, which may compromise healing. In such cases, the benefits of being upright in a chair (especially on the pulmonary and neurological systems) need to be weighed up against the difficulty of mobilisation and the limited functional benefits of a simple sheet transfer for a patient. Modern electric beds can be positioned to simulate a chair and early during the patient's stay in the ICU this may be the technique of choice (Hall and Brody, 2005).
- In patients who have sustained brachial plexus injury and present with muscle paralysis, traction through the shoulder joint must be avoided, especially when moving the patient in bed or assisting with transfers in and out of bed. Passive shoulder joint ROM must be carefully maintained for all joints of the upper limb.
- If a vascular or nerve repair was undertaken, the repaired artery or nerve may allow for only limited ROM of the associated joints. Range of motion exercises and muscle stretching must be limited to prevent any strain on the graft. It is vital to maintain joint ROM and muscle length without stressing an injured or repaired artery or nerve while it recovers; therefore precautions to movement must be discussed with the surgeon.
- Fractures of the shoulder girdle are often treated with a sling or brace. Minor displacement at the fracture site would necessitate a period of two weeks in a sling. Major displacement may necessitate wearing a sling for up to five weeks.

- Type A (stable) pelvic fractures are treated symptomatically. Mobilisation is performed as pain allows, with weight-bearing according to level of pain experienced.
- Type B1 (open book unstable) pelvic fractures are managed with bed rest for four weeks if the patient has additional injuries, after which mobilisation using partial or full weight-bearing can be performed. Where the symphysis pubis gap is less than 2.5 cm, patients require bed rest for four weeks and then the fracture is treated as stable. If the fracture was stabilised surgically, patients are allowed to mobilise earlier.
- Type B2 and B3 (ipsilateral and contralateral unstable) pelvic fractures are managed with external fixators or plates. In such cases hip flexion should be limited to 45° for four weeks. If a pelvic sling is used no sitting is permitted for four weeks. As with all complex fractures, guidance should be sought from the orthopaedic surgeon on when sitting and mobilisation may begin, as this may vary between patients.
- Type C (rotationally and vertically unstable) pelvic fractures are usually managed with external fixation. Patients are on bed rest for six weeks and may only sit up to 45° hip flexion after three weeks. After the initial six weeks bed rest, they should mobilise non-weight bearing for a further six weeks. Guidance should be sought from the orthopaedic surgeon, as mentioned above.
- Joint dislocations may require a period of bed rest or non-weight bearing, the duration of which should be determined through communication with the orthopaedic surgeon.
- It is essential to elevate injured limbs to minimise oedema, as previously mentioned. This is especially relevant in injured lower limbs following mobilisation to prevent oedema that is exacerbated by gravity. Swelling of a limb can lead to excessive pain and compromise the healing process.
- When deep vein thrombosis is suspected, patients are generally placed on anticoagulation therapy. Thrombo-embolic disease (TED) stockings are a standard of care together with anticoagulation and mobilisation in many hospitals nowadays. Patients must mobilise while wearing the stockings, but they can be slippery on smooth floors; therefore patients must wear slippers or shoes. Alternatively, the TED

stockings may be rolled up around the ankle, with the proviso that it is unrolled following mobilisation, as ankle pressure is increased tremendously if the stocking is not used as a single layer.

- Malunion, delayed union or non-union of fractures may be avoided in part by ensuring that the correct amount of weight-bearing is used during mobilisation. The physiotherapist should be aware that in a patient who has concomitant traumatic brain injury (with cognitive impairment), mobilisation may result in excessive weight-bearing of a fracture site.
- If a patient presents with intense pain during passive stretching of the joints distal to a fracture, it is possible that compartment syndrome has developed. The physiotherapist should immediately inform the surgeon regarding this possibility.
- In cases of myositis ossificans and heterotopic ossification, vigorous passive mobilisation will increase muscle damage and worsen the condition. Joints should be passively moved only in the ROM where no resistance is felt.

7.9.2.2. *Paediatric patients*

- In addition to the precautions described above, the physiotherapist managing a child with orthopaedic injuries should be aware that the presence of an open fracture is not protective against the development of compartment syndrome in children, which most often occurs in the leg and forearm (Abdelgawad and Kanlic, 2011). The limb should not be elevated above the heart, as this can further decrease limb perfusion (Abdelgawad and Kanlic, 2011).
- Times to weight bearing of fractured limbs in children may differ from adults, so discussion with the orthopaedic surgeon is essential before mobilising.
- The developmental stage of the child must be considered before prescribing walking aids.

7.10. Physiotherapy Intervention

Polytrauma patients may present very differently from each other. Patient response to rehabilitation interventions may be related to the site and number of fractures or compromised joints, pain intensity and presence of premorbid conditions. Recommendations provided here are based on evidence as well as expert opinion in the absence of research evidence.

7.10.1. *Respiratory system*

As mentioned earlier in this chapter, patients who present with multiple extremity fractures often present with injuries to other bodily organs and systems.

The reader is referred to:

- Chapter 5 (Section 5.6.1) for the physiotherapy management of the pulmonary system of a patient who presents with abdominal or thoracic injuries;
- Chapter 6 (Section 6.8.3) for the pulmonary physiotherapy management of a patient with burn injuries to the thorax;
- Chapter 8 (Section 8.9.1) for physiotherapy interventions used for pulmonary system care in patients who present with spinal cord injury; and
- Chapter 9 (Section 9.8.1) for the physiotherapy management of patients with traumatic brain injury to prevent and treat respiratory system complications.

7.10.2. *Neuromusculoskeletal system*

7.10.2.1. *Pain*

Pain is one of the most common complaints from patients following orthopaedic injury. The origin of pain in the early phase after injury is usually from the bone and soft tissue affected by the traumatic event. Joint stiffness in the latter phases following injury may also contribute to pain.

In the acute care setting, pain in adult patients is managed with the administration of pharmacological agents. Pain may be under-treated in critically ill patients who are unresponsive. Pain should always be considered as a causative factor for raised heart rate and blood pressure levels in these patients, and the dosage of analgesic medication administered should be reviewed on a daily basis. Non-pharmacological therapy such as cold and heat therapy may also be used to reduce swelling around the fracture site and to encourage the relaxation of muscle fibres, respectively, in alert patients. Heat therapy should only be used when haemorrhage from the initial injury is no longer a concern. Elevation of the limb(s) to reduce oedema may also contribute to a reduction in the level of pain experienced by the patient. When the patient is awake and cooperative and the fracture site stabilised, active exercises can be used to reduce joint stiffness and therefore level of pain.

Pain in children can be difficult to diagnose, particularly in young patients and in those with reduced levels of consciousness, and consequently it is recognised that pain in children is often under-treated. Various scales can be used to assess levels of pain in these groups. Children of three years and older have been shown to be able to identify and report pain intensity accurately. In the context of orthopaedic injury, both the injury itself and the treatment can cause the child pain (Ali *et al.*, 2010). Various pharmacological and non-pharmacological strategies for pain management are available for children, similar to adults. Non-pharmacological strategies include icing, appropriate immobilisation and positioning of the affected limb, preparatory information, relaxation and distraction, breathing techniques, emotional support, music therapy and positive reinforcement (Ali *et al.*, 2010).

7.10.2.2. *Joint range of motion*

Patients with multiple traumatic injuries may be very unwell at hospital admission and require close observation and care in the ICU. At this stage, treatment of the orthopaedic injuries may not be the most important component of overall patient management and treatment may simply be focused on preserving fracture stabilisation or joint stability.

7.10.2.2.1. Sedated patient in the ICU

After the patient's condition has stabilised, early and effective rehabilitation should be initiated in the ICU setting. Passive ROM exercises, within the limitations posed by the orthopaedic injuries, can be used to prevent joint stiffness and loss of ROM. A continuous passive motion device or passive bed cycling may be used to maintain joint ROM within the limitations posed by the patient's injuries. Functional bracing may also reduce joint complications. Maintaining maximum possible and permissible ROM in all joints is paramount.

Ligaments of the knee and ankle might be disrupted with traumatic injuries to the lower extremity. These injuries are frequently diagnosed by physiotherapists during passive ROM exercises. Typically, ligament repairs might be performed later, once the patient is stable. Depending on the ligament and the type of repair, patients may wear a ROM brace to limit motion at the joint. Exercise programmes should focus on maintaining ROM of the joint as allowed (McRae, 2006).

7.10.2.2.2. Cooperative intubated or spontaneously breathing patient

As soon as the patient is able to respond to commands, active-assisted and active ROM exercises should be introduced as part of their care in the ICU. Accessory joint mobilisations may be used if indicated. Exercise must be performed within the limits of pain and comfort. Exercise programmes must be controlled and progressive to increase ROM without exacerbating injury or compromising healing. Active bed cycling is an effective means of encouraging patient participation in rehabilitation.

Handling is important with those patients that have had a dislocation, as they are at risk from subsequent dislocations. Guidance should be sought from the orthopaedic surgeon on limitations to movement and when exercise may begin. Muscle strengthening and joint stabilisation retraining are important components of the rehabilitation of patients with dislocated joints. The reader is referred to Section 7.12 for further information.

7.10.2.3. *Muscle strength*

If a patient is awake and cooperative, the physiotherapist should progress to using active and active-resisted exercises to maintain the patient's strength in the unaffected limbs and improve the strength of all muscles affected by the traumatic injury (Fig. 7.9).

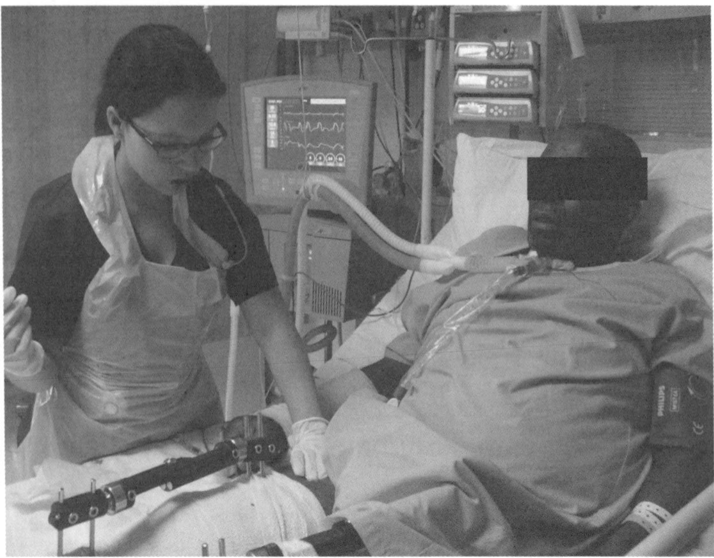

Fig. 7.9: Intubated cooperative patient with bilateral tibial plateau fractures, managed with external fixation, performing active muscle contraction to improve quadriceps strength with supervision of a physiotherapist.

Each patient's exercise programme should be individualised according to their needs. Strengthening exercises for deconditioned patients may begin with isometric muscle contractions around the injured area, which should be progressed to isotonic exercises as soon as it is safe to do so. Rehabilitation is further progressed with the application of gentle resistance (when appropriate) to active exercises, followed by more resistance as the patient's condition allows. Moderate resistance exercise counteracts decreases in muscle protein synthesis, which often develops due to inflammation and critical illness and immobility (Hopkins and Spuhler, 2009; Jakob and Takala, 2009). Regaining and maintaining muscle strength in the affected joint, unaffected limbs and core muscles is therefore an important component of any rehabilitation programme to counteract the loss of muscle power and muscle mass and to improve functional ability (Schweikert *et al.*, 2009; Pohlman *et al.*, 2010; Pattanshetty and Gaude, 2011). The reader is referred to Chapter 4 (Section 4.1.2) for information on exercise prescription for resistance exercise training in the acute care setting.

In patients with multiple orthopaedic injuries, it is important to maintain global body conditioning to ensure that they have adequate muscle strength in their unaffected limbs to perform ADL while they are not allowed to bear weight through the injured limbs, e.g. patients with multiple lower limb fractures need great upper body strength in order to perform transfers if bearing full weight on their lower extremities is not permissible. Pre-gait exercise training is important, and focus should be placed on strength training of, in particular, the gluteus maximus and quadriceps muscle groups to ensure adequate strength for full weight-bearing on one leg if the other is to be partial or non-weight bearing. Optimal upper limb strength is essential for safe mobilisation with walking aids (Schweikert *et al.*, 2009; Pohlman *et al.*, 2010; Pattanshetty and Gaude, 2011).

Any patient on prolonged bed rest (e.g. those with pelvic fractures or on traction) is at risk of developing pressure sores, deep vein thrombosis, joint contractures and general deconditioning. They require an individualised bed exercise programme that focuses particularly on upper body and trunk strength and strengthening of the non-affected leg. These patients must be encouraged to assist in daily functional activities and be shown ways to perform pressure relief. Nursing staff caring for such patients should also be orientated by the physiotherapist as to the extent to which the patient can assist with functional activities.

7.10.2.4. Functional activity, mobilisation and exercise endurance

Rehabilitation should be based on the needs of each individual patient, as previously mentioned, taking into consideration the patient's orthopaedic and other associated injuries. For all injuries, the site and extent of injury will determine the extent of rehabilitation and the type of approach used.

With clearance from the orthopaedic surgeon and guidance on acceptable weight-bearing status depending on the type and stability of the fracture, early mobilisation should be a constant consideration for any patient (Dubov *et al.*, 2008). The possibility of initiation of activity and mobilisation should be assessed daily. Such mobilisation includes bed mobility, sitting over the edge of the bed, transfers to a chair and ambulation. Early mobilisation and restoration of gait with walking aids, if appropriate, should be part of rehabilitation in the acute care setting (Schweikert *et al.*, 2009; Pohlman *et al.*, 2010; Pattanshetty and Gaude, 2011). Weight-bearing and muscle activity are more effective at promoting bony union than fixator stiffness (Hipp and Hayes, 2009). Gait and balance re-education should therefore start as soon as possible when a patient is awake, cooperative and able to follow commands, to such an extent that this can be done safely without compromising healing (Hall and Brody, 2005).

Patients with ligament repairs to the knee or ankle are often allowed to mobilise with a walking aid wearing a ROM brace, if other injuries allow. Ambulation is with some degree of weight-bearing of the affected joint (McRae, 2006).

As the patient's ability to perform functional activities and ambulation improves, the frequency and duration of daily treatment sessions can be increased. This will assist with improving the patient's exercise tolerance. The reader is referred to Chapter 4 (Section 4.1.2) for guidelines on aerobic exercise prescription for patients in the acute care setting. Activities such as stair climbing and equipment such as stationary bicycles or a treadmill in the physiotherapy in-hospital department may be used for cardiovascular exercise training, if permitted in view of the patient's injuries.

In addition, education and advice to the patient and caregivers regarding treatment, exercises, contraindications and precautions, as well as prognosis and time to recovery, should be undertaken early in the patient's rehabilitation (Hall and Brody, 2005).

7.10.2.5. *Paediatric considerations*

Post-cast care does not usually require physiotherapy intervention, as most children will move and weight-bear as soon as union occurs. The child should be allowed to spontaneously return to activity and mobilisation but vigorous play should be limited for one month (Staheli, 2006). Muscle strengthening is accomplished in young children using play activities, graded as to levels of resistance and assistance. Strengthening can be done in combination with neurodevelopmental facilitation and play therapy, which can also be used to maintain or improve ROM. Graded active mobilisation at an age-appropriate level should be encouraged. This is usually much easier in children than in adults, as they will generally move if they are able. For older children able to follow commands, the same principles as for adult rehabilitation apply. The emotional and chronological age of the child must be taken into account when considering the facilitation of ADL and improving levels of function.

7.10.3. *Patient response to treatment*

Outcome measures for patients with multiple orthopaedic injuries are highly variable and depend on the site of the injury and the number of areas involved. Irrespective of this, the ultimate outcome measure for all patients should be function and to what degree they can return to their premorbid status. Some outcome measures may be more useful than others at particular stages of recovery. The reader is referred to Chapter 4 (Section 4.3) for a list of subjective and objective markers, as well as outcome measurement tools to use during the evaluation of the effectiveness of treatment interventions used for the rehabilitation of patients with multiple orthopaedic injuries.

7.11. Clinical Case Scenarios

7.11.1. *Case scenario of an adult patient*

A healthy 28-year-old man works in a factory and packs goods into boxes from the conveyor belt. The filled boxes are then moved to the storage area of the factory by fork lift. The driver of the fork lift was coming around a corner inside the factory at high speed, lost control of the vehicle and crashed into the conveyor belt worker, pinning him between the conveyor belt and the vehicle. An ambulance was called and the man was brought to the emergency department of your trauma centre. During the primary and secondary surveys it was found that he sustained an open book pelvic fracture (Tile type B1), open fracture of the left tibia and fibula with extensive soft tissue damage and periosteal stripping (Type IIIB Gustilo-Anderson classification) and blunt trauma to the lower abdomen, with significant abdominal distension due to internal bleeding. He did not sustain any head trauma. He was immediately taken to theatre for exploratory laparotomy to control the internal bleeding, and external fixators were placed on his pelvis as well as the left tibia and fibula to stabilise the fractures. After surgery he was transferred to the ICU for continued MV, observation and care.

On day three following admission to the ICU he was taken back to theatre for closure of the abdominal wound and debridement of the wound at the fracture site on the left lower leg. After a few days his general condition deteriorated and he was diagnosed with sepsis originating from the contaminated wound on the left lower leg. He developed acute renal failure and was treated with daily dialysis until kidney function was restored. After a week in the ICU a tracheostomy was performed, as prolonged ventilation was anticipated due to the severity of his illness. A below knee amputation was performed on day 13 of his ICU stay. Afterwards his condition gradually improved and he was successfully extubated on day 27.

- What precautions and contraindications would you adhere to during physiotherapy management of this patient while he is intubated and ventilated?
- What impairments in relation to activity and participation (according to the international classification of function) would you expect this patient to present with?

7.11.1.1. *Discussion*

7.11.1.1.1. Precautions and contraindications to physiotherapy intervention

- Adherence to universal infection control principles when working in the ICU is an essential component of this patient's physiotherapy management. Physiotherapists work in close contact with patients and diligence in hand washing, removal of protective clothing and cleaning of equipment used during treatment are important to prevent infection from spreading to other patients in the ICU.
- The physiotherapist should liaise with the nursing staff to ensure adequate analgesia is administered to the patient prior to physiotherapy treatment.

- If secretion retention is detected in this patient's anterior basal lung segments, the physiotherapist should be cautious to apply only gentle manual chest clearance techniques when treating these segments, as the patient is likely to experience pain from his swollen abdomen following laparotomy. Careful observation of the patient's response to treatment is advised, and if he seems to be in too much pain and discomfort, alternative methods for mobilisation of secretions should be used.
- The physiotherapist should apply support to the laparotomy incision site when the patient coughs to facilitate a more effective cough effort. As the patient wakes up from sedation, the physiotherapist should teach him how to support his own wound when coughing.
- Before the patient is suctioned, preoxygenation should be applied through the ventilator to avoid episodes of hypoxaemia during the procedure. Between suction passes the patient should be reconnected to the ventilator circuit or the manual hyperinflation (MHI) circuit to ensure adequate provision of oxygen therapy.
- Suction of the artificial airway should be performed in an aseptic manner.
- The physiotherapist should take care not to allow the ventilator circuit to pull on the tracheostomy tube during position changes in bed. Excessive pulling on the tracheostomy can lead to displacement of the tube as well as enlargement of the stoma wound and delayed wound closure after extubation.
- Generally a four-week period of bed rest is prescribed for a Tile type B1 pelvic fracture. As the patient regains consciousness in the ICU, the physiotherapist should discuss the benefits and risks of him sitting up in bed with the orthopaedic team.
- The physiotherapist and nursing staff should be aware of the dimensions of the external fixator in the pelvis to ensure that no pressure is applied to the fixator when turning the patient in bed.
- In an attempt to reduce the amount of pain experienced by the patient during turning, the physiotherapist should try to log roll the patient by limiting the amount of shoulder girdle and hip dissociation during the turn.
- There is a strong possibility that the patient will present with oedema of the left leg following the amputation. The physiotherapist may elevate the limb onto one or two pillows placed length-wise under the leg to reduce swelling, but must ensure that the whole leg is supported.

If the knee is not supported by the pillow it will hyperextend and cause severe patient discomfort. Pillows placed only under the knee will encourage shortening of the hamstring muscles and result in loss of knee extension ROM. This will have negative consequences on the patient's ability to mobilise with a prosthetic leg in future.

- A pillow or two should be placed as support under the amputated limb when turning the patient.

7.11.1.1.2. Limitations related to activity and participation

The patient's severity of illness following the traumatic event, prolonged inflammation and sepsis and prolonged period of immobility would put him at risk of developing ICU-acquired weakness. ICU-acquired weakness is characterised by muscle protein breakdown and general muscle weakness, which involves the muscles of respiration and the extremities. Muscle weakness for this patient would be further exaggerated due to pain from his orthopaedic injuries and the surgical procedures that he underwent. Respiratory muscle weakness leads to decreased lung volumes and lung capacities. These result in less diffusion of oxygen molecules across the alveolar-capillary membranes and therefore less oxygen delivery at tissue level; as a result, the patient is likely to suffer from shortness of breath and fatigue. Blood lost from the patient's circulatory system after the amputation will lead to changes in his cardiac output, which will contribute to poorer oxygen delivery at tissue level and, consequently, shortness of breath and fatigue.

Fatigue, muscle weakness and the limitation caused by his injuries negatively impact his ability to perform ADL such as moving in bed, sitting up over the side of the bed, performing sit-to-stand and mobilising away from the bedside. His balance in sitting and standing will be influenced by pain from the pelvic fracture as well as the left below knee amputation. He is likely to experience low levels of exercise endurance, which will affect his ability to mobilise independently with a walking aid in the ICU and in the ward.

The ICU physiotherapist should give a detailed handover of the patient to the ward physiotherapist to ensure progression of rehabilitation. Before discharge to a rehabilitation facility or home, a discussion should be held between the physiotherapist and other members of the interdisciplinary team regarding the patient's eligibility for receiving a prosthetic leg, as this will influence his rehabilitation as well as him returning to his job. A prosthetic leg will make is easier for this patient to use public transportation or to drive his own car, be more independent with regards to ADL at home and reintegrate well back into the community.

7.11.2. *Case scenario of a paediatric patient*

A seven-year-old girl was admitted to the paediatric ICU directly on arrival to the hospital via ambulance, after a motor vehicle-pedestrian accident. She was hit by a taxi whilst walking on the pavement. She sustained the following injuries:

- closed head injury with Glasgow coma scale score of six out of 10 (eye response two, verbal response two, motor response two) on admission and moderately raised intracranial pressure;
- pulmonary contusion of the right lung;
- rib fractures on the right thoracic cage (no flail segments);
- right mid-shaft open femur fracture with severe soft tissue damage; and
- right closed humeral fracture (stabilised in the emergency department using a U-slab).

Her spine was cleared clinically and radiologically. She was intubated and ventilated with brain and lung protective strategies with appropriate levels of sedation and analgesia. On day one following admission, surgical reduction, debridement and external fixation of the right femur were performed. Her level of consciousness improved rapidly and on day three the intracranial pressure (ICP) monitor was removed. From day three she was actively weaned with reduced sedation levels and she was extubated on day four. Whilst on the ventilator the nursing staff reported suctioning fresh blood, but by extubation the secretions were reported as thick and brown (old blood) or creamy. She was discharged from the paediatric ICU on day five and had a cast placed on her right arm to stabilise the humeral fracture. Mobilisation was challenging, with the humeral fracture restricting use of crutches and the need for non-weight bearing activity for five weeks.

- How would you manage this child in the ICU and in the ward during the non-weight bearing phase of recovery?

7.11.2.1. *Discussion*

Sufficient analgesia must be given. It would not be appropriate to treat the chest until active bleeding from the pulmonary contusion was resolved (e.g. while fresh blood was suctioned). Raised ICP is a precaution to chest physiotherapy and mobilisation, so active prophylactic intervention would be limited during the acute phase (first two to three days). During the acute phase, physiotherapy management would be focussed on maintaining available ROM within the constraints of the fracture sites. Positioning with the head of bed raised would be desirable, with regular turning to prevent pressure sores and respiratory complications. Elevation of the right leg and arm would be beneficial to reduce oedema.

Once the ICP stabilised and the secretions were no longer containing fresh blood, it would be appropriate to position the child to optimise ventilation and oxygenation, determined on an individual basis (Chapter 4), taking into account the limits imposed by the fixed and unstable fractures, respectively. If secretion retention was assessed as a problem, gentle vibrations over the contused lung using a vibromat would be appropriate, followed by endotracheal suctioning to clear the secretions.

It is important to obtain a history of previous levels of motor and cognitive functioning from a parent or caregiver in order to determine appropriate aims of therapy. The external fixator site should be assessed for possible infection and both limbs with fractures should be assessed for the possibility of compartment syndrome. Functional ability and voluntary movement should be assessed on an ongoing basis to determine muscle strength, ROM, cognition and the presence of concomitant nerve injuries.

After moving to the ward, graded mobilisation can occur whilst continuing active exercises to maintain ROM and strengthen muscles. Mobilisation must be non-weight bearing through the right leg, so use one-leg transfers, standing on one leg to start with. Once the surgeon has given approval, crutch walking could be considered, using a gutter crutch for the right arm. The ability to follow commands and understand risks, as well as establishment of the patient's developmental stage, is imperative before starting this part of rehabilitation. Most seven-year-olds should be able to accomplish this, but the head injury may limit compliance and this must therefore be carefully assessed. If the child does not understand the instructions, or is not capable of following them, it is preferable to continue bed exercises, transfers, one-legged standing with support, and sitting out of bed; but wait until partial weight bearing is permitted before resuming crutch walk education.

In the ward, chest physiotherapy should continue in order to prevent complications of immobility. Techniques such as deep breathing exercises, positive expiratory pressure (PEP) therapy (bubble PEP bottle or blowing games), forced expiratory technique (huffing) and supported coughing (preferably in sitting) could be used.

7.12. Suggested Reading Material for Further Study

Ventilator-induced lung injury (PulmCCM, 2012; Slutsky and Ranieri, 2013); rehabilitation guideline for rotator cuff repair (Van der Meijden *et al.*, 2012); rehabilitation guidelines for joint dislocations (Wilk *et al.*, 2006; Gammons, 2014); hand and wrist injuries (Adams and Hamblen, 2005); and amputation and prosthetics (Smith *et al.*, 2004).

7.13. Conclusion

The patient with critical illness due to multiple orthopaedic injuries poses a challenge to physiotherapists who work in acute care, as they need to incorporate orthopaedic rehabilitation in their patient management plan together with other forms of therapy. A patient's pre-morbid state will directly affect the intensity of therapy that a patient is able to undertake; for example, a patient with AIDS and newly fractured pelvis and femur would need a different approach to rehabilitation than a previously healthy patient with similar injuries. The information in this chapter should assist the physiotherapist in providing effective and safe care for patients with multiple orthopaedic injuries during the acute phase of management, until they are transferred to a rehabilitation setting or home with outpatient referral for continued rehabilitation.

Bibliography

Abdelgawad, A.A., and Kanlic, E.M. (2011). Orthopedic management of children with multiple injuries, *J. Trauma,* **70**, 1568–2574.

Adams, J.C., and Hamblen, D.L. (2005). *Outlines of Fractures*, 11th edn,, Churchill Livingstone, Edinburgh.

Ali, S., Drendel, A.L., Kircher, J., *et al.* (2010). Pain management of musculo-skeletal injuries in children. Current state and future directions, *Pediatr. Emerg. Care,* **26**, 518–527.

American Academy of Pediatrics and Pediatric Orthopaedic Society of North America. (2008). Management of pediatric trauma, *Pediatrics,* **121**, 849–854.

American Association of Orthopaedic Surgeons (AAOS). (2010). *Calcaneus (Heel Bone) Fractures*. OrthoInfo. [Online] Available at: http://orthoinfo.aaos.org/topic.cfm?topic=A00524 [Accessed 24 May 2014].

Augat, P., Burger, J., and Schorlemmer, S. (2003). Shear movement at the fracture site delays healing in a diaphyseal fracture model, *J. Orthop. Res.,* **21**, 1011–1017.

Bosse, M.J., and Kellam, J.F. (2009). 'Damage control orthopaedic surgery: a strategy for the orthopaedic care of the critically injured patient', in Browner, B.D., Levine, A.M., Jupiter, J.B., *et al.* (eds), *Skeletal Trauma: Basic Science, Management and Reconstruction*, 4th edn., Saunders Elsevier, Philadelphia, PA, pp. 197–218.

Boyd, A.S., Benjamin, H.J., and Asplund, C. (2009). Principles of casting and splinting, *Am. Fam. Physician,* **79**, 16–24.

Brautigam, R.T., Sheppard, R., Robinson, K.J., *et al.* (2009). 'Evaluation and treatment of the multiple-trauma patient', in Browner, B.D., Levine, A.M., Jupiter, J.B., *et al.* (eds), *Skeletal Trauma: Basic Science, Management and Reconstruction*, 4th edn., Saunders Elsevier, Philadelphia, PA, pp. 177–195.

Carroll, E.A., Schweppe, M., Langfitt, M., *et al.* (2012). Management of humeral shaft fractures, *J. Am. Acad. Orthop. Sur.,* **20**, 423–433.

Clements, J.R., and Schopf, R. (2013). Advance in forefoot trauma, *Clin. Podiatr. Med. Surg.,* **30**, 435–444.

Cordey, J., Borgeaud, M:., and Perren, S.M. (2000). Force transfer between the plate and the bone: relative importance of the bending stiffness of the screws and the friction between plate and bone, *Injury,* **31**, 21–28.

Dandy, D.J., and Edwards, D.J. (2009). *Essential Orthopaedics and Trauma*, 5th edn., Churchill Livingstone Elsevier, Edinburgh.

Deitch, E.A., and Dayal, S.D. (2006). Intensive care unit management of the trauma patient, *Crit. Care Med.,* **34**, 2294–2301.

De Jonghe, B., Lacherade, J.C., Sharshar, T., *et al.* (2009). Intensive care unit-acquired weakness: risk factors and prevention, *Crit. Care Med.,* **37** [Suppl], S309–S315.

Dubov, W., Badellino, M.M., and Pasquale, M.D. (2008). 'Trauma rehabilitation', in Asensio, J.A., and Trunkey, D.D. (eds), *Current Therapy of Trauma and Surgical Critical Care*, Elsevier Mosby, London, pp. 751–757.

Ebraheim, N.A., Martin, A., Sochacki, K.R., *et al.* (2013). Nonunion of distal femoral fractures: a systematic review, *Orthop. Surg.,* **5**, 46–50.

Fragomen, A.T., and Rozbruch, S.R. (2007). The mechanics of external fixation, *HSS Journal,* **3**, 13–29.

Gammons, M. (2014). *Hip Dislocation Treatment and Management*. Medccape. [Online] Available at: http://emedicine.medscape.com/article/86930-treatment [Accessed 24 May 2014].

Gao, Y.S., Ai, Z.S., Zhu, Z.H., *et al.* (2013). Injury-to-surgery interval does not affect postfracture osteonecrosis of the femoral head in young adults: a systematic review, *Eur. J. Orthop. Surg. Traumatol.,* **23**, 203–209.

Gaston, M.S., and Simpson, A.H.R.W. (2007). Inhibition of fracture healing: a review article, *J. Bone Joint Surg. (Br).,* **89B**, 1553–1560.

Green, N.E., and Swiontkowski, M.F. (2009). *Skeletal Trauma in Children*, 4th edn., Elsevier, London.

Groenewald, P., Bradshaw, D., Daniels, J., *et al.* (2008). *Cause of Death and Premature Mortality in Cape Town, 2001–2006.* Cape Town: South African Medical Research Council. [Online] Available at: http://www.mrc.ac.za/bod/premort_cpt.pdf [Accessed 25 July 2014].

Gupta, A., and Reilly, C.S. (2007). Fat embolism, *Cont. Educ. Anaesth. Crit. Care Pain,* **7**, 148–151.

Gustilo, R.B., Mendoza, R.M., and Williams, D.N. (1984). Problems in the management of type III (severe) open fractures: a new classification of type III open fractures, *J. Trauma,* **24**, 742–746.

Hall, C.M., and Brody, L.T. (2005). *Therapeutic Exercise: Moving Toward Function*, 2nd edn., Lippincott, Williams and Wilkins, Philadelphia, PA.

Hayek, T.E., Daher, A.A., Meouchy, W., *et al.* (2004). External fixators in the treatment of fractures in children, *J. Pediatr. Orthop.,* **13**, 103–109.

Henrichs, A. (2004). A review of knee dislocations, *J. Athl. Train.,* **39**, 365–369.

Hernandez, R.K., Do, T.P., Critchlow, C.W., *et al.* (2012). Patient-related risk factors for fracture-healing complications in the United Kingdom general practice research database, *Acta Orthop.,* **83**, 653–660.

Hipp, J.A., and Hayes, W.C. (2009). 'Biomechanics of fractures', in Browner, B.D., Levine, A.M., Jupiter, J.B., *et al.* (eds), *Skeletal Trauma: Basic Science, Management and Reconstruction*, 4th edn., Saunders Elsevier, Philadelphia, PA, pp. 51–82.

Hopkins, R.O., and Spuhler, V.J. (2009). Strategies for promoting early activity in critically ill mechanically ventilated patient, *AACN Adv. Crit. Care,* **20**, 277–289.

Ip, D. (2008). 'Trauma to the lower extremities', in Ip, D. (ed.), *Orthopaedic Traumatology — A Resident's Guide*, 2nd edn., Springer, Philadelphia, PA, pp. 355–495.

Jakob, S.M., and Takala, J. (2009). Physical and occupational therapy during sedation stops, *Lancet,* **373**, 1824–1826.

Jayakumar, P., Barry, M., and Ramachandran, M. (2010). Orthopaedic aspects of paediatric non-accidental injury, *J. Bone Joint Surg. [Br],* **92**, B189–B195.

Kay, R.M., and Skaggs, D.J. (2006). Pediatric polytrauma management, *J. Pediatr. Orthop.,* **26**, 268–277.

Kemp, A., Dunstan, F., Harrison, S., *et al.* (2008). Patterns of skeletal fractures in child abuse: systematic review, *Br. Med. J.,* **337**, a1518. [Online] Available at: http://www.bmj.com/content/337/bmj.a1518.long [Accessed 15 November 2014].

Khoshhal, K.I., and Kiefer, G.N. (2005). Physeal bridge resection, *J. Am. Acad. Orthop. Sur.,* **13**, 47–58.

Kim, H.T., Ahn, J.M., Hur, J.O., *et al.* (2011). Reconstruction of acetabular posterior wall fractures, *Clin. Orthop. Surg.,* **3**, 114–120.

Kinner, B., Tietz, S., Müller, F., *et al.* (2011). Outcome after complex trauma of the foot, *J. Trauma,* **70**, 159–169.

Kool, D.R., and Blickman, J.G. (2007). Advanced trauma life support. ABCDE from a radiological point of view, *Emerg. Radiol.,* **14**, 135–141.

Lee, J.J., Patel, R., Biermann, J.S., *et al.* (2013). The musculoskeletal effects of cigarette smoking, *J. Bone Joint Surg. Am.,* **95**, 850–859.

Li, J., Ahmad, T., Spetea, M., *et al.* (2001). Bone reinnervation after fracture: a study in the rat, *J. Bone Miner. Res.,* **16**, 1505–1510.

Lindaman, L.M. (2001). Bone healing in children, *Clin. Podiatr. Med. Surg.,* **18**, 97–108.

Lundy, D.W., and Johnson, K.D. (2001). Floating knee injuries: ipsilateral fractures of the femur and tibia, *J. Am. Acad. Orthop. Sur.,* **9**, 238–245.

McRae, R. (2006). 'Fractures and dislocations', in McRae, R. (ed.), *Pocketbook of Orthopaedics and Fractures*, Churchill Livingstone Elsevier, Edinburgh, pp. 211–268.

Mejaddam, A.Y., and Velmahos, G.C. (2012). Randomized controlled trials affecting polytrauma care, *Eur. J. Trauma Emerg. Surg.,* **38**, 211–221.

Mooney, J.F. (2012). The use of 'damage control orthopedics' techniques in children with segmental open femur fractures, *J. Pediatr. Orthop.,* **B21**, 400–403.

Musgrave, D.S., and Mendelson, S.A. (2002). Pediatric orthopedic trauma: principles in management, *Crit. Care Med.,* **30** [Suppl], S431–S443.

National Institute of Health and Care Excellence (NICE). (2009). *Rehabilitation after Critical Illness. Clinical Guideline 83*. NICE. [Online] Available at: http://www.nice.org.uk/guidance/cG83 [Accessed 25 July 2014].

National Trauma Data Bank Report. (2013). *American College of Surgeons Trauma Registry*. National Trauma Data Bank. [Online] Available at: www.facs.org/trauma/ntdb.html [Accessed 20 May 2014].

Pandya, N.K., Baldwin, K., Wolfgruber, H., *et al.* (2009). Child abuse and orthopaedic injury patterns: analysis at a level 1 pediatric trauma center, *J. Pediatr. Orthop.,* **29**, 618–625.

Pattanshetty, R.B., and Gaude, G.S. (2011). Critical illness myopathy and polyneuropathy — a challenge for physiotherapists in the intensive care units, *Indian J. Crit. Care Med.,* **15**, 78–81.

Penn-Barwell, J.G. (2011). Outcomes in lower limb amputation following trauma: a systematic review and meta-analysis, *Injury,* **42**, 1474–1479.

Pohlman, M.C., Schweikert, W.D., Pohlman, A.S., *et al.* (2010). Feasibility of physical and occupational therapy beginning from initiation of mechanical ventilation, *Crit. Care Med.,* **38**, 2089–2094.

PulmCCM. (2012). *Mechanical Ventilation in ARDS: 2014 Update*. PulmCCM. [Online] Available at: http://pulmccm.org/main/2012/review-articles/mechanical-ventilation-in-ards-2012-update/ [Accessed 25 July 2014].

Ratini, M. (2014). *Understanding Bone Fractures*. WebMD. [Online] Available at: http://www.webmd.com/a-to-z-guides/understanding-fractures-basic-information [Accessed 21 May 2014].

Rennie, L., Court-Brown, C.M., Mok, J.Y., *et al.* (2007). The epidemiology of fractures in children, *Injury,* **38**, 913–922.

Ricci, W.M., Gallagher, B.G., and Haidukewych, G.J. (2009). Intramedullary nailing of femoral shaft fractures, *J. Am. Acad. Orthop. Sur.,* **17**, 296–305.

Roberts, C.S., Pape, H.C., Jones, A.L., *et al.* (2005). Damage control orthopaedics, *J. Bone Joint Surg.,* **87**, 434–449.

Schweikert, W.D., Pohlman, M.C., Pohlman, A.S., *et al.* (2009). Early physical and occupational therapy in mechanically ventilated, critically ill patients: a randomized controlled trial, *Lancet,* **373**, 1874–1882.

Skaggs, D.L., and Flynn, J.M. (2006). *Staying out of Trouble in Pediatric Orthopaedics*, Lippincott & Williams, Philadelphia, PA.

Slutsky, A.S., and Ranieri, V.M. (2013). Ventilator-induced lung injury: review article, *N. Engl. J. Med.,* **369**, 2126–2136.

Smith, D.G., Michael, J.W., and Bowker, H.J. (2004). *Atlas of Amputations and Limb Deficiencies. Surgical, Prosthetic and Rehabilitation Principles*, 3rd edn., American Association of Orthopaedic Surgeons, Rosemont, IL.

South African Medical Research Council. (2008). *Frequently Asked Questions. Are the Cause of Death Statistics Reliable?* MRC South Africa. [Online] Available at: http://www.mrc.ac.za/bod/faqstatistics.htm [Accessed August 2013].

Staheli, L.T. (2006). *Practice of Pediatric Orthopaedics*, 2nd edn., Lippincott Williams & Wilkins, Philadelphia, PA.

Thim, T., Krarup, N.H.V., Grove, E.L., *et al.* (2012). Initial assessment and treatment with the airway, breathing, circulation, disability, exposure (ABCDE) approach, *Int. J. Gen. Med.,* **5**, 117–121.

Uniform Data System for Medical Rehabilitation. (2004). *Annual Inpatient Rehabilitation Facilities Report 2004 (2003–2004).* UDS. [Online] Available at: http://www.udsmr.org/WebModules/DOC/Doc_About.aspx [Accessed August 2012].

Van der Meijden, O.A., Westgard, P., Chandler, Z., *et al.* (2012). Rehabilitation after arthroscopic rotator cuff repair: current concepts review and evidence-based guidelines, *Int. J. Sports Phys. Ther.,* **7**, 197–218.

Weatherford, B. (2014). *Acetabular Fractures*. Orthobullets.com [Online] Available at: http://www.orthobullets.com/trauma/1034/acetabular-fractures [Accessed 21 May 2014].

Wheeless, C.R. (2012). *Wheeless' Textbook of Orthopaedics*. Wheelessonline. [Online] Available at: www.wheelessonline.com [Accessed 21 May 2014].

Wilk, K.E., Macrina, L.C., and Reinold, M.M. (2006). Non-operative rehabilitation for traumatic and atraumatic glenohumeral instability, *N. Am. J. Sports Phys. Ther.,* **1**, 16–31.

Wilkins, K.E. (2005). Principles of fracture remodeling in children, *Injury,* **36** [Suppl], A3–A11.

World Health Organisation. (2004). *Global Burden of Disease Report*. World Health Organisation. [Online] Available at: http://www.who.int/healthinfo/global_burden_disease/GBD_report_2004update_full.pdf [Accessed August 2013].

Chapter 8

Spinal Cord Injury

Written by W. Mudzi, H. van Aswegen and B.M. Morrow

Spinal cord injuries remain a major health concern the world over, with an annual incidence of 12.1–57.8 cases per million in developed and 2.1–130.7 cases per million in developing countries (Rahimi-Movaghar *et al.*, 2013); up to 10% of these injuries will occur in children (Clarke, 2012). In developing countries, spinal cord injury (SCI) often involves young adults (aged 20–30) in the prime of their economically productive lives; whereas in developed countries the reported mean age (40–60 years) tends to be higher, possibly due to higher mean population age and better medical care systems (Ackery *et al.*, 2004; Rahimi-Movaghar *et al.*, 2013). Spinal cord injury is not a notifiable disease and hence figures relating to the cost to the individual and the health care system, especially in the developing world, are difficult to find (Ackery *et al.*, 2004; Wyndaele and Wyndaele, 2006; Cripps *et al.*, 2011). What are not in dispute are the causes and mechanisms of SCI, which will be discussed later in this chapter.

This chapter contains information about:

- The structure of the spinal cord.
- The causes and mechanisms of SCI.
- Spinal cord lesions and classification of the level of injury.
- Respiratory system complications following SCI and changes in respiratory muscle function.
- The complications related to other bodily systems following SCI.
- The medical and surgical management of a patient who sustained SCI.
- The physiotherapy aims for the management of a patient who has sustained SCI in the intensive care unit and the spinal ward.
- The contraindications and precautions related to the physiotherapy management of a patient with SCI.
- The physiotherapy interventions for patients who have suffered SCI.
- Adult and paediatric clinical case scenarios.

8.1. Structure of the Spinal Cord

The spinal column consists of 33 vertebrae and is divided into four regions: cervical, thoracic, lumbar and sacral (Gondim, 2013). Intervertebral discs separate the vertebrae and each vertebra has a vertebral arch, inside which the spinal cord is located. The spinal cord functions as a conduction pathway for impulses to and from the brain and, together with the brain, forms the central nervous system. It also serves as the centre for all spinal reflexes. The spinal cord is a cylindrical structure of nervous tissue that extends from the foramen magnum in the skull to the level of the second lumbar vertebra. It is surrounded by dura mater, arachnoid and pia mater connective tissue membranes and is made up of white and grey matter (Kahle and Frotscher, 2003; Gondim, 2013) (Fig. 8.1).

Nerve roots, which form 31 pairs of spinal nerves with motor and sensory nerve fibres, connect the spinal cord with all bodily structures. There are eight cervical, 12 thoracic, five lumbar and five sacral nerves (Fig. 8.2).

The collection of nerves at the bottom of the spinal column is called the cauda equina, with the conus medullaris at the inferior end of the spinal cord. At the intervertebral foramen of each vertebral body, dorsal

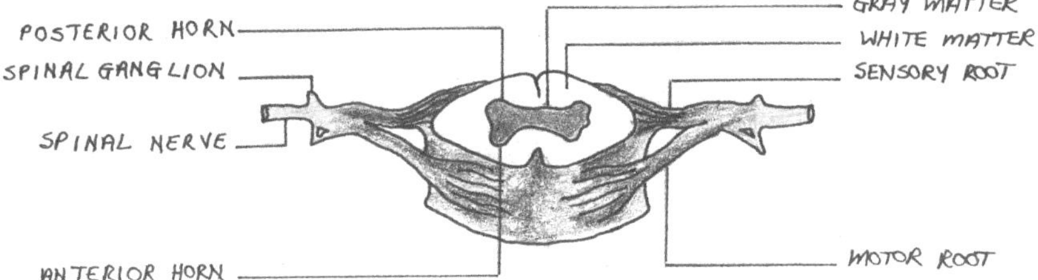

Fig. 8.1: Diagram of a transection of the spinal cord, illustrating the white and grey matter and sensory and motor spinal nerve roots.

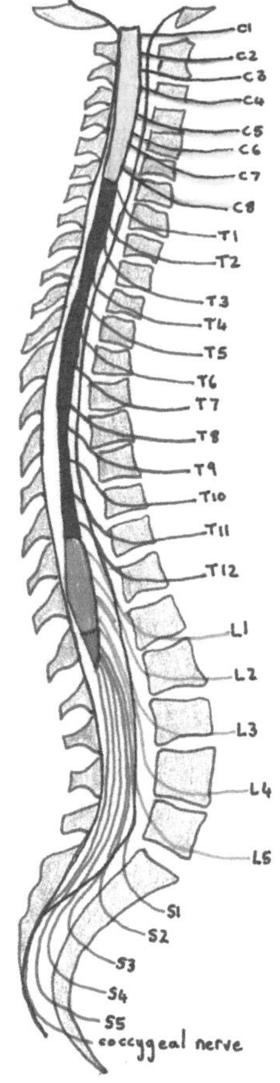

Fig. 8.2: Diagram of the spinal nerve roots.

nerve roots exit the cord posteriorly and ventral nerve roots enter the cord anteriorly. The nerve roots that leave the spinal cord contain motor fibres and those that enter the spinal cord contain sensory fibres (Fig. 8.1). Spinal nerves C1–C7 exit above their corresponding vertebrae, whereas C8 and the rest of the spinal nerves exit below the level of their corresponding vertebrae (Marieb, 1992; Gondim, 2013).

The internal structure of the spinal cord, as viewed transversely, shows a central point of cerebral spinal fluid accumulation, which is surrounded by grey matter (in the shape of an H). The grey matter contains neuronal cell bodies. The outer portion of the spinal cord consists of white matter, which contains nerve fibres (axons) (Kahle and Frotscher, 2003; Gondim, 2013) (Fig 8.1).

Dermatomes are areas of the skin that are innervated by the nerve roots of each spinal nerve. Dermatomes can be mapped fairly accurately on the surface of the body (Fig 8.3).

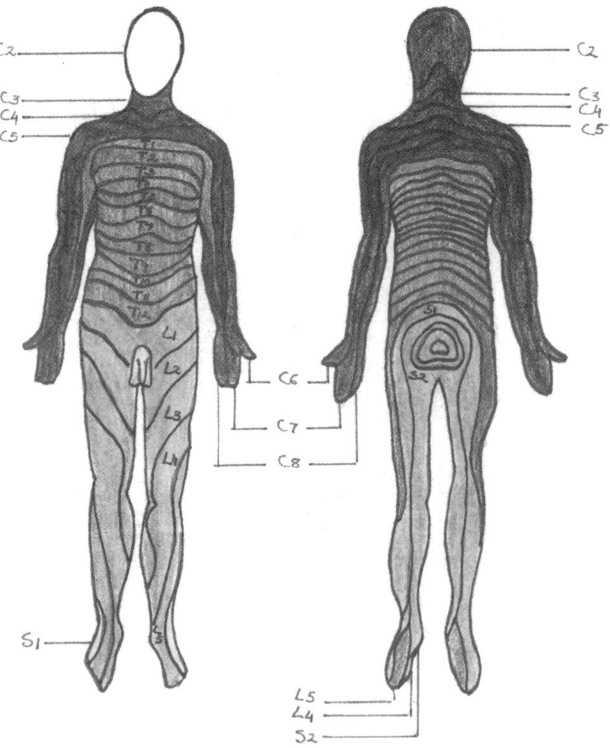

Fig. 8.3: Diagram depicting dermatomes of the human body.

Table 8.1: Ascending and descending tracts of the spinal cord and their functions.

Name	Location	Function
Ascending tracts		
Lateral spinothalamic	Lateral white columns	Pain and temperature sensation as well as proprioception and exteroception (sensation of impulses that originate outside the body)
Anterior spinothalamic	Anterior white columns	Crude touch and pressure sensation
Posterior spinocerebellar	Lateral white columns	Proprioceptive impulses from joints, tendons and muscle spindles
Fasciculi gracilis and cuneatus	Posterior white columns	Location and quality of tactile stimulation as well as limb position and body posture
Descending tracts		
Lateral corticospinal	Lateral white columns	Voluntary movement and muscle contraction of hands, fingers, feet and toes on the opposite side
Anterior corticospinal	Anterior white columns	Similar to the above but muscle function on the same side
Lateral reticulospinal	Lateral white columns	Facilitatory action on motor neurons to skeletal muscles
Medial reticulospinal	Anterior white columns	Inhibitory action on motor neurons to skeletal muscles

Loss of sensation in a dermatome therefore acts as an indication of the level of SCI. The dermatomes of the trunk do overlap and are not as clearly defined as the dermatomes on the extremities (Marieb, 1992; Gondim, 2013).

The term myotome refers to a group of muscles that are innervated by the motor fibres of a single nerve root and is referred to as the motor equivalent of a dermatome. Myotome testing, using isometric muscle contraction, can assist with determination of the level of SCI.

The impulse conduction function of the spinal cord is facilitated through spinal cord tracts. The ascending tracts conduct impulses from the body up to the brain and the descending tracts conduct impulses from the brain down to the different parts of the body. Many spinal cord tracts exist, and only the most important ones are listed in Table 8.1 (Kahle and Frotscher, 2003).

A visual summary of these tracts is provided in Fig. 8.4.

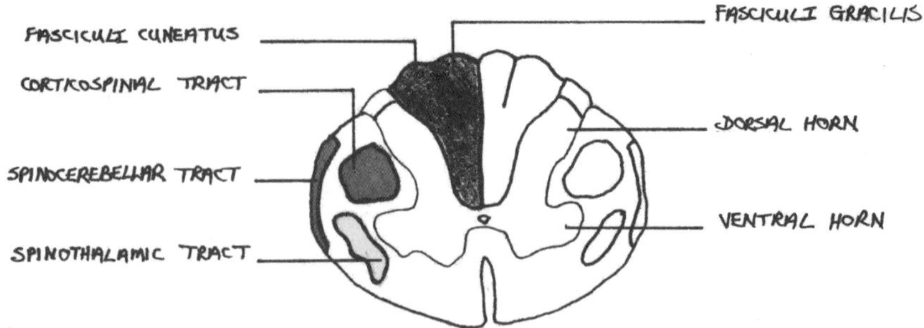

Fig. 8.4: Diagram of spinal cord tracts.

Blood supply to the spinal cord is provided by the anterior spinal artery and two posterior spinal arteries. The anterior spinal artery supplies blood to two-thirds of the anterior aspects of the spinal cord. The posterior spinal arteries supply blood to most of the posterior aspects of the spinal cord. In addition to these arteries, segmental arteries that arise from various blood vessels in the cervical, thoracic and lumbar areas of the spine assist with blood supply to the spinal cord. The segmental arteries form anterior medullary and posterior medullary arteries. The great anterior medullary artery supplies blood to the lumbar enlargement of the spinal cord (Newton, 2008).

The reader is referred to Section 8.11 for further reading that offers more detailed information on the structure of the spinal cord.

8.2. Causes and Mechanisms of Injury

8.2.1. *Causes of injury in*

In developing countries, males are more likely to suffer from traumatic SCI than females (4.8:1), as females are traditionally more involved with home-based activities which place them at a lower risk for SCI (Rahimi-Movaghar *et al.*, 2013). In developed countries the male to female ratio is more equal (3:4) due to females being more involved in competitive sporting and social activities (Rahimi-Movaghar *et al.*, 2013). The causes of SCI can be traumatic or non-traumatic. Traumatic causes of SCI account

Table 8.2: Direct and indirect causes of traumatic SCI*.

Direct causes	Indirect causes
Nerve injury: • Penetrating injury such as gunshot or stab wounds	Injury to the bone, soft tissue or vessels of the spinal cord: • Fracture dislocations: o Motor vehicle accidents and falls (40–56%) o Industrial accidents (10–26%) o Sporting activities (10–25%) o Accidents at home (10%) • Haematoma formation • Ischaemia

*Sekhon and Fehlings (2001); Ackery *et al.* (2004); Pickett *et al.* (2006); Rahimi-Movaghar *et al.* (2013).

for 70–80% of injuries through fractures or dislocations. Dislocations account for approximately 25% of trauma cases alone (Pickett *et al.*, 2006; Cripps *et al.*, 2011). Traumatic causes of SCI can be either direct or indirect and are summarised in Table 8.2. Non-traumatic causes of SCI fall outside the scope of this text and will not be discussed.

Generally, the most vulnerable areas for SCI through trauma are:

- upper (C1–C2) and lower cervical regions (C5–C7);
- mid-thoracic region (T4–T7); and
- thoracolumbar junction (T10–L2).

These will be discussed below.

8.2.2. *Mechanisms of injury in adults*

8.2.2.1. *Primary mechanisms of injury to the spinal cord*

The primary mechanism of injury refers to the initial mechanical trauma to the spinal cord. In cases of violence, the spinal cord may be severed (missile penetration), but more commonly neurological compromise following SCI is the result of ischaemic injury to the cord. Injury to the grey matter occurs within one hour after injury and is irreversible; injury to the white matter becomes irreversible 72 hours after injury (Dumont *et al.*, 2001).

8.2.2.1.1. Dislocation of vertebral bodies

This may occur anywhere in the cervical spine. Most commonly, dislocation occurs between C1 and C2 and C5 and C7 as a result of the lack of a solid vertebral body at C1 (which makes that section of the spine more vulnerable), anatomical curvature of the cervical spine and relative mobility of the lower cervical spine, which attaches to the stiff thoracic spine (Middleditch and Oliver, 2005). Dislocations can also occur in the lower thoracic segments, T11 and T12, but are normally rare in the thoracic region due to stabilisation from the rib cage.

The degree of dislocation does not necessarily parallel the degree of damage to the spinal cord. The degree of injury is influenced by other factors, which include pre-existing degenerative changes in the vertebral spine, blood vessel damage, swelling and disruption of the anterior longitudinal ligament (Sekhon and Fehlings, 2001). Spinal dislocation can also damage nerve roots, intervertebral discs and blood vessels (Baydur *et al.*, 2001).

8.2.2.1.2. Fracture of vertebrae

Vertebral fracture can occur with or without displacement. The fracture may involve vertebral bodies (wedge compression or burst fractures), laminae or pedicles. Bony fragments may be pushed into the spinal canal and impinge on the spinal cord or nerve roots. Table 8.3 summarises the mechanisms involved with various types of vertebral fractures.

Upper cervical spine fractures (C1–C3) occur regularly, with a reported rate of up to 25% (Longo *et al.*, 2010) (Fig. 8.5). Causes of injury to the odontoid or atlas in young adults include motor vehicle accidents and penetrating neck injuries. In the elderly, odontoid peg fractures occur as a result of falls. Traumatic spondylolisthesis of the axis is often referred to as hangman's fracture. Stable odontoid fractures (fracture of the tip of the odontoid) are managed conservatively, but unstable fractures (fracture at the junction of the odontoid with the body of the axis) might need surgical intervention, where appropriate, as not all elderly people are able to undergo surgery (Longo *et al.*, 2010).

Table 8.3: Mechanisms involved in fractures of the vertebrae*.

Type of fracture	Mechanism of injury
Compression	
• Anterior wedge	• Anterior flexion
• Lateral wedge	• Lateral flexion
Burst	
• Grade A	• Axial load
• Grades B	• Axial load with flexion
• Grade C	• Axial load with rotation
• Grade D	• Axial load with lateral flexion
Fracture-dislocation	
• Flexion-rotation	• Flexion-rotation
• Shear	• Anterior-posterior or posterior-anterior

*Magerl *et al*. (1994).

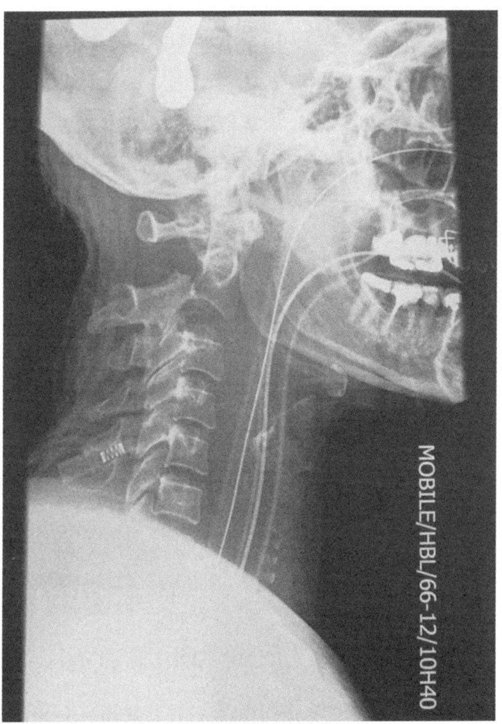

Fig. 8.5: Fracture of C2 vertebral body with dislocation on C3 following motor vehicle accident.

Thoracic spine fractures in young adults are associated with high-energy trauma and the patient often presents with additional injuries (e.g. fractures of the rib cage, pelvis or peripheries; abdominal injury). In the elderly, underlying osteoporosis may result in thoracic spine fractures from low-energy trauma such as falling out of bed. Thoracic spine fractures have a higher incidence of SCI due to the narrower spinal canal and sparse blood supply in the thoracic region in relation to other areas of the spine (Marré *et al.*, 2011).

8.2.2.1.3. Spinal epidural haematoma

Although uncommon, haematoma formation results from bleeding from the traumatic incident but can occur in patients with a coagulation defect following anticoagulation therapy (Binder *et al.*, 2004). It may be acute or chronic, spontaneous, posttraumatic, iatrogenic, or associated with specific medications and disease states (Binder *et al.*, 2004; Cha *et al.*, 2011). Spinal epidural haematoma is mostly localised to the cervical or thoracic spine (Cha *et al.*, 2011). If a patient with spinal epidural haematoma presents with abnormal neurological signs, prompt spinal decompression is performed surgically through evacuation of the haematoma (Cha *et al.*, 2011).

8.2.2.1.4. Spinal subdural haematoma

This is a rare cause of acute spinal cord compression. It can occur with minor trauma and normally presents with what can be termed dramatic symptoms. Paraplegia is preceded by severe back pain in cases of acute spinal subdural haematoma and emergency surgery is often required; however, there are reports of cases in which spontaneous resolution has occurred (Oh *et al.*, 2009).

8.2.2.1.5. Indirect trauma of the spinal cord

This type of injury can result from blows to the head which then result in energy transmission along the brainstem and spinal cord, causing haemorrhages in the grey matter of the upper cervical region.

8.2.2.1.6. Laceration of the spinal cord

Severe injury may lead to laceration of the spinal cord. The most common causes of laceration of the spinal cord (partial or complete) include stab wounds, gunshot wounds and fracture dislocations. Surgical error may also lead to partial laceration of the cord. The continuity of the spinal cord is disturbed and there will be oedema and haemorrhage of meninges and cord followed by scarring of nervous tissue (Dumont *et al.*, 2001).

8.2.2.1.7. Haematomyelia

This can occur as a complication of a fracture dislocation or whiplash injury. It produces a spindle-shaped haemorrhage within the substance of the spinal cord located in the grey matter (Pullarkat *et al.*, 2000). It is usually followed by loss of function below the level of the lesion. As oedema subsides and the clot is slowly absorbed, there is a return of function in the posterior and lateral white columns (Rodesch *et al.*, 2004). The patient usually has a flaccid paralysis in muscles supplied by the anterior horn cells at the level of the lesion. There is gradual development of spastic paralysis, with loss of pain and temperature sensation over segments affected by the clot. Pain and temperature sensation are preserved below the level of the haematomyelia and posterior column function is normal. Haematomyelia is managed surgically either through aggressive (urgent clot evacuation) or less aggressive approaches (plateau of neurologic deficit prior to clot removal), depending on the preference of the attending surgeon. Regardless of the management approach used, the underlying cause for the haematomyelia should be adequately addressed (Oskouian, 2012).

8.2.2.2. *Secondary mechanisms of injury to the spinal cord*

Secondary mechanisms of injury to the spinal cord set in within minutes of the primary injury and involve a cascade of vascular, cellular and biochemical events that extend from the primary mechanism of injury. The secondary mechanisms of injury may last for weeks or months after the initial injury, and during this phase the area of trauma enlarges (Oyinbo, 2011). Fewer inflammatory mediators are released with mild SCI and may result in less secondary cord injury compared to that caused by moderate or severe primary SCI (Oyinbo, 2011). Delayed specialised management of the patient with acute SCI may further contribute to a worsened outcome due to the ensuing secondary damage to the cord (Oyinbo, 2011).

Secondary SCI occurs when blood flow at the site of injury is reduced due to local vascular injury to the venules and capillaries, vasospasm and intravascular thrombosis, which lead to ischaemia. Over the ensuing hours hypoperfusion and ischaemia spread outwards from the injury site, up and down the spinal cord. Spinal cord autoregulation is lost and cord injury is exacerbated by systemic hypotension (Dumont *et al.*, 2001; Kwon *et al.*, 2004). Other causative factors of ischaemia of the spinal cord include oedema, inflammation and cord compression. The ischaemic area encourages the release of inflammatory mediators such as reactive oxygen species. These inflammatory mediators cause oxidative cell membrane damage, which may eventually lead to apoptosis and cell death (Dumont *et al.*, 2001; Kwon *et al.*, 2004). An in-depth discussion of the complex intracellular mechanisms that contribute to apoptosis and cell death following SCI is beyond the scope of this text. Readers are referred to Section 8.11 for further suggested reading.

8.2.2.2.1. Neurogenic shock

Neurogenic shock results from central nervous system injury such as cervical or high thoracic SCI. It causes hypotension and inadequate tissue perfusion due to sudden loss of sympathetic vasomotor function, which leads to severe disruption of the balance between vasodilator and vasoconstrictor functions of the arterioles and venules, hence decreased systemic and vascular resistance and pooling of blood in the peripheries (Denton and McKinlay, 2009). Bradycardia develops and the patient is unable to increase cardiac output by changes in heart rate (Denton and McKinlay, 2009). This shock state leads to ischaemia, which may contribute to secondary injury of the spinal cord (Dumont *et al.*, 2001).

8.2.2.2.2. Spinal shock

Spinal shock is not related to the circulatory system. Depressed spinal reflexes inferior to the level of injury is referred to as spinal shock. Those with mild SCI may not develop spinal shock, whereas those with more severe injury will. The four phases of spinal shock reported in the literature include the following (Ditunno *et al.*, 2004).

8.2.2.2.2.1. *Areflexia or hyporeflexia.* In this phase the patient presents with absent deep tendon reflexes (e.g. ankle jerk or knee jerk) below the level of injury up to one day after injury. As a result muscles are flaccid and paralysed. Patients present with bradycardia, atrioventricular block and hypotension.

8.2.2.2.2.2. *Initial reflex return.* One to three days following injury deep tendon reflexes start to return in children and the elderly but remain absent in adults. The faster return of deep tendon reflexes in children is ascribed to descending supraspinal tracts that are still developing. In the elderly, underlying subclinical myelopathy (pathology of the spinal cord) may contribute to the recovery of reflexes.

8.2.2.2.2.3. *Early hyperreflexia.* Four days to one month following SCI, deep tendon reflexes return fully for all ages, but the timing of reflex return varies between individual patients. Ankle jerk reflexes precede knee jerk. Babinsky sign appears soon after recovery of the ankle jerk reflex. Less episodes of bradycardia, cardiac arrhythmias and hypotension are observed and episodes of autonomic dysreflexia may begin to emerge in patients with injuries above T6 (see further information in Section 8.2.2.2.3).

8.2.2.2.2.4. *Spasticity or hyperreflexia.* Vasovagal-induced cardiovascular abnormalities resolve in three to six weeks. Orthostatic hypotension in patients with tetraplegia may persist for weeks or months following SCI. One to 12 months following injury, cutaneous and deep tendon reflexes become hyperactive and respond to minimal stimuli.

During spinal shock, a patient's neurological deficit may present at a higher spinal level than the original injury due to cord swelling. In the initial period of spinal shock the patient is nursed in a supine position to minimise secondary injury to the spinal cord. Over the course of the following weeks the patient is gradually brought into a head-up position; however, if this position leads to deterioration of the patient's neurological function, the supine position is resumed. As the swelling eventually subsides, the patient's deep tendon reflexes will begin to return and this signifies the end of the spinal shock period.

8.2.2.2.3. Autonomic dysreflexia

Partial or complete elimination of supraspinal sympathetic control of cardiovascular functions (e.g. coronary blood flow, cardiac contractility and heart rate) occur with moderate to severe SCI. Autonomic dysreflexia is a potentially life-threatening condition that may occur in patients with SCI above level T6 (Furlan, 2013; Stephenson, 2013), whereby an inciting stimulus (not necessarily noxious) below the level of the lesion causes an uninhibited sympathetic reflex and unbalanced physiological response. This sympathetic over-activity causes vasoconstriction and severe hypertension and is also known as hyperreflexia.

An inciting stimulus (originating most commonly from the bladder and bowel) is generated below the level of the lesion and impulses are sent via the spinal cord to the brain. These impulses are prevented from reaching the brain by the cord injury (Stephenson, 2013). However, the sympathetic nervous system is stimulated by the receptors located at the sympathetic ganglion at T5–T6 and a massive sympathetic response is generated, causing widespread vasoconstriction and peripheral arterial hypertension (Stephenson, 2013). The brain detects this sudden increased blood pressure (BP) through the baroreceptors located in the carotid artery and aortic arch; subsequently the parasympathetic nervous system is stimulated via the vagal nerve. Again the SCI (at T6 or above) prevents the inhibitory effect of the parasympathetic descending impulses below the lesion, which normally would cause peripheral vasodilation (Stephenson, 2013); however, there is a parasympathetic response above the level of the lesion that results in the patient presenting with flushed features. Through the vagal nerve, parasympathetic cardiac responses remain intact as the only supraspinal control of the heart. This leads to the development of heart rate irregularities and cardiac arrhythmias. The brain attempts to lower the peripheral arterial hypertension through slowing the heart rate using stimulation of the vagal nerve; however, this compensatory bradycardia is often unsuccessful and the patient's hypertensive state continues (Stephenson, 2013). The reflex hypertension only resolves once the inciting stimulus is removed (Furlan, 2013; Stephenson, 2013).

Untreated autonomic dysreflexia can result in intracranial bleeding, retinal detachments, myocardial infarction, pulmonary oedema, renal insufficiency, coma and death (Furlan, 2013; Stephenson, 2013).

Episodes of autonomic dysreflexia may occur during the sub-acute (recovery from spinal shock) and chronic stages after severe SCI (Furlan, 2013) and have a higher incidence in complete spinal cord lesions (91%) than incomplete lesions (27%) (Stephenson, 2013). Patients with SCI above T6 present with systolic blood pressure (SBP) and diastolic blood pressure (DBP) values well below the norm during the acute stage of injury. Normal SBP for such patients is 90–110 mmHg (Stephenson, 2013). During episodes of autonomic dysreflexia, SBP rises by more than 30 mmHg and DBP by more than 20 mmHg. Therefore it may seem as though the patient's BP had stabilised to normal values; however, a life-threatening situation has developed (Furlan, 2013; Stephenson, 2013). At the onset of an episode of autonomic dysreflexia, bradycardia or tachycardia develops together with the signs and symptoms summarised in Table 8.4 (Furlan, 2013; Stephenson, 2013).

Preventive strategies for autonomic dysreflexia include proper bowel and bladder care and the prevention of pressure sore formation. Short-acting anti-hypertensive medication may be used to lower BP during an

Table 8.4: Signs and symptoms associated with an episode of autonomic dysreflexia.

Signs and symptoms	Reason for development
Headache and seizures	Elevated BP
Visual disturbances	Elevated BP
Altered heart rate or rhythm	Vagal nerve response to elevated BP
Flushing, diaphoresis, and profuse sweating (above the level of the lesion)	Vasodilation in response to elevated BP
Nasal congestion	Vasodilation in response to elevated BP
Pallor, cold extremities and piloerection (gooseflesh) (below the level of the lesion)	Sympathetic tone and the lack of descending inhibitory parasympathetic tone
Chills without fever, muscle spasm, penile erection	Sympathetic tone and the lack of descending inhibitory parasympathetic tone
Bronchospasm	Increased vagal nerve tone

episode of autonomic dysreflexia if non-pharmacological measures (e.g. loosening of tight clothing, unblocking or repositioning the indwelling urinary catheter and removal of faecal impaction) are ineffective (Furlan, 2013; Stephenson, 2013).

The reader is referred to Section 8.11 for further suggested reading on this topic.

8.2.3. *Causes and mechanisms of injury in paediatrics*

The causes of SCI are similar between adults and children, with motor vehicle accidents and falls being the most common (Mortavazi *et al.*, 2011; Clarke, 2012). Sports injuries are also a common cause of SCI in older children (Mortavazi *et al.*, 2011). Non-accidental injuries and penetrating injuries (such as gunshot and stab wounds) have also been reported in small numbers (Mortavazi *et al.*, 2011), along with other rare causes such as high cervical injuries related to skeletal dysplasias (e.g. achondroplasia), juvenile rheumatoid arthritis and Down's syndrome or Trisomy 21 (Zidek and Srinivasan, 2003).

Distraction forces that stretch the spinal cord, such as flexion, extension, rotation or dislocation, may cause SCI in children. The mechanism of injury, however, is profoundly different between adults and children. Whereas the mechanism of SCI in adults is most commonly that of vertebral fracture, the most common mechanisms for SCI in children younger than 10 years are vertebral dislocations without fracture and SCI without radiological abnormality (SCIWORA). Children younger than eight years are significantly more likely to sustain SCIWORA than older children and adolescents (Pang and Wilberger, 1982; Clarke, 2012). Spinal cord injury without radiological abnormality presents clinically as an SCI, but plain x-ray shows normal alignment and no vertebral fracture; although magnetic resonance imaging (MRI) may show ligament rupture. It is believed that SCIWORA is caused by vertebral displacement followed by re-alignment with stretching, tearing or contusion of the spinal cord and is extremely rare in the adult population (Pang and Wilberger, 1982; Clarke, 2012).

Factors related to immaturity, such as ligament laxity, shallow horizontal facet joints, underdeveloped spinous processes and relatively weak neck muscles, predispose the child to SCI as a result of increased flexibility under fairly low-loading conditions (Dumont *et al.*, 2001; Mortavazi *et al.*, 2011; Clarke, 2012). The most common level of SCI in children is the cervical spine, with up to 80% of paediatric SCI being cervical (compared to about 55% in adults) (Patel *et al.*, 2001). Younger children more commonly sustain upper cervical spine injury (C2–C3) compared to C4–C5 in adults and adolescents (Patel *et al.*, 2001). This high rate of cervical injury in children is likely a result of increased flexibility in the cervical spine compared to the thoracic and lumbar regions, as well as the relatively large head size in children (Clarke, 2012). Injury patterns approach an adult pattern from eight years of age (Mortavazi *et al.*, 2011).

8.3. Spinal Cord Lesions and Classification of the Level of Injury

8.3.1. *Types of spinal cord lesions*

The clinical effects of SCI depend on the extent and location of the damage to the spinal cord. The extent of the damage to the spinal cord may result in either a complete or incomplete lesion. The location of the SCI may result in either paraplegia or tetraplegia.

8.3.1.1. *Complete lesion of the spinal cord*

This type of lesion is characterised by loss of both the motor and sensory abilities of the patient below the neurological level, including the sacral segments S4 and S5 (Kirshblum *et al.*, 2004).

8.3.1.2. *Incomplete lesion of the spinal cord*

There is preservation of either sensory and/or motor function below the neurological level with an incomplete lesion of the spinal cord. It is now globally agreed that the presence of any sensation in the lower sacral segments of S4–S5 means that the lesion is incomplete. This preservation is a good predictor of improved outcome, especially if there is pinprick sensation 72 hours to one week after injury (Kirshblum *et al.*, 2004).

Syndromes associated with incomplete lesions of the spinal cord are below.

8.3.1.2.1. Anterior cord syndrome

This syndrome occurs due to injury to the anterior two-thirds of the spinal cord. It often results from compression of the anterior spinal artery caused by flexion injuries, direct damage by bone fragments or disc compression. The resultant neurological deficits are usually due to damage of the corticospinal and spinothalamic tracts. The neurological manifestation includes muscle weakness, incomplete sensory loss, loss of sensitivity to pain and temperature below the level of the lesion with preservation of posterior column function (McKinley *et al.*, 2007; Scivoletto and Di Donna, 2009).

8.3.1.2.2. Central cord syndrome

This is the most common of the incomplete traumatic cervical cord syndromes. It is typically seen in older patients with cervical spondylosis and in certain ethnic groups who present with a tight cervical canal (Harrop *et al.*, 2006). In these patients, hyperextension from minor trauma will result in spinal cord compression. This injury can cause ischaemia within the grey matter in the central portion of the cord, but the peripheral area of the cord remains relatively unaffected. The result is that the patient presents with significant loss of function in their upper limbs but relatively preserved function in their lower limbs. Young adults may develop central cord syndrome due to severe spinal column injury from high-energy trauma such as motor vehicle accidents, falls and diving accidents (Harrop *et al.*, 2006). Low-energy traumatic injury that leads to acute central cervical disc herniation may also cause central cord compression (Harrop *et al.*, 2006). The pathogenesis of central cord syndrome suggests the involvement of the lateral white matter columns and corticospinal tracts, which have a great influence on hand function. Patients present with flaccid paralysis of the upper limbs and relatively strong but spastic leg function. This is due to the fact that the cervical tracts are located more centrally within the cord. Sacral sensation and bowel and bladder function are usually partially spared (Harrop *et al.*, 2006; McKinley *et al.*, 2007).

Neurologic recovery is influenced by age, with patients younger than 50 years regaining function faster and in a shorter time period than older patients. Recovery of function tends to start in the legs, followed by the bladder, arms and lastly the hands (Harrop *et al.*, 2006; McKinley *et al.*, 2007; Scivoletto and Di Donna, 2009).

8.3.1.2.3. Posterior cord syndrome

Posterior cord syndrome is a very rare incomplete lesion of the spinal cord. This syndrome is seen in hyperextension injuries and causes contusion of the posterior spinal cord columns. The trauma to the posterior tracts results in loss of proprioception, deep touch and vibration sense. The patient presents with good motor function, pain and temperature sensation, but at times with profound loss of proprioception, which can make walking very difficult and results in an ataxic-type gait (McKinley *et al.*, 2007).

8.3.1.2.4. Brown Sequard syndrome

Brown Sequard syndrome refers to injury in one hemi-section of the spinal cord. It usually occurs in stab or gunshot wound trauma. Contralaterally (opposite the side of the injury), there is a loss of sensitivity to pain, temperature and crude touch below the lesion from interruption of the spinothalamic tracts. The spinothalamic tracts cross or intersect at the level of the spinal cord; hence the hemi-section of the cord preserves pain, temperature and crude touch sensation on the side of the injury.

Ipsilaterally (the same side as the injury), interruption of the corticospinal tracts results in paralysis of voluntary movements below the level of the lesion, spasticity, positive Babinski sign and hyperreflexia. Interruption of the posterior columns results in loss of vibration, form perception, two-point discrimination and proprioception (McKinley *et al.*, 2007; Scivoletto and Di Donna, 2009). Patients who present with more upper limb weakness than lower limb weakness are likely to be able to ambulate before discharge from the hospital (McKinley *et al.*, 2007).

8.3.1.2.5. Compression of the conus medullaris and cauda equina

The spinal cord ends at the level of L1–L2 vertebrae. Compression of the conus medullaris usually results from a compression fracture of L1, which causes contusion and haemorrhage with damage to sacral segments of the cord. Injuries above the conus are predominantly upper motor neuron lesions, although anterior horn cells of lower motor neurons can be damaged at the site of the injury. Damage to the conus can involve both upper and lower motor neurons (McKinley *et al.*, 2007; Lavy *et al.*, 2009).

Simultaneous compression of several lumbar and sacral nerve roots in the lower lumbar region (L4–S1) lead to the development of cauda equina syndrome. Injuries involving the cauda equina are lower motor neuron injuries and will therefore result in flaccid paralysis. The patient also typically presents with neuromuscular and urogenital symptoms such as low back pain, sciatica (usually bilateral), saddle sensory disturbances, bladder and bowel dysfunction and sensory loss in the lower limbs that may differ in severity from one patient to the next (McKinley *et al.*, 2007; Lavy *et al.*, 2009).

8.3.2. *Location of injury*

8.3.2.1. *Paraplegia*

Paraplegia refers to damage to spinal cord levels T1 and below. Consequently the resulting paralysis can affect the lower limbs, bladder and bowel function and, depending on the level, the trunk. Thoracic spine injury affects intercostal and abdominal muscle innervation, which impairs ventilation and may lead to respiratory muscle fatigue and failure (refer to Section 8.4) (Kirshblum *et al.*, 2004).

8.3.2.2. *Tetraplegia*

Tetraplegia refers to loss of motor and/or sensory function as a result of damage to the cervical segment of the spinal cord. There is paralysis of the upper and lower limbs, trunk, bowel and bladder function. As this injury affects both inspiratory and expiratory muscles of respiration and the sympathetic nervous system, it has a greater negative impact on cardiovascular system and respiratory system stability than paraplegia, leading to the development of cardiac arrhythmia, hypotension and respiratory distress and failure (refer to Section 8.4) (Kirshblum *et al.*, 2004).

8.3.3. *Classification of the level of injury*

In the 1970s a method of classification of SCI was developed by Frankel in the UK. This system classified the patient as having a lesion A, B, C or D. The Frankel classification system caused some confusion among clinicians, and the American Spinal Injury Association (ASIA) refined Frankel's classification to alleviate this confusion. More and more countries and major trauma centres have adopted the ASIA classification scale for SCI (Ditunno *et al.*, 1994) (Table 8.5). This classification now supersedes the Frankel classification system. The term 'neurological level' in the ASIA scale refers to the spinal roots that enter and exit the spinal column between the vertebral bodies. Classification of the level of injury differs between clinicians, with neurologists classifying the level of SCI as the first spinal segmental level with abnormal neurological loss, orthopaedic surgeons classifying it as the level of bony involvement, and rehabilitation specialists classifying it as the lowest spinal segmental level with preserved function.

Table 8.5: The ASIA impairment scale*.

Grade	Description
A	Complete lesion: no motor or sensory function is preserved in the sacral segments S4–S5
B	Incomplete lesion: sensory but not motor function is preserved below the neurological level and includes the sacral segments S4–S5
C	Incomplete lesion: motor function is preserved below the neurological level and the majority of key muscles below the neurological level have a muscle grade of less than three
D	Incomplete lesion: motor function is preserved below the neurological level and at least half of the key muscles below the neurological level have a muscle grade greater than or equal to three
E	Motor as well as sensory function is normal

*Adapted from American Spinal Cord Injury Association (2003) and Eng and Chan (2013).

Using the ASIA impairment scale, if there are no reflexes in the affected region within 48 hours, the patient will be diagnosed with complete cord lesion; however, there are patients who will recover even after 48 hours. The ASIA scale further determines that the lack of voluntary control of the anal sphincter (sacral sparing) must be present for a lesion to be considered complete (American Spinal Cord Injury Association, 2003). A person with an ASIA A classification has more neurological deficits than a person with an ASIA D classification. It therefore follows that a patient with a C6 ASIA D classification has potential for a more functional lifestyle than one with a C6 ASIA A classification.

The ASIA includes bilateral assessment of 28 dermatomes using pinprick and light touch sensation and manual muscle testing of 10 key muscles. Total motor and sensory scores are calculated based on these results and are used in combination with anal sphincter sensory and motor function to determine ASIA classification (Eng and Chan, 2013). It is important to note that, in SCI rehabilitation, short-term and long-term goals are established based upon the patient's neurological level and degree of preserved function below the level of injury.

8.4. Respiratory System Complications following Spinal Cord Injury and Changes in Respiratory Muscle Function

8.4.1. *Spinal cord injury and respiratory muscle function*

Trauma to the spinal cord results in a loss of motor neurons, interneurons, myelin insulation and ascending and descending long tract axons within the injury zone, which can result in neurological deficits spanning many segments. Depending on the level of the lesion, loss of innervation will lead to paralysis or paresis of respiratory muscles and consequently altered lung mechanics (Tables 8.6 and 8.7). Spinal shock can severely impact the patient's ability to breathe spontaneously (due to muscle paralysis) and hence might necessitate intubation and mechanical ventilation (MV). Hypoxaemia may lead to secondary injury to the spinal cord and should be avoided at all cost.

Table 8.6: Muscles of respiration*.

Muscle	Innervation	Function related to respiration
Diaphragm	Phrenic nerve through segmental nerve roots C3–C5	Primary muscle of inspiration and active during tidal and forced inspiration
External intercostals	Segmental nerve roots T1–T11	Primary muscles of inspiration and active during tidal and forced inspiration
Scalenes	Segmental nerve roots C4–C8	Accessory muscle of inspiration and only active during forced inspiration to facilitate elevation of the upper rib cage
Sternocleidomastoid and trapezius	Segmental nerve roots C1–C4 and accessory nerve XI	Accessory muscles of inspiration and only active during forced inspiration to facilitate elevation of the upper rib cage
External oblique	Segmental nerve roots T6–T12 and subcostal nerve	Forced expiration
Pectoralis major	Segmental nerves C5–T1	Forced expiration
Internal intercostals	Segmental nerve roots T1–T11	Forced expiration
Internal oblique and transverse abdominis	Segmental nerve roots T6–T12	Forced expiration
Rectus abdominis	Thoracoabdominal nerve through nerve roots T7–T11	Forced expiration

*Terson de Paleville *et al.* (2011).

The function of the respiratory muscles below the level of injury may be permanently impaired as a result of the primary injury; however, the function of the respiratory muscles above the level of injury may be temporarily impaired due to the presence of oedema fluid and blood in the spinal canal, as mentioned in Section 8.2.2.2.2. These patients often require intubation and MV in the intensive care unit (ICU) until the oedema fluid and amount of haemorrhage in the spinal canal has subsided in order for nervous supply to be restored to the muscles that were not affected by the injury. As the swelling in the spinal canal subsides, the

Table 8.7: Level of spinal cord injury and its effects on respiratory muscle function and vital capacity*.

Level	Effect on respiratory muscles	Vital capacity in acute stage
C1–C2	• Partial innervation of accessory inspiratory muscles • Likely to be ventilator-dependent	5–10% of normal (500–600 ml)
C3–C6	• Innervation of accessory inspiratory muscles • Partial innervation of primary inspiratory muscles	20–30% of normal (1 litre)
C7–T4	• Innervation of sternocleidomastoid, trapezius and scalene muscles • Innervation of diaphragm • Partial innervation of intercostal muscles	30–50% of normal (1.4–2.3 litres)
T5–T10	• Innervation of primary and accessory inspiratory muscles • Partial innervation of intercostal muscles • Partial innervation of expiratory muscles	75–100% of normal (4–5 litres)

*Chin (2014).

patient may be able to resume spontaneous breathing and may eventually be weaned from the ventilator. When muscle paralysis changes to spasticity, respiratory function improves due to the development of chest wall rigidity (Berney *et al.*, 2011; Vásquez *et al.*, 2013). Although MV is life-saving, it does have negative consequences on respiratory function, such as weakening of the preserved muscles. Acquiring a nosocomial lung infection in addition to muscle weakness increases ventilation time and ICU length of stay and eventually leads to difficulty in weaning patients from MV.

8.4.2. *Respiratory complications following spinal cord injury*

Respiratory complications are a leading cause of morbidity and mortality in patients with SCI, being more severe in patients with high-level and complete injuries (Cotton *et al.*, 2005; Brown *et al.*, 2006; Shavelle *et al.*, 2006; Kawu *et al.*, 2011; Vásquez *et al.*, 2013). Serious complications such as pneumonia, atelectasis and ventilatory failure are experienced by up to 83% of patients with cervical lesions and 50% of patients with high-thoracic spinal cord lesions (T1–T6) in the acute phase (first five days) of injury (Berlly and Shem, 2007; Berney *et al.*, 2011; Terson de Paleville *et al.*, 2011). The level of SCI and the degree of motor function loss correlates directly with the development of respiratory complications. Age, pre-existing medical illness and smoking history may be additional predisposing factors to the development of respiratory complications over the first five days following SCI (Berlly and Shem, 2007). Intensive chest physiotherapy management during this acute phase after injury is advocated to prevent the development of respiratory complications (Berney *et al.*, 2011).

8.4.2.1. *Complications encountered in the early phase after spinal cord injury*

Respiratory complications encountered by patients in the acute stage after SCI include the overproduction of pulmonary secretions, bronchospasm, atelectasis, ventilator-associated pneumonia, pulmonary oedema or respiratory failure.

8.4.2.1.1. Overproduction of pulmonary secretions

Hypersecretion of mucus after SCI is thought to be caused by the loss of sympathetic control and unopposed vagal activity in the first few weeks after injury. Overproduction of secretions is worsened by pre-existing factors such as smoking, chronic obstructive pulmonary disease, asthma and ageing (Berlly and Shem, 2007; Sheel *et al.*, 2008). Mucus hypersecretion can occur within one hour after cervical SCI and goes hand-in-hand with changes in the chemical content of mucus. Tenacious secretions lead to the formation of mucus plugs in the lung periphery. Weakness or paralysis of the muscles of inspiration and forced expiration leads to the generation of inefficient inspiratory volumes and poor peak expiratory flow rate and results in a poor cough effort. The presence of an additional chest wall injury, in patients with thoracic SCI, may further impair the patient's ability to cough and clear retained secretions effectively (Berlly and Shem, 2007). All of these factors contribute to the development of atelectasis or pneumonia and subsequent respiratory failure. The chemical content of mucus returns to normal only months after injury (Berlly and Shem, 2007).

8.4.2.1.2. Bronchospasm

Patients with cervical SCI often suffer from bronchospasm, even in the absence of a history of asthma, due to autonomic nervous system dysfunction seen in the acute phase after injury. Resting airway tone is increased due to the interruption of sympathetic nervous system supply to the lungs in the presence of intact parasympathetic nervous system activity, as mentioned previously. Bronchospasm contributes to secretion retention and respiratory distress. Therefore the patient will be in need of bronchodilator therapy before physiotherapy treatment is initiated during the acute phase (Berlly and Shem, 2007; Vásquez *et al.*, 2013).

8.4.2.1.3. Atelectasis

Atelectasis may occur due to poor lung expansion as a result of weak or paralysed inspiratory muscles, retained bronchial secretions, weak cough effort, cephalad movement of abdominal content and decreased production of surfactant in lung segments that have lost volume. These changes can also lead to the development of pneumonia and respiratory failure (Berlly and Shem, 2007).

8.4.2.1.4. Respiratory failure

Respiratory complications after cervical SCI include hypoventilation, hypercapnia, reduction in surfactant production, atelectasis, increased work of breathing and respiratory muscle fatigue (Wong *et al.*, 2012). Patients with lesions above C3 are at particular risk for the development of respiratory failure. Patients with SCI at level C3 or below may be able to breathe spontaneously following the injury, but evidence shows that respiratory failure occurs in some of these patients by the fourth day after hospital admission and may last for up to five weeks (Wong *et al.*, 2012). Risk factors for the development of respiratory failure have been mentioned in the previous paragraphs and are summarised in Table 8.8.

Table 8.8: Risk factors for the development of respiratory failure in patients with spinal cord injury.

Spinal shock
Decreased lung expansion due to impaired innervation of the inspiratory muscles
Impaired cough effort due to impaired innervation of the expiratory muscles
Increased secretion production
Decreased surfactant production resulting in lung volume loss

Respiratory failure has a direct influence on the patient's mortality and therefore patients with cervical or thoracic SCI (especially above T6) should be closely monitored for signs of respiratory distress, which is a precursor to respiratory failure, in the acute phase after injury.

8.4.2.1.5. Ventilator-associated pneumonia

Similar to other patients who are intubated and mechanically ventilated, patients with SCI are at risk of developing ventilator-associated pneumonia (VAP) due to the presence of the endotracheal tube (ETT) and impaired mucociliary function and cough ability (Mietto *et al.*, 2013). Ventilator-associated pneumonia is associated with increased mortality, hospital length of stay and health care cost (Mietto *et al.*, 2013). Patients with SCI and weaning and extubation failure face a high risk for the development of VAP (Call *et al.*, 2011).

8.4.2.1.6. Pulmonary oedema

Up to 50% of patients with tetraplegia present with pulmonary oedema during the acute stage following injury (Berlly and Shem, 2007). Pulmonary oedema may arise due to a variety of factors, such as direct trauma to the lung tissue, acute respiratory distress syndrome and fluid overload, or may be neurogenic in origin (Berlly and Shem, 2007). Overhydration may occur in instances in which low BP is misinterpreted as traumatic hypovolaemic shock (instead of a normal feature of spinal shock) and treatment with fluid resuscitation is erroneously performed. Careful fluid resuscitation is important to avoid overhydration, particularly in the polytrauma patient, where a balance between treatment for hypovolaemia and the natural reduction in BP after SCI is vital.

The information shared in this section highlights the need for early respiratory treatment provided by physiotherapists, the main aim being the prevention of atelectasis and respiratory infections (Vásquez *et al.*, 2013). It has been shown that comprehensive clinical pathways and structured respiratory protocols reduce respiratory complications in patients with tetraplegia. It limits cost to the patient and hospital as it plays a role in altering the patient's need for intubation and MV (Berney *et al.*, 2011). The reader is referred to Section 8.9 for detailed information on physiotherapy intervention strategies that should be used in the management of patients with SCI in the acute phase after injury. Section 8.11 suggests further reading on clinical practice guidelines for the respiratory management of patients with SCI.

8.4.2.2. *Complications encountered in the later stages following spinal cord injury*

In the later stages following SCI, patients develop changes in respiratory pattern, chest wall and lung compliance, lung capacity and lung volumes, and may also develop aspiration pneumonia or pulmonary thromboembolism.

8.4.2.2.1. Changes in respiratory pattern

Anatomically, the diaphragm is positioned in apposition (side-by-side) to the rib cage. The area extending from the origin of the diaphragm on the rib cage to the dome of the diaphragm is referred to as the zone of apposition. During diaphragmatic contraction in individuals without SCI, intra-abdominal pressure rises as the dome of the diaphragm moves caudally and assists with the elevation of the rib cage through the zone of apposition (Brown *et al.*, 2006). In patients with cervical SCI, however, the abdomen is highly compliant, which leads to no or minimal increase in intra-abdominal pressure at the onset of inhalation. The lack of increased intra-abdominal pressure causes the lower ribs to be pulled inwards as the orientation of the diaphragm fibres is not conducive towards the elevation of these ribs (Brown *et al.*, 2006). The reader is referred to

Sections 8.4.2.2.3 and 8.9.1.1 for information on the effect of body positioning on respiration.

In cervical SCI, during spontaneous inhalation the upper anterior chest wall moves inwards when the diaphragm contracts due to the lack of innervation of the external intercostal muscles. This gives rise to an abnormal breathing pattern commonly called 'paradoxical' breathing, which is isolated diaphragmatic action with retraction of the chest wall (Berlly and Shem, 2007).

A patient with cervical SCI and diaphragm weakness may suffer from episodes of breathlessness when spastic contractions of the abdominal muscles occur. During spastic abdominal muscle contraction, gastric and oesophageal pressures increase. This increase in pressure needs to be overcome by the patient for inspiration to take place; hence resulting in breathlessness (Terson de Pavilles *et al.*, 2011).

8.4.2.2.2. Changes in compliance

Within one month following SCI, reductions in lung compliance is observed. The exact cause of reduced lung compliance in this early stage after injury is unknown. It is suggested that reductions in lung volumes due to respiratory muscle weakness and changes in the mechanical properties of the lung from alterations in surfactant production in areas of atelectasis may be contributing factors to the reduction in lung compliance (Brown *et al.*, 2006; Harvey, 2008).

A reduction in chest wall compliance is observed in patients with tetraplegia due to the rigidity of the chest wall from muscle spasticity. Articular changes occur over time at the costosternal and costovertebral joints due to poor inspiratory muscle performance, which restricts the stretching of the chest wall to the level of total lung capacity (TLC) (Brown *et al.*, 2006; Harvey, 2008).

8.4.2.2.3. Changes in lung capacity and lung volumes

Muscle weakness or paralysis and spastic muscle contractions have a significant impact on lung capacity (functional residual capacity (FRC), TLC, vital capacity (VC) and forced vital capacity (FVC)) and lung volume (expiratory reserve volume (ERV), forced expiratory volume in one second (FEV_1), tidal volume (TV) and residual volume (RV)) following SCI. The higher the lesion, the more severely it affects lung capacity and lung volumes (Baydur *et al.*, 2001; Terson de Paleville *et al.*, 2011).

Patients with complete cervical lesions below C2 experience decreases in VC of 20–50% of predicted values due to changes in lung compliance and impairments in inspiratory and expiratory muscle function (Brown *et al.*, 2006; Berlly and Shem, 2007). This drastic reduction in VC leads to inefficient ventilation and poor cough ability. Gaseous exchange is affected by reductions in VC, TLC and VT as hypoventilation leads to carbon dioxide retention and hypoxaemia (Harvey, 2008). Reductions in mean values for FEV_1 and FVC to 40–50% of predicted values have also been reported (Brown *et al.*, 2006). Over time, there seems to be an improvement in VC, FEV_1 and FVC values by approximately 10–15% as a result of improved diaphragmatic efficiency (Brown *et al.*, 2006).

Changes in body positioning influence lung volume and lung capacity in patients with tetraplegia. When a person without SCI moves from a seated to supine position, VC reduces by approximately 7% and inspiratory capacity (IC) increases by approximately 55%. These changes in lung capacity are attributed to fluid shifts in and out of the thorax, resulting in a larger intrathoracic volume in the supine position (Baydur *et al.*, 2001). In tetraplegia, movement into the supine position leads to increases in VC and IC, not only because of increased intrathoracic volume but also due to the effect of gravity on the abdominal contents (Baydur *et al.*, 2001). This explains why patients with tetraplegia report less breathlessness and greater ability to cough without an abdominal binder in a supine position compared to seated position.

8.4.2.2.4. Aspiration pneumonia

Patients with SCI are at high risk for developing aspiration pneumonia (Chin, 2014). Table 8.9 lists the risk factors for aspiration pneumonia in this patient population (Paralyzed Veterans of America, 2005).

The reader is referred to Section 8.6.3.3.9 for information on preventive strategies used for aspiration pneumonia.

Table 8.9: Risk factors for the development of aspiration pneumonia following spinal cord injury.

Spinal shock
Supine position
Cervical spinal cord injury with dysphagia
Slowing of gastro-intestinal tract function, e.g. development of paralytic ileus
Nausea and vomiting
Neck swelling from recent anterior cervical spine surgery
Impaired cognitive state
Poor cough effort or inability to expectorate secretions
Presence of a tracheostomy

8.4.2.2.5. Pulmonary thromboembolism and deep venous thrombosis

Patients with SCI have a three times higher risk for the development of pulmonary embolism and deep venous thrombosis than the general population from 72 hours following injury onwards (Miranda and Hassouna, 2000; Berlly and Shem, 2007). Pulmonary embolism develops in approximately 5% of patients with SCI and deep venous thrombosis in 15% of these patients (McKinney, 2013). Deep venous thrombosis develops as early as 72 hours following injury and the risk remains high until two weeks after SCI (McKinney, 2013).

Possible explanations offered for this increased incidence of thrombosis include metabolic changes in blood vessels due to the interruption of neurologic impulses and resultant paralysis, decreased venous distensibility and increased resistance to venous blood flow, sluggish vasomotor tone and, lastly, vascular adaptations to inactivity and muscle atrophy (Miranda and Hassouna, 2000; McKinney, 2013). Prophylactic therapy in the form of low molecular weight heparin and the use of intermittent pneumatic compression devices as precautionary methods are recommended for a minimum of eight weeks following SCI (Berlly and Shem, 2007). Regular screening of the patient for sudden onset of shortness of breath, difficulty breathing and hypoxia or limb pain, limb swelling, limb tenderness, limb discolouration and increased skin temperature is of vital importance.

8.4.3. *Recovery of respiratory function following spinal cord injury*

Respiratory function improves spontaneously in patients with low level tetraplegia or paraplegia within the first year after injury, and only a small percentage of patients require further ventilatory support. This improvement is ascribed to small improvements in general motor function. Very little improvement is noted after the first year, and in some cases loss of function is even observed (Zimmer *et al.*, 2007). Breathlessness is a symptom that many patients with chronic SCI report and seems to be more prominent in patients with tetraplegia than in those with paraplegia. Environmental factors, such as exposure to hot air, or lifestyle choices, e.g. exposure to direct or second-hand smoke and increased body mass index, may increase the sensation of breathlessness in tetraplegic patients (Stepp *et al.*, 2008; Schilero *et al.*, 2009). Increased body mass index leads to decreased TLC, FRC and RV. Patients with thoracic SCI between T1 and T6 have permanently altered lung mechanics, but have a greater chance of recovering from future lung infections than those with tetraplegia. In those with thoracic lesions below T6, lung mechanics are less altered and their ability to recover from future lung infections is greater.

8.4.4. *Spinal cord injury not associated with respiratory compromise*

Not all SCIs result in respiratory function abnormalities. Patients with central cord syndrome present with minimal to no respiratory system involvement if they are mobilised early during their admission. Posterior cord syndrome does not affect the respiratory system much and hence chest complications are rare. The effects of Brown Sequard syndrome on the chest are minimal, and if the patient does not develop other complications they are unlikely to develop respiratory complications. If a patient with compression of the conus medullaris and cauda equina is mobile, there should not be any complications concerning the respiratory system. Early mobilisation, in patients with stable SCI, or prophylatic chest physiotherapy should help prevent any respiratory system complications.

Table 8.10: Bodily system complications secondary to spinal cord injury.

Bodily system	Complications
Digestive system and gastro-intestinal tract	• Cholecystitis • Upper gastro-intestinal tract bleeding • Stool incontinence • Constipation • Haemorrhoids
Integumentary system	• Pressure ulcers
Musculoskeletal system	• Muscle weakness • Atrophy • Spasticity • Osteoporosis • Hypercalcemia
Psychological	• Pain • Depression
Renal and urinary systems	• Hydronephrosis • Urinary tract infections
Reproductive system	• Male infertility • Erectile dysfunction
Vascular system	• Thromboembolism

8.5. Complications Related to Other Bodily Systems following Spinal Cord Injury

Patients with SCI are at a higher risk of developing complications related to the integumentary, musculoskeletal, vascular, gastrointestinal, digestive and renal systems. A short summary of complications commonly reported are listed in Table 8.10 (Wuermser *et al.*, 2007; Rahimi-Movaghar *et al.*, 2013). The development of any one of these complications increases patient morbidity and hospital length of stay and therefore high quality care should be provided by the interdisciplinary team members to any patient with SCI to avoid its development as far as possible.

8.6. Medical and Surgical Management

On admission to the emergency department, the patient with suspected acute SCI undergoes assessment through use of primary and secondary survey procedures; thereafter, definitive care is provided.

Key Message

At the scene of the accident, a patient with suspected SCI undergoes triple immobilisation. This involves placing the patient in a hard cervical collar, head restraints with sand bags and strapping to a long spinal board. The patient is kept in a flat supine position and log rolled, when necessary, until the spine is cleared of fractures through clinical and radiological investigations in the emergency department.

8.6.1. *Primary survey and resuscitation of vital functions*

The primary survey consists of using the internationally accepted 'airways, breathing, circulation, disability, exposure' (ABCDE) approach to advanced trauma life support, as described in Chapter 5. Important aspects of the ABCDE approach to patients with suspected SCI include (Schmidt *et al.*, 2009; Thim *et al.*, 2012; Chin, 2014) the following.

- *Airway* patency with protection of the cervical spine. If an artificial airway is needed this is put into position through the 'stiff-neck' procedure in unconscious patients or conscious patients who complain of neck pain. The 'stiff-neck' procedure refers to using a jaw-thrust technique while the patient's spine is kept in a stable in-line position.
- *Circulation*. Patients with tetraplegia or high level (above T6) thoracic SCI often present with low BP due to neurogenic shock (see Section 8.2.2.2.1). This is a normal occurrence and intravenous volume replacement is monitored carefully in the emergency department to maintain mean arterial pressure at 85–90 mmHg to minimise secondary damage to the spinal cord through ischaemia; however, overhydration and resultant pulmonary oedema should be avoided. Hypotension in patients with SCI below T6 is caused by haemorrhage, the origin of which should be determined as a matter of priority.
- *Disability*. Motor and sensory examination as well as the establishment of the presence or absence of reflexes and sphincter control is performed; this examination may be hindered in the unconscious patient.

This will allow any potential neurological impairment to be identified as a baseline measure, as this may change with the development of spinal shock. Assessment for the presence of fractures or deformities, abdominal injuries or other neurological injuries is also performed.

- Injuries identified by *exposing* the patient through the removal of clothes in order to visualise the skin and identify injuries. The patient is log rolled during examination of the dorsal spine for bruising. In this position the spinous processes are palpated for fractures or widened spaces, which would indicate spinal trauma.

The type of radiological investigations performed and care provided to the patient is similar to that described in Chapter 5. If thoracic trauma is suspected in addition to SCI, the patient will be screened for the presence of the 'lethal six injuries' related to thoracic trauma, as discussed in Chapter 5 (Section 5.3.1.1).

8.6.2. *Secondary survey as adjunct to primary survey*

The secondary survey consists of a 'head-to-toe' evaluation of the patient as well as detailed history taking, as discussed in previous chapters. Whole body spiral computed tomography (CT) scan from 'head-to-toe' is often used to diagnose spinal trauma. If a person was ejected from a motor vehicle in the event of a motor vehicle accident, their likelihood to have sustained spinal trauma is 26 times greater than for a person who was restrained in the vehicle with a seatbelt (Schmidt *et al.*, 2009).

If the patient sustained additional thoracic injuries, screening for the presence of the 'hidden six injuries' will be performed at this stage (Chapter 5, Section 5.3.2.1). If the patient's condition is stable, placement of arterial and central venous pressure lines is performed. Stable patients are transferred to the spinal ward for monitoring and care. In the case of an unstable spinal injury, the patient may be referred for emergency surgery and the placement of lines is performed in theatre. After surgery, the patient may be admitted to a high care unit or ICU for observation and care until their condition stabilises. Patients with unstable spinal injuries who are either deemed too unstable for immediate surgery or are being managed conservatively are admitted to the ICU for specialised care.

8.6.3. *Definitive care*

Definitive care is initiated once the patient is transferred either to theatre, the ICU or the spinal ward. In the context of SCI, surgical or conservative interventions as well as the care provided to the patient in the ICU are discussed below.

8.6.3.1. *Surgical interventions*

8.6.3.1.1. Early stage after spinal cord injury

Indications for surgery include neurological impairment, mechanical instability due to disruption of the posterior tension band or rotational instability, spinal canal encroachment by more than 50%, vertebral body wedging by more than 50% or kyphosis more than 25° at the injury level (Marré *et al.*, 2011).

Not all patients will require surgical stabilisation; however, when appropriate, spinal decompression surgery is performed on patients with unstable spinal fractures within the first 24 hours after injury in order to preserve as much neurological function as possible. This is the case even in the polytrauma patient (Schmidt *et al.*, 2009). Decision making regarding early surgical intervention is, however, based on individual patient assessment, as early surgical intervention may pose more risks than benefits for some patients.

Decompression surgery of the cervical, thoracic or lumbar spine is performed with the aim of freeing up space for nerves in the spinal canal. A variety of techniques may be used, such as discectomy, laminectomy, laminotomy, laminoplasty or foramenotomy. The technique used depends on the level of the spinal lesion and the structures causing the compression (Farcy and Schwab, 2009). Instrumentation may also be used to provide additional stabilisation to the spine and is made of metal, stainless steel or titanium. The types of instrumentation used include (Farcy and Schwab, 2009; Marré *et al.*, 2011):

- plates,
- screws, rods or hooks,
- wiring, and
- interbody cages.

An anterior or posterior surgical approach may be used for early decompression surgery (Farcy and Schwab, 2009; Schmidt *et al.*, 2009). Consideration for surgery must include the need for a tracheostomy. If an anterior approach to surgery is used, this may impact on tracheostomy placement due to the sites of incisions. Patients who present with signs of shock, hypothermia, coagulopathy and acidosis have a high risk for mortality and undergo a staged procedure of initial stabilisation of the spine. Secondary surgery for further stabilisation of the spine is performed when the patient's condition stabilises. Secondary surgery is often scheduled between days seven and 10 of the patient's stay in the ICU. The decision to take the patient to theatre is influenced by the presence of infection or acute respiratory distress syndrome, which prolongs the hyperinflammatory state of the patient and thus patient outcome. An anterior surgical approach may be used for secondary surgery (Schmidt *et al.*, 2009).

Surgical management of an odontoid fracture includes a posterior fusion of C1 and C2 vertebrae with wire, cable or screw instrumentation to prevent subluxation of C1 vertebra on C2 (Shears and Armitstead, 2010). Posterior fusion has a high success rate, but the patient's quality of life (QOL) is severely affected, as a reduction of up to 50% in rotational movement at the atlanto-axial joint occurs after surgery, together with a 10% reduction in flexion and extension of the upper cervical spine (Longo *et al.*, 2010). Anterior fusion of odontoid fractures may preserve rotational movement at the atlanto-axial joint, more so than posterior fusion, but can lead to several complications, such as neural or vessel injury, oesophageal injury or airway obstruction (Longo *et al.*, 2010). The reader is referred to Section 8.6.3.2 for more information on the non-operative approach to high cervical SCI.

After decompression surgery, the patient may be required to wear a brace for a number of weeks to allow for joint immobilisation to limit movement and prevent further damage during the healing process. A variety of cervical braces (Section 8.6.3.2.3) or thoraco-lumbar-sacral orthosis (TLSO) may be prescribed, depending on the type of surgery that was performed (Fig. 8.6). A variety of brands of TLSO are available and, depending on availability, different brands may be used in different countries.

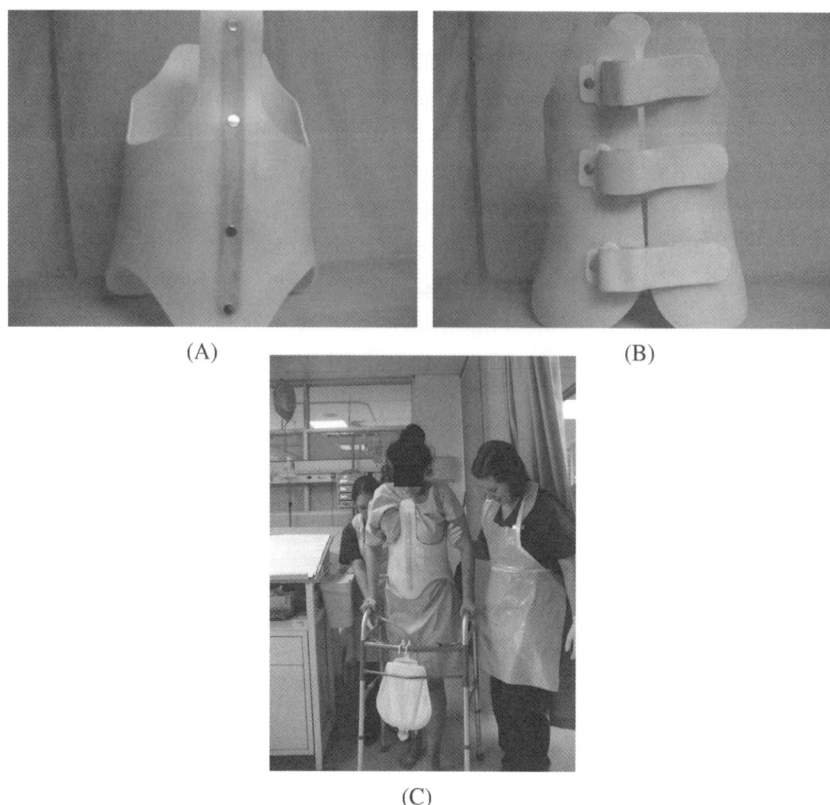

Fig. 8.6: Thoraco-lumbar-sacral orthosis. (A) Anterior view; (B) Posterior view; (C) Postoperative patient mobilising with TLSO, walking frame and minimal assistance of one physiotherapist in the ICU.

8.6.3.1.2. Surgical management approaches in the later stages after spinal cord injury

8.6.3.1.2.1. *Diaphragm pacing*. Patients with high-level SCI, who are chronically dependent on MV, may benefit from diaphragm pacing to assist with weaning from ventilation. Diaphragmatic pacemaker implantation can be performed laparoscopically and is considered for patients who have a diaphragm that will respond to stimulation and has preserved phrenic nerves (Tedde *et al.*, 2012). The electrodes are implanted into the motor points of the branches of the left and right hemi-diaphragms. After

Table 8.11: Advantages associated with a diaphragm pacing device.

Greater patient mobility
Elimination of fear of disconnection from the ventilator
Elimination of embarrassment and social stigma associated with connection to a ventilator
Improved speech
Reduced requirements for nursing assistance
Improved sense of well-being

placement of the pacemaker, the patient is placed back onto their previous level of respiratory support. Condition training of the diaphragm is initiated soon after surgery through intermittent use of the pacing device. This is done for progressively longer time periods over the following days. Diaphragmatic pacing allows for the generation of adequate VT and VC, which enables breathing without ventilator support for a certain time period. Some patients manage to wean off MV altogether, while others manage to breathe for up to 16 hours per day with the diaphragm pacemaker (Tedde *et al.*, 2012). The advantages of diaphragm pacing are summarised in Table 8.11 (DiMarco, 2005). The costs associated with the pacing device and its surgical implantation makes this option available only to a select number of patients with SCI.

8.6.3.1.2.2. *Other methods of spinal cord stimulation.* Techniques such as phrenic nerve pacing, intercostal pacing and combined intercostal and unilateral diaphragm pacing may also be used to facilitate weaning of patients with high cervical SCI from MV. A thoracotomy procedure is necessary for phrenic nerve pacing to implant the electrodes on the phrenic nerve. Some complications associated with phrenic nerve pacing include a high risk of nerve damage or deterioration associated with the placement of the electrodes. Clinical trials have shown that patients with diaphragm pacing or phrenic nerve pacing have significantly improved lung volumes, which assist with weaning from MV (DiMarco, 2005; Zimmer *et al.*, 2007).

Sharma *et al.* (2012) state that expiratory muscle function in patients with SCI can be improved through the use of functional electrical stimulation in order to produce a stronger cough effort. In a small trial that consisted of only nine patients with cervical SCI, the effect of lower thoracic

(T9–L1) spinal cord stimulation on expiratory muscle function was assessed. Surgery was performed on each patient to place the implantable electrical stimulation system. The authors reported good activation of the expiratory muscles, which resulted in higher peak expiratory flow rates and improved cough effort (DiMarco *et al.*, 2009). The results of this study are promising but need to be verified in larger trials.

8.6.3.2. *Conservative management*

Conservative management of cervical SCI aims to provide stabilisation to the spine in the early stage after injury prior to surgery, postoperatively or as the definitive method of treatment (Lauweryns, 2010). Skeletal skull traction, halo vest or cervical braces can be used.

8.6.3.2.1. Skeletal skull traction

Skeletal skull traction is used in patients with subluxation or dislocation of facet joints, burst-type fractures or upper cervical fractures (Lauweryns, 2010). Gardner-Wells tongs are used for skeletal skull traction and should be placed into position by an experienced team. X-rays, fluoroscopic equipment and MRI are used to determine if the tongs are correctly placed in order to stabilise and re-align the cervical spine. A halo ring can be used instead of tongs in patients where halo vest treatment will be the choice of definitive management (Lauweryns, 2010). After the placement of skeletal skull traction, the patient is confined to bed rest for a period of six weeks; thereafter, treatment might be changed to halo vest traction for a further three to four months (Lauweryns, 2010).

8.6.3.2.2. Halo vest immobilisation

This type of immobilisation can be used as a definitive treatment or adjunct to surgical intervention (O'Dowd, 2010). A halo traction ring is attached to the patient's head with titanium screws that are screwed into the skull. A vest is made for each individual patient and is attached to the ring through wiring to ensure adequate stabilisation of the cervical spine during sitting (Fig. 8.7).

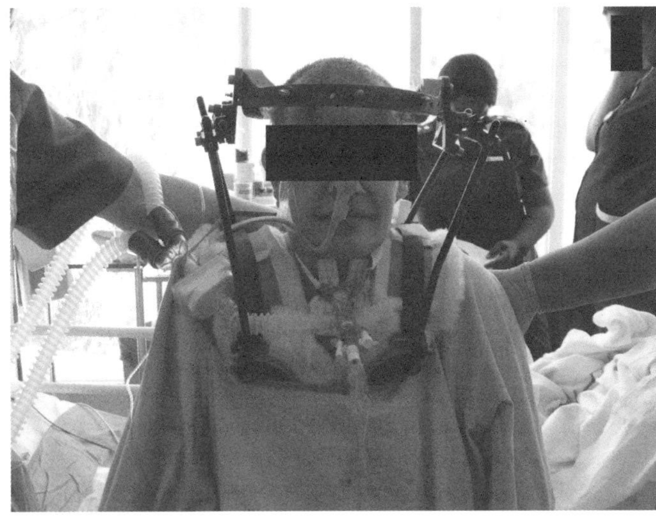

Fig. 8.7: A ventilated patient with C2 on C3 fracture dislocation sits up over the side of the bed in the ICU wearing a halo vest with the assistance of a physiotherapist and nursing sister.

The halo vest is more effective in stabilising the spine than cervical braces, as it restricts flexion-extension motion in the upper cervical spine by up to 75% (Lauweryns, 2010). It is superior to cervical braces as it controls the amount of lateral bending and rotation of the neck more effectively (Lauweryns, 2010). The halo vest is associated with a shorter duration of hospital stay and is less costly to the patient. This type of management can be used for patients with a variety of upper cervical fractures, except for hangman's fractures (O'Dowd, 2010). No evidence exists to show that surgical management of an odontoid fracture is superior to the conservative management of these fractures (Shears and Armitstead, 2010). Halo vest immobilisation is also recommended for patients with atlas fractures, although those who present with persistent pain or non-union should undergo surgery (Longo *et al.*, 2010).

The complications reported from halo vest immobilisation are listed in Table 8.12 (Longo *et al.*, 2010).

Children younger than eight years old with upper cervical spine injuries are usually managed with halo immobilisation, as they tend to have poor compliance with wearing cervical braces (Lauweryns, 2010). When

Table 8.12: Complications associated with halo vest immobilisation.

Patient discomfort	Dural penetration
Pin-site infection	Cerebrospinal fluid leakage
Nerve injury	Intracranial abscesses
Osteomyelitis	Dysphagia
Pin-site scar formation	Loss of reduction
Restriction of pulmonary function	

Table 8.13: Cervical braces commonly used in the management of patients with spinal cord injury.

Type	Function	Application
Soft cervical collar	• Uses sensory feedback to limit motion of the cervical spine • Provides no significant control of cervical motion	• Soft tissue injuries of the neck (whiplash)
Hard cervical collar (Fig. 8.8)	• Provides more restriction to neck flexion, extension, lateral bending and rotation than soft collars • It extends from the occiput and lower jaw down to the upper region of the thorax	• Soft tissue injuries (including ligamentous injury) • Stable bony injury • Used when weaning patients off a more restrictive orthosis
Cervico-thoracic orthosis	• Provides more restriction to neck flexion, extension, lateral bending and rotation than hard cervical collars • It is lighter in weight than a halo vest orthosis but provides less restriction of motion than the halo vest	• Moderately stable cervical fractures • Postsurgical fusions

indicated, wiring and fusion is used in children older than eight years, as their vertebrae are developed more like that of an adult (Duhem *et al.*, 2008).

8.6.3.2.3. Cervical braces

A variety of cervical braces are available to assist with spinal immobilisation, and Table 8.13 offers a summary of their functions and applications (Uustal and Baerga, 2004; Lauweryns, 2010).

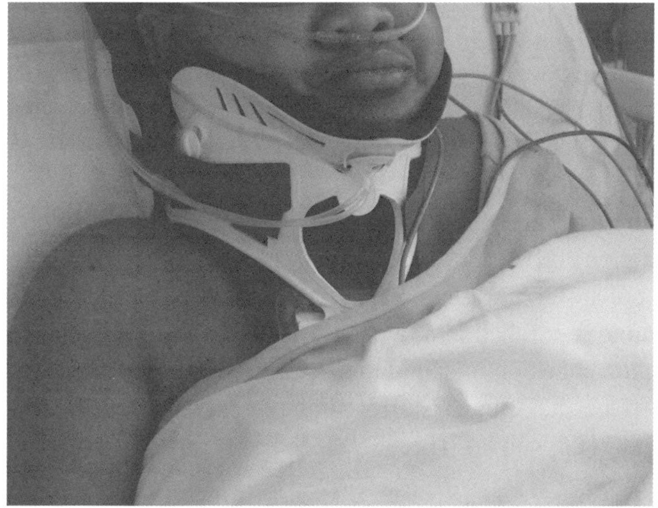

Fig. 8.8: Hard cervical collar.

Reported complications related to long-term use of cervical collars include skin irritation or skin breakdown, muscle atrophy, pain and psychological dependence (Lauweryns, 2010).

8.6.3.3. *Care provided in the ICU or the spinal unit*

Adult or paediatric patients with high-level SCI, haemodynamic instability or additional injuries that warrant specialised care are admitted to the ICU. Treatment provided in the ICU includes the following.

8.6.3.3.1. Pain control

Pharmacological pain management in the acute care setting includes the use of non-steroidal anti-inflammatory drugs, non-narcotic muscle relaxants, psychotropic (antidepressant and anti-convulsant) drugs, anaesthetic drugs, anti-spasticity drugs and opioids. Most of these drugs have been reported to reduce neuropathic as well as musculoskeletal pain after SCI (Mehta *et al.*, 2014).

8.6.3.3.2. Management of hypoxaemia

Hypoxaemia in patients with SCI is a risk factor for secondary damage to the cord and is counteracted by the administration of oxygen therapy using devices such as nasal cannula, face mask or partial rebreathing or non-rebreathing oxygen masks.

Non-invasive pressure ventilation devices can also be used for oxygen administration and, in addition, applying pressure to the airways to recruit partially collapsed lung segments. Non-invasive ventilation is also useful in preventing re-intubation of a patient with SCI after weaning from invasive MV. It can be administered in the form of continuous positive airway pressure (face mask interface) or biphasic airway pressure (face mask interface or chest cuirass) (Fig. 8.9).

8.6.3.3.3. Respiratory failure

As mentioned in earlier sections of this chapter, patients with SCI above T6 are more at risk of developing respiratory failure due to spinal shock, inability

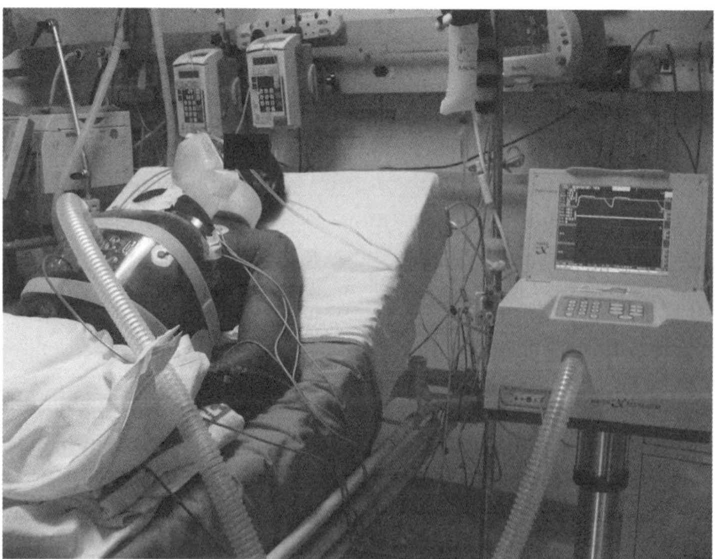

Fig. 8.9: A postoperative patient with fusion for C4 on C5 dislocation managed with non-invasive biphasic airway pressure ventilation (applied using chest cuirass) and a partial rebreathing oxygen mask.

to clear secretions effectively, loss of lung volumes and poor inspiratory muscle strength. In these situations, endotracheal intubation and MV can be life-saving. Patients with ASIA A SCI above C5 are managed with intubation and MV and all of these patients will require tracheostomy. Tracheostomy will also be required for 50% of those with ASIA A lesions below C6 and in only 7% of those with incomplete SCI (Berlly and Shem, 2007).

Advantages associated with tracheostomy include greater comfort for the patient, easier access for airway suction and easier weaning from MV due to the reduction in dead space breathing compared to an endotracheal tube (Berlly and Shem, 2007). Tracheostomy in patients with cervical SCI has been shown to reduce ICU and hospital length of stay, duration of MV and mortality rates (Call *et al*., 2011). Not all patients with cervical SCI require tracheostomy and can be successfully weaned and extubated from MV using a carefully executed protocol (Call *et al*., 2011). Tracheostomy performed within seven to 10 days from intubation leads to significant reductions in MV duration and ICU length of stay when compared to tracheostomy insertion after day 10 (Romero *et al*., 2009; Berney *et al*., 2011; Markandaya *et al*., 2012; Choi *et al*., 2013). No significant differences in the rates of VAP or patient mortality were reported when early tracheostomy was compared to late tracheostomy (Romero *et al*., 2009; Choi *et al*., 2013). The reader is referred to Chapter 5 (Section 5.3.4.1) for information on tracheostomy care.

Suctioning of the airways as part of pulmonary hygiene is important to assist with the prevention of respiratory infections. The reader is referred to Chapter 4 (Section 4.2.7) for information on suction procedures used for artificial airways, as well as how to perform oronasal and nasotracheal suction.

Key Message

Suction of the airways may lead to bradycardia and even cardiac arrest in patients with cervical SCI within the first four weeks after injury due to spinal shock and the development of autonomic dysreflexia. Pre-oxygenation prior to suction and close monitoring of the patient during the procedure is of great importance.

8.6.3.3.4. Haemodynamic support

To maintain perfusion to the spinal cord and further minimise secondary damage to the cord, mean arterial BP is maintained at 85–90 mmHg with the administration of intravenous fluids, as mentioned previously. Patients with severe cervical SCI are at risk of developing arrhythmias (especially bradycardia or tachyarrhythmia) and need close monitoring and pharmacological intervention if indicated (McKinley, 2014). Vasopressor medication may also be administered for patients with cervical SCI, as some may present with persistent mean arterial BP below 85 mmHg (Casha and Christie, 2011).

8.6.3.3.5. Regulation of body temperature

Patients with SCI above T6 are unable to self-regulate their body temperature (Denton and McKinlay, 2009; McKinley, 2014) and therefore monitoring of core and peripheral temperatures and the use of warming devices form part of ICU care (Denton and McKinlay, 2009).

8.6.3.3.6. Genitourinary care

The bladder is flaccid in the acute stages after SCI and the insertion of an indwelling urinary catheter is required to facilitate emptying of the bladder. Bladder flaccidity is followed by bladder spasticity with long-term impairment in bladder emptying and the development of recurrent urinary tract infections. The indwelling catheter is removed after three weeks and intermittent straight catheterisation of the bladder is performed.

8.6.3.3.7. Corticosteroids

Corticosteroids such as methylprednisolone, when administered in high doses within eight hours of injury, leads to significant improvement in motor and sensory function in adult patients with complete or incomplete SCI (Kwon *et al.*, 2004; Markandaya *et al.*, 2012; Chin, 2014). There is currently insufficient evidence for the use of neuroprotective approaches such as hypothermia and steroids for the treatment of SCI in children (Parent *et al.*, 2011).

8.6.3.3.8. Prophylaxis for deep venous thrombosis

Deep venous thrombosis prophylaxis is an important element of ICU management of both adult and paediatric patients with SCI, as deep venous thrombosis can lead to pulmonary embolism and death. An aggressive approach to prophylaxis should be followed and should include baseline and serial screening of blood clotting factors, Doppler ultrasonography of the lower extremities, anti-embolism stockings and administration of low molecular weight heparin or placement of an inferior vena cava filter (McKinley, 2014). Continuation of thromboprophylaxis therapy and compression stockings is recommended for a duration of three months following injury (Zidek and Srinivasan, 2003; Casha and Christie, 2011).

8.6.3.3.9. Gastro-intestinal care

Patients with cervical or high thoracic SCI suffer from delayed gastric emptying and paralytic ileus often develops, which can last for three weeks after injury (Denton and McKinlay, 2009). As a result, gastric distension and vomiting may occur and lead to the development of aspiration pneumonia. Gastro-intestinal care in the ICU involves the administration of laxatives to avoid constipation and daily rectal examination to identify and reduce faecal impaction. Prokinetic drug therapy is used to promote feeding and a nasogastric or orogastric tube, placed during the primary survey, is used for gastric emptying to prevent aspiration of feed into the lungs (Denton and McKinlay, 2009).

8.6.3.3.10. Nutrition

In the acute stage after SCI, patients present with lower metabolic activity and a negative nitrogen balance (Thibault-Halman *et al.*, 2011). Enteral feeding is performed using a nasogastric or orogastric tube. If the nasogastric route is unsuccessful, feeding is done through a nasojejunal tube or percutaneous endoscopic gastrostomy tube (Denton and McKinlay, 2009; Thibault-Halman *et al.*, 2011).

8.6.3.3.11. Spasticity

Spasticity may develop as spinal shock resolves. Spasticity in adults and children can be treated pharmacologically with antispastic medication, e.g. baclofen, tizanidine, diazepam, dantrolene or clonidine. Splinting or casting may also be beneficial to avoid contracture formation (Denton and McKinlay, 2009).

8.7. Physiotherapy Aims of Management

Physiotherapists are essential members of the interdisciplinary team involved in the management of patients with SCI. The accepted standards of care that form the basis of physiotherapeutic management of the patient with SCI includes the importance of team work, continued education of patients and caregivers, evaluation and re-evaluation throughout the continuum of care and the use of outcome measures. Daily re-evaluation of the patient's condition and response to treatment given is essential, as each patient differs and therefore treatment intervention should be tailored to individual needs. The reader is referred to Chapter 5 (Section 5.4) for information on the National Institute of Health and Care Excellence (NICE) clinical practice guidelines on rehabilitation of patients after critical illness. The interdisciplinary team approach to patient rehabilitation in the ICU with regard to regular communication between team members and treatment planning that involves all team members is of utmost importance for the management of patients with SCI. As mentioned previously in this chapter, the use of a comprehensive clinical pathway and structured respiratory care protocol reduces the development of respiratory complications in patients with acute cervical or high thoracic SCI (Berney *et al.*, 2011).

Physiotherapy-specific aims of intervention for patients with SCI are listed in Table 8.14. These suggested aims of management should be tailored to the needs of each individual patient with SCI in the acute care setting.

Table 8.14: Aims of physiotherapy management for patients with SCI in the ICU.

- Adequate humidification of the airways to limit the development of thick tenacious secretions
- Mobilisation and removal of excessive retained secretions from the airways of patients who are intubated in order to prevent the development of secondary chest infections
- Augment the patient's cough effort in order to assist with effective secretion clearance
- Increase posterior and basal lung volumes of patients who are intubated and sedated in order to prevent the development of atelectasis
- Increase chest wall and lung compliance in order to optimise and restore lung function
- Increase oxygenation
- Improve the strength of respiratory muscles that are still innervated following spinal cord trauma as soon as the patient becomes conscious and cooperative in order to assist with weaning from MV
- Maintain or restore passive range of motion (ROM) of all limbs in order to prevent or reduce joint stiffness in patients who are intubated and sedated
- Maintain or restore the length of two-joint muscles through the use of positioning and splinting to prevent contracture formation
- Improve muscle power to innervated muscles following SCI as soon as the patient regains consciousness and is able to participate
- As the patient regains consciousness and their condition stabilises, aim to improve functionality in order for them to gain as much independence with activities of daily living (ADL) within the limitations posed by the SCI and postoperative care protocols

Important aims for the progression of the patient's physiotherapy management on the ward are listed in Table 8.15. These aims should be tailored to each individual patient's needs.

8.7.1. *Paediatric considerations*

The aims of physiotherapy intervention are similar for adults and children with SCI, but the pre-morbid functional and developmental level of the child must be taken into account when devising short-term and long-term aims of treatment.

Despite their injury level, cognisance must be taken of the fact that children continue to grow and develop physically, cognitively and emotionally. Family-centred care that includes the child and the family in setting treatment goals and priorities, and the involvement of the family in the treatment itself, is imperative. Considering the increased

Table 8.15: Aims for the progression of management for patients with SCI in the ward setting.

- Continue with humidification of the airways for as long as the patient receives oxygen therapy
- Enhance the patient's independence by teaching them and the nursing staff assisted coughing techniques to mobilise and clear excessive retained secretions
- Optimise lung volumes and lung compliance during the patient's stay in the ward within the limitations posed by the level of SCI
- Improve the patient's independence through encouragement of active and active-resisted ROM exercises of the limbs, as can be reasonably expected following the injury
- Joint end-of-range motion should be maintained for all affected joints at least once per day. An exception to this rule applies to patients with C6 SCI, in which finger flexion contracture is encouraged to enable the patient to have a functional hand grip (passive grip and release) when performing wrist extension with finger tenodesis
- Optimise muscle power in all functional peripheries, especially the upper limbs, within the limits of the injury
- Education and rehabilitation of the patient and their family regarding functional activities (e.g. wheelchair use and transfers) on the ward
- Increase cardiorespiratory exercise endurance in order to obtain the health benefits of exercise

prevalence of upper cervical SCI in young children, they are more likely to suffer widespread impairment than adults. However, a greater proportion of children improve neurologically with improved functional ability following SCI than adults (Parent *et al.*, 2011; Clarke, 2012). This may in part be due to neuroplasticity of the immature nervous system (Pape, 2012).

Scoliosis is a particularly common complication of SCI in children, occurring in almost all children who sustain an injury more than a year before reaching skeletal maturity (Zidek and Srinivasan, 2003; Parent *et al.*, 2011). Spinal deformities can lead to pelvic obliquity, pressure ulcers, pain and severe respiratory complications. Therefore careful attention to orthoses and supported seating with correct postural alignment is essential to minimise the complication of skeletal deformities.

For more information about the rehabilitation of patients with SCI after discharge from the acute care setting, refer to Section 8.11.

8.7.2. *Functional assessment prior to discharge*

Prior to discharge from the acute care facility, every adult and paediatric patient with SCI should undergo a functional assessment (Chapter 5, Section 5.4.2). The impact of the functional assessment outcomes on the patient's ability to perform ADL should be assessed. Based on these findings, the rehabilitation goals for post-discharge care should be discussed with the patient and their family and agreed upon.

8.8. Precautions and Contraindications Related to Physiotherapy Management

Recommendations provided here are mostly based on expert opinion derived from clinical practice due to paucity in the literature in certain aspects of patient care in the acute care setting.

8.8.1. *General precautions related to physiotherapy in intensive care*

The reader is referred to Chapter 5 (Section 5.5.1) for a list of general precautions that should be adhered to during the treatment of any trauma patient in the acute care setting.

8.8.2. *Specific precautions and contraindications related to physiotherapy in patients with spinal trauma*

8.8.2.1. *Adult patient*

- It is the physiotherapist's duty to check the patient's operation notes regularly to ascertain safe, effective treatment in light of the type of surgical procedure performed and any surgical requests.
- The head-down tilt position for postural drainage is contraindicated in patients with acute spinal cord trauma due to the presence of oedema around the cord lesion and inefficiency of the diaphragm, as these might lead to further haemodynamic instability.

- Log rolling of any patient with unstable SCI is of vital importance during position changes for physiotherapy treatment and the performance of nursing activities such as pressure care and washing the patient.
- Manual cough assistance manoeuvres are contraindicated in patients with SCI who have inferior vena cava filters, as such manoeuvres can dislodge the filter (Roth *et al.*, 2010). In the case of cervical SCI, manually assisted coughs should only be considered after spinal stabilisation or if a second person is available to stabilise the spine during the manoeuvre.
- It is recommended that a hard cervical collar is worn during the day for a period of six weeks after cervical surgery. The patient should be educated that a soft cervical collar should be worn at night. Postoperative care protocols may differ in various settings and should be discussed with the local attending surgeon.
- In some countries, the physiotherapist educates the patient, family and nursing staff on the correct placement and positioning of the TLSO brace before the patient is mobilised after surgery. In other countries, such education is performed by the orthotist.
- The TLSO brace is usually worn for a period of eight to 12 weeks after thoracic spine surgery. The exact duration should be discussed with each patient's surgeon.
- Throughout physiotherapy sessions with patients that have T6 lesions or above, the therapist should monitor the urinary catheter for possible twisting or blockage. If the patient develops an episode of autonomic dysreflexia during physiotherapy treatment, the physiotherapist should immediately place them in an upright position to encourage pooling of blood in the lower extremities to reduce BP (Stephenson, 2013). The patient's BP must be monitored and the cause of the painful stimulus identified. The physiotherapist should treat this as a medical emergency and terminate the treatment session until the patient stabilises. The physiotherapist should follow the established protocols in their local place of work for alerting the medical team to the incident and ensuring appropriate management is given to the patient.

8.8.2.2. *Paediatric patient*

The precautions to physiotherapy intervention are similar between adults and children with SCI. In addition, the following paediatric-specific factors should be considered.

- Heterotopic ossification has been reported in some children following SCI, with the hip most commonly involved. Limited joint ROM, with or without pain and swelling, is the most common sign in children. If ossification is related to muscle trauma, the joint should be immobilised for a period of five to seven days, after which active movement should be encouraged (Staheli, 2001).
- Manual cough assistance should not be performed using an abdominal thrust in young children. This manoeuvre may cause damage to abdominal organs and vascular structures (especially the descending aorta), which are not as well protected by muscle and adipose tissue in children. Bilateral chest wall compression techniques (Chapter 4, Sections 4.2.5.1 and 8.9.1.3.1) should rather be used.

8.9. Physiotherapy Interventions

Similar to the management of other patients with traumatic injuries, physiotherapy management focuses on support of the respiratory system in the acute stage after SCI. Mortality rate is significantly reduced in patients with SCI if a structured respiratory care protocol is used by physiotherapists and nurses looking after such patients in the acute setting (see Section 8.11 for further information). Patients, however, will only benefit from such an approach when a combination of techniques are included in a respiratory care protocol and applied frequently (Berney *et al.*, 2011). Examples of such techniques are discussed in this section. As the patient's condition stabilises and they wake up from sedation in the ICU and become more cooperative, active rehabilitation is immediately commenced.

In several developed countries, patients with SCI who have stabilised but are still intubated and ventilated are transferred from the level one trauma centre to other 'step down' rehabilitation units that specialise in the management of patients on long-term ventilation. Interventions such as respiratory and peripheral muscle training and retraining of functional activities would be implemented as part of patient care in these rehabilitation units and may be interpreted as 'later stage management' of these patients. In other countries, patients with SCI who have been stabilised remain in the ICU of the trauma centre to which they were originally admitted while they are on MV, until such time that they are weaned and successfully extubated and transferred to a rehabilitation hospital. Some that cannot be weaned from MV may be transferred to a nursing home facility for long-term care. The interventions mentioned above form part of the acute care setting daily management of SCI patients in these countries until the time of their discharge from the ICU to a rehabilitation setting or nursing home. The discussion of physiotherapy interventions provided below has taken into consideration both of these scenarios. It starts with interventions used for respiratory system management and is followed by musculoskeletal system management. Recommendations provided here are based on evidence and, in the absence of research evidence, expert opinion has been used.

8.9.1. *Respiratory system*

8.9.1.1. *Oxygenation*

In the previous chapters of this book the use of body position changes as part of physiotherapy patient management in acute care is advocated in order to improve oxygenation and FRC. Use of the upright position in particular is emphasised to achieve these goals. These principles do, however, not apply to patients with SCI, especially those with cervical cord lesions.

Expiratory reserve volume is less in patients with SCI than able-bodied persons, regardless of the level of injury to the spine (Schilero *et al.*, 2009). In the supine position patients with cervical SCI experience an increase in VC due to a reduction in RV as a result of the effect of gravity on the abdominal contents. The abdominal contents rest against the diaphragm, increasing the zone of apposition, and as the diaphragm contracts it has a greater downwards excursion because the diaphragm fibres function at a more favourable portion of their length-tension curve (Schilero *et al.*, 2009). In the seated position these patients experience significantly lower FVC and FEV_1 values due to the loss of tension in the abdominal wall (decreasing the zone of apposition) as a result of the spinal cord trauma. This loss of abdominal wall tension causes the abdominal contents to fall forward and downwards. The use of an abdominal binder for a patient with tetraplegia is reported to alleviate these symptoms somewhat and improvements in VC, inspiratory capacity and TLC in sitting have been found (Schilero *et al.*, 2009; Reid *et al.*, 2010).

In the acute stage after SCI, the seated position is contraindicated due to the presence of spinal shock and cord oedema. Therefore, in the acute stage, the optimal position to improve oxygenation for a patient with tetraplegia is the supine position. In the later stages after injury a seated position and abdominal binder may be used to further improve oxygenation.

8.9.1.2. *Humidification*

The same methods, described in Chapter 5 (Section 5.6.1.2), may be used to provide humidification of the airways of intubated and non-intubated patients with SCI.

8.9.1.3. *Management of pulmonary secretions*

8.9.1.3.1. Intubated patient

Pulmonary secretion mobilisation and clearance can be achieved through the use of modified postural drainage positions, manual chest clearance techniques, suction and manual hyperinflation (MHI). The reader is referred to Chapter 4 (Section 4.2) for information on the safe and effective performance of these techniques. Low-level evidence exists to support the use of manual percussion, vibrations, chest wall shaking and postural drainage to mobilise and clear retained secretions from the airways of patients with SCI (Reid *et al.*, 2010). Principles regarding the use of saline during suction and the use of open versus closed suction systems in the management of patients with SCI are similar to that described in Chapter 5 (Section 5.6.1.3).

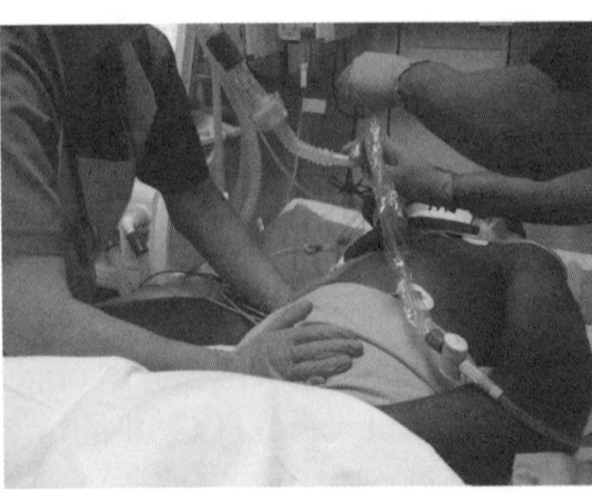

(A)

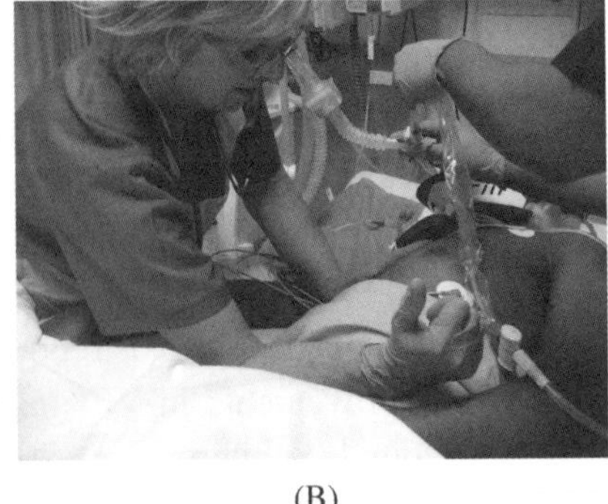

(B)

Fig. 8.10: Manually assisted cough manoeuvres utilising abdominal compression. (A) A physiotherapist applies abdominal compression with one hand while the other hand is stabilised on the patient's chest wall; (B) Abdominal compression applied using forearm pressure over the upper abdomen with the therapist's other hand stabilised on the patient's chest wall.

Peak expiratory cough flow and cough effectiveness are decreased in most patients with cervical and high-thoracic SCI due to denervation of expiratory muscles, as discussed earlier. Strong evidence supports the use of manually assisted cough manoeuvres to increase cough expiratory flow and therefore cough efficacy and secretion clearance in patients with high SCI lesions (Reid *et al.*, 2010). A variety of manually assisted cough manoeuvres can be used to achieve this goal. One example is bilateral chest wall compression applied by one or two physiotherapists to the lower lateral aspects of the chest wall to improve expiratory flow from the lungs and enhance cough effectiveness (Chapter 4, Section 4.2.5.1). Alternatively, manual abdominal compressions applied by one or two people can be performed and similarly result in improved expiratory flows and cough effort (Kang *et al.*, 2006) (Figs 8.10A and B and Figs 4.9A and B in Chapter 4).

Key Message

The physiotherapist should be aware that assisted cough manoeuvres may lead to adverse events such as perforation of the small bowel. This type of injury would necessitate surgical repair. Therefore the amount of pressure applied by the physiotherapist to a tetraplegic patient's abdomen, in order to improve cough effort, should be carefully regulated.

8.9.1.3.2. Spontaneously breathing patient

Manual therapy techniques, postural drainage and assisted cough manoeuvres, as described above, should also be employed for secretion mobilisation and clearance in spontaneously breathing patients with SCI. In the absence of a tracheostomy, airway suction using oral or nasal airways may be useful to assist with airway clearance. It is very important to be aware that the whole approach towards achieving secretion removal can exhaust a tetraplegic patient. Rest periods should be provided frequently, especially after assisted cough or suctioning. Providing respiratory muscle rest with intermittent positive pressure breathing (IPPB) or MHI bags can be helpful for these patients to prevent fatigue and respiratory failure.

The use of insufflation-exsufflation devices has an important role to play in the management of patients with SCI. It has been reported that insufflation, followed by manually assisted cough manoeuvres, is successful in the removal of retained secretions. The positive insufflation pressure creates larger inspiratory volumes than the patient is able to create on their own. This enables loosening of retained secretions. The negative exsufflation pressure creates increased expiratory flow rates and, applied together with manually assisted cough manoeuvres, improves the patient's ability to expectorate secretions (Reid *et al.*, 2010; Wong *et al.*, 2012). It should be noted that, despite clinical reports of its effectiveness, limited research evidence exists for the use of insufflation-exsufflation devices in patients with tetraplegia, mostly due to the poor methodological quality of trials that have been performed in this patient population (Berney *et al.*, 2011). There are also no prospective clinical trials that have assessed its effectiveness in the acute care management of patients with SCI undergoing MV (Vásquez *et al.*, 2013). When using mechanical insufflation-exsufflation devices in patients with SCI, it is important to remember that anatomical differences exist between adults and children; therefore the pressures applied to the airways of such individuals should be carefully monitored to avoid adverse effects, such as cardiovascular instability and pneumothorax (Morrow *et al.*, 2013).

As mentioned previously, the use of abdominal binders in the seated position for patients with tetraplegia in the later stages after injury has been reported to improve maximal expiratory pressure and FVC

(Boaventura *et al.*, 2003). The improvement in maximal expiratory mouth pressure and FVC enables the patient to cough more effectively.

Clinical studies have reported that strength training of the pectoralis major muscle significantly increases cough effectiveness in patients with cervical SCI. Contraction of the pectoralis major muscle causes dynamic airway compression during expiration and thus improves cough efficacy (Van Houtte *et al.*, 2006; Schilero *et al.*, 2009). Therefore, after the patient has been stabilised, strengthening of the pectoralis major muscles should form part of the rehabilitation of patients with SCI.

In the longer term, electrical stimulation of muscles of the lower thoracic and lumbar areas can be used to improve expiratory pressures and peak flow rates, and hence cough efficacy (Gollee *et al.*, 2008; Lee *et al.*, 2008). Electrical stimulation was performed through surface functional electrical stimulation (FES) of abdominal wall muscles in Gollee *et al.*'s (2008) study, and via a commercially available stimulator (Multi-tems Pty Ltd, Sydney, Australia) in Lee *et al.*'s (2008) study. What is not clear, however, is the frequency and duration of the stimulation required for effective results. Some studies have reported frequency of up to 60 times daily for a period of three months (DiMarco *et al.*, 2006, 2009).

8.9.1.4. *Lung capacity and volumes*

Pulmonary function may be decreased in any patient with SCI and the degree of reduction in volume and capacity is dependent on the level of the lesion. Patients with tetraplegia and high-level paraplegia present with a restrictive disease pattern due to neuromuscular weakness that leads to significant reduction in most lung volumes as well as VC, TLC and IC. Residual volume increases and FRC remains unchanged (Schilero *et al.*, 2009). The inability of patients with high-level SCI to sigh to prevent airway collapse predisposes them to the development of partial or complete atelectasis (Schilero *et al.*, 2009). Furthermore, a reduction in chest wall compliance develops due to rib cage stiffness as a result of the inability to inhale deeply or as a result of spasticity of the intercostal muscles (Schilero *et al.*, 2009; Sharma *et al.*, 2012).

Physiotherapists may use various methods to increase IC and inspiratory volumes in patients with SCI. These methods will be discussed in more detail below. The effectiveness of these methods will be dependent on the level of the lesion of each individual patient.

8.9.1.4.1. Intubated patient

The use of different body positions in bed, with consideration to the contraindications posed by the level of the SCI, directs air to the non-dependent lung regions and is a very useful method to ventilate areas of atelectasis and reduced air entry.

In patients with complete high-cervical SCI, increasing the amount of pressure support delivered by the ventilator, together with body position changes, will further augment lung volumes.

Manual hyperinflation (ambubagging) can be used to increase lung capacity, lung volumes and lung compliance in patients with SCI. The application of and precautions and contraindications related to the use of MHI in patients with SCI are similar to those discussed in Chapter 4 (Section 4.2.6.1.2). Manual hyperinflation used in combination with changes in body position further increases lung volumes and lung compliance in segments that are partially collapsed.

Deep breathing and breath stacking may be taught to patients with incomplete SCI to increase lung volumes as soon as they regain consciousness; however, the level of SCI will influence the effectiveness of the patient's spontaneous breathing efforts. It is also important to note that the patient's ventilation mode will affect their ability to augment their tidal volume. Patients need to be on a pressure ventilation mode in order for them to increase their lung volumes. Patients with lower-thoracic SCI may be able to perform the different components of the active cycle of breathing technique (ACBT). Biofeedback, using the graphics on the ventilator screen, with ACBT could be useful to encourage such patients to increase their inspiratory lung volumes as far as they are able.

8.9.1.4.2. Spontaneously breathing patient

Physiotherapists worldwide use IPPB in the management of patients with SCI. The beneficial effects of IPPB in this population have been reported from the clinical setting; however, there is currently little research evidence to support the effectiveness of IPPB as a standalone treatment. If clinicians decide to use IPPB, it should be implemented as part of a treatment package in order to have a beneficial effect on lung volume (Berney *et al.*, 2011). The need for well-designed studies on this technique cannot be overemphasised, given its potential to increase respiratory compliance and lung volumes and reduce secretion retention and re-intubation rates for patients with SCI (Reid *et al.*, 2010; Berney *et al.*, 2011).

Non-invasive ventilation in the form of bi-level positive airway pressure or continuous positive airway pressure ventilation or mechanical insufflation-exsufflation, given continuously or intermittently during the day, is useful to maintain optimal lung volumes and oxygenation in patients with cervical SCI to avoid the need for intubation (Wong *et al.*, 2012). Various interfaces, such as nasal, mouth or full face masks, can be used for the administration of non-invasive ventilation (Zimmer *et al.*, 2007). In intubated patients with SCI the duration of MV is, however, not reduced through the use of non-invasive ventilation (Berney *et al.*, 2011).

In the later stages after SCI, the use of glossopharyngeal (FROGG) breathing by patients with complete high-cervical lesions has been reported to increase inspiratory lung volumes to such a degree that the patient is able to cough more effectively. It is also used as a survival technique, in which the patient is taught how to use these muscles to stay off the ventilator for some time. Currently, low-level research evidence exists to support the use of FROGG breathing (Reid *et al.*, 2010). The reader is referred to Chapter 4 (Section 4.2.1.4) for more information on how to perform this technique.

8.9.1.5. *Respiratory muscle training*

The focus of clinical research in patients with SCI has increasingly been on the role of inspiratory and expiratory muscle training and its effectiveness on coughing in the reduction and prevention of respiratory complications. The rationale behind this research drive is that increases in inspiratory muscle strength should enhance inspiratory volumes, which could lead to better cough efficacy; increases in expiratory muscle strength should increase expiratory mouth pressure, and therefore the driving force for forced expiration, resulting in a stronger cough (Van Houtte *et al.*, 2006).

Methods that can be used for respiratory muscle training in the cooperative intubated patient include:

- temporary reduction in the level of pressure support or trigger sensitivity supplied by the MV, and
- spring-loaded inspiratory muscle-trainer devices (Threshold® IMT, supplied by Respironics Incorporated, or PowerBreathe®).

The reader is referred to Chapter 4 (Section 4.2.1.5) for a description on how to apply these techniques.

The first step in respiratory muscle training in the acute phase after injury, when a patient with an incomplete lesion regains consciousness and is able to cooperate, is to teach the patient to trigger more spontaneous breaths through the ventilator. The physiotherapist should ensure that the patient's ventilation mode permits spontaneous breathing and volume augmentation and then the ventilator graphics can be used for biofeedback. Following successful achievement of spontaneous breathing, the techniques listed above can be employed for further respiratory muscle training. Define a time for the training session and avoid more than a 20% increase in the patient's vital signs during training. As the patient's respiratory muscles grow accustomed to the training, the duration of the training session can be gradually increased. It is important not to fatigue the respiratory muscles with training, as patients would need 48 hours of rest to recover from fatigue and this would delay their weaning from MV.

The physiotherapist should be alert to identify when a patient's condition is deteriorating during a training session. Table 8.16 summarises the

Table 8.16: Signs and symptoms of patient deterioration.

- Decline in peripheral oxygen saturation that requires increased levels of oxygen administration
- Respiratory rate changes very early when a patient is unwell, but as a patient tires respiratory rate may start to slow due to fatigue and muscle failure
- Confusion and drowsiness
- Deterioration in arterial partial pressure of carbon dioxide ($PaCO_2$), pH and arterial partial pressure of oxygen (PaO_2) values on arterial blood gas analysis
- Deterioration in peak expiratory flow rate
- Initial moderate or strong cough effort that becomes weak and ineffective

common signs and symptoms of patient deterioration. The physiotherapist should immediately alert the patient's medical team if any of these signs or symptoms develops.

Van Houtte *et al.* (2006) performed a systematic review on the effects of respiratory muscle training in patients with tetraplegia three months after injury. They reported tendencies towards improved expiratory muscle strength, VC and decreased RV after respiratory muscle training; however, there was insufficient support for improved inspiratory muscle strength and endurance after respiratory muscle training. Reid *et al.* (2010), in a more recent systematic review, reported that high-level evidence exists for the use of respiratory muscle training in patients with SCI, and that a drastic reduction in the occurrence of respiratory infections is seen as a result. Other researchers support these reports (Zimmer *et al.*, 2007; Roth *et al.*, 2010). Systematic reviews performed to date found the major impediment to meta-analysis of the data to be differences in study designs, type of subjects used and treatment protocols that were followed (Van Houtte *et al.*, 2006; Sheel *et al.*, 2008). There is clear evidence of the need to conduct research using standardised treatment protocols for respiratory muscle training to enable comparisons and pooling of data to generate stronger evidence.

8.9.1.6. *Paediatric considerations*

There is little scientific evidence for chest physiotherapy in paediatric patients with traumatic SCI and therefore the recommendations below are based on expert opinion and physiological plausibility.

The goals of respiratory physiotherapy are the same in children as adults with regard to clearing pulmonary secretions, improving ventilation and chest wall expansion, increasing lung volumes, strengthening available respiratory muscles, improving respiratory compliance and educating the patient and their caregiver. These goals can be met in children by using age-appropriate physiotherapy techniques, outlined in Chapter 4. These include positioning (with no head-down postural drainage positioning), regular changes in position or mobilisation, breathing exercises, respiratory muscle training, chest manipulations (vibrations and shaking) and assisted coughing, with suctioning if necessary. Manually assisted coughing should be performed by a chest wall compression technique instead of abdominal compression, owing to the potential hazards of abdominal injury and exacerbation of reflux in children (Finder, 2010).

Manual hyperinflation should not be standard practice in intubated children after SCI, but inflation to normal, deep inspiratory levels may be appropriate via an appropriately sized self-inflating resuscitator bag to facilitate the inspiratory phase of an effective cough. Manual insufflation may be performed via a tracheostomy, ETT or face mask interface (Boitano, 2009). Similarly, whilst there is no clear evidence for the safety or efficacy of mechanical insufflation-exsufflation in children, this intervention may be beneficial for a child with SCI with respiratory muscle weakness.

In paediatrics, it is preferable to do frequent, short treatment sessions, as the child tires quickly.

8.9.2. *Neuromusculoskeletal system*

8.9.2.1. *Pain*

In the later stages after SCI, the physiotherapeutic contribution to pain management may include the administration of heat therapy to encourage muscle relaxation to manage pain with a musculoskeletal origin. Regular exercise significantly reduces post-SCI pain. Shoulder pain is a complaint of many patients after SCI due to the fact that the patient is very reliant on the use of the upper limb. A strength exercise and stretch protocol for the shoulder has been reported to significantly reduce the intensity of shoulder pain following SCI (Mehta *et al.*, 2014).

The effect of transcutaneous electrical nerve stimulation (TENS) on the management of neuropathic pain in patients with SCI has not been well researched over the years. Only one study could be found that investigated the effect of low-frequency TENS on pain in patients with SCI using a randomised controlled study design (Celik *et al.*, 2013). All patients received pharmacological interventions for their pain as well as low-frequency TENS four times a day. The duration of each TENS session was 30 minutes for those in the experimental group over a period of 10 days. Those in the control group received sham TENS for the same duration and length of time. Results showed that subjects in the low-frequency

TENS group had significantly lower scores on the visual analogue scale at the end of the trial than those who received sham TENS (Celik *et al.*, 2013). There may be a place for the use of low-frequency TENS, in addition to pharmacological treatment of neuropathic pain, in this patient population.

8.9.2.2. *Joint range of motion*

Patients with tetraplegia and paraplegia will be very dependent on their upper limb function for activities such as transfers, wheelchair mobility and ADL. In order to optimise upper limb function, joint ROM should be unrestricted.

8.9.2.2.1. Uncooperative intubated patient

Daily stretches of the upper limb and lower limb joints through full ROM should be performed while the patient is sedated (Figs 8.11 and 8.12). Care should be taken not to overstretch the joints and cause soft tissue injury. Resting splints for the hands and ankles may be used for joint protection.

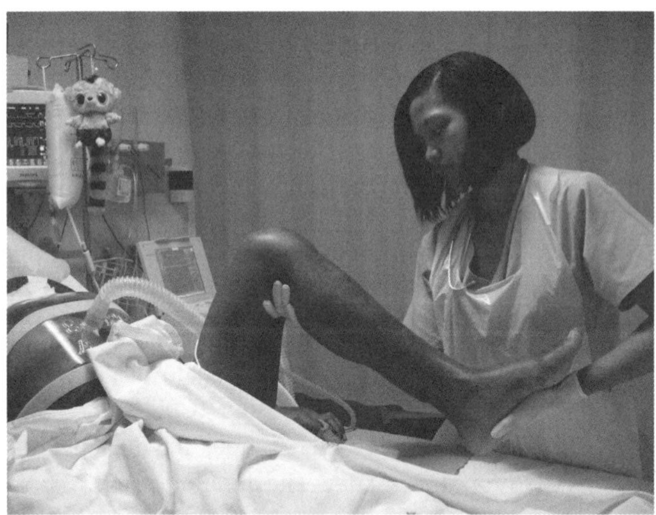

Fig. 8.11: Passive ROM exercises performed by a physiotherapist in the ICU for a patient with C4–C5 dislocation.

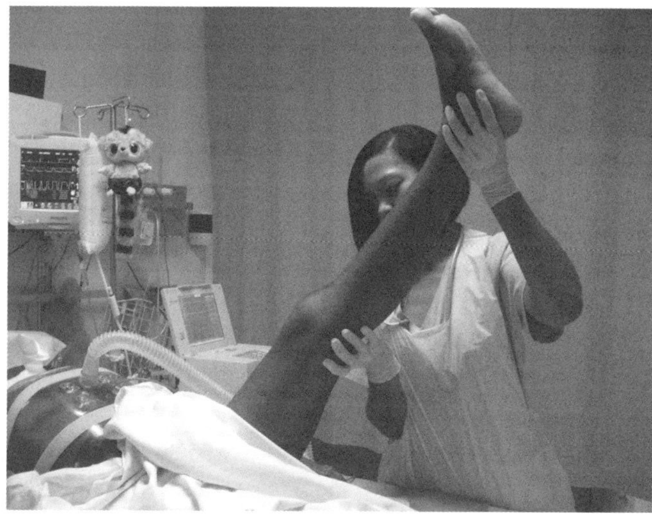

Fig. 8.12: Passive stretch of the hamstring muscles performed in the ICU for the same patient.

An exception to this rule is the purposeful shortening of finger flexors in patients with C6 lesions for the formation of tenodesis (Section 8.8).

8.9.2.2.2. Cooperative intubated or spontaneously breathing patient

As soon as consciousness is regained, active-assisted and free active ROM exercises should be initiated. Optimal ROM in the lower limbs should be preserved for patients with incomplete lesions. Active-assisted and active ROM exercises (depending on the patient's ability to cooperate) for the lower limbs, and upper limbs when applicable, should be performed daily.

In patients with complete SCI, full passive ROM of the lower limbs should be maintained in order to prevent contracture formation. This should allow the patient to assume different body positions in a comfortable manner. Cosmetically, maintenance of full passive ROM is beneficial for any patient with complete SCI.

If the patient has any additional orthopaedic injuries, precautions and contraindications to the movement of the affected limbs should be adhered to (Chapter 7, Section 7.9.2).

8.9.2.3. *Muscle strength*

The ability of a patient with SCI to function independently is determined by the level of the lesion and also by the patient's muscle strength. As mentioned previously, upper limb strength is vitally important to support the body during ADL, wheelchair mobility, seated pressure relief, transfers in and out of bed, on and off the toilet or in and out of a car. For patients with incomplete lesions, lower limb strength should be adequate to support the body during walking. Keeping these long-term goals in mind, strength training should form part of the acute care management of any patient with SCI as early as possible during their stay in the ICU, depending on their level of consciousness and ability to cooperate. A baseline assessment of muscle strength (using a muscle chart and ASIA) should be done as soon as the patient is cooperative, and re-assessment of muscle strength to detect changes in function should be performed regularly.

Active-resisted exercises may be performed, utilising manual resistance from the physiotherapist, resistance bands, water bottles or small weights. Strength training should be performed daily, and even twice daily as the patient's condition improves, to ensure that optimal upper limb strength is obtained. Neuromuscular stimulation-assisted exercise has been reported to improve upper limb muscle strength more than conventional exercise in all phases of rehabilitation (Connolly *et al.*, 2014). Arm cycle ergometry may also be used to improve the muscle strength of triceps, biceps and anterior deltoids in the acute care setting (Connolly *et al.*, 2014).

Lower limb strength training in the acute care setting may include active-resisted exercises similar to those described above for the upper limb. In the later stages of rehabilitation, electrical stimulation (patterned electrical stimulation and FES) of lower limb muscles has been reported to improve strength and endurance and reduce the amount of muscle atrophy often observed in patients with tetraplegia (Domingo *et al.*, 2014). Patterned electrical stimulation (PES) aims to produce muscle contraction used to generate muscle force, such as an isometric contraction. Functional electrical stimulation aims to produce purposeful movement such as cycling or walking (Domingo *et al.*, 2014). In patients with incomplete SCI, PES may be used initially to condition and prepare the lower limbs for FES. Another approach to strength training of the lower limbs is task-specific training activities such as transfers and walking (Domingo *et al.*, 2014).

The use of thumb opponens splints in patients with tetraplegia does seem to improve pinch strength and functional use of the hand, but very little research is available to ascertain whether the use of these splints reduces the occurrence of thumb web-space contractures (Connolly *et al.*, 2014).

In the polytrauma patient with SCI, strength training should be performed within the limitations of precautions and contraindications to movement for limb fractures (Chapter 7, Section 7.9.2).

8.9.2.4. *Functional activity, mobilisation and exercise endurance*

When spinal shock had subsided, prior to activities in and out of bed, the deconditioned patient with SCI (especially those with T6 lesions or above) may benefit from time spent in a tilt table (even in the ICU) to accustom them to the upright position. Initially a tilt table test with BP monitoring should be performed to establish the severity of orthostatic hypotension, which the patient may present with. Standing in the tilt table should be performed daily, if appropriate, and the angle to which the tilt table is inclined should be gradually increased, according to each patient's level of tolerance, to reduce episodes of light-headedness.

Functional rehabilitation of the spinal cord-injured patient in the ICU and ward setting is focused on task-specific activities and may include training in rolling in bed, transfers in and out of bed to a chair or wheelchair and on and off the toilet from a wheelchair. The use of an electronic hoist may assist nursing and physiotherapy staff with transferring the patient to a chair safely. A patient with an incomplete lesion or low thoracic lesion may eventually become strong enough to assist with their transfers. Stable patients with incomplete lesions may benefit from standing in a standing frame with braces around the legs to support their body weight. The duration of standing can be progressed daily according to the patient's ability. This will help with improvements in exercise endurance.

Arm cycle ergometry can be used, while the patient is on MV, to improve exercise endurance. The duration and intensity of exercise should be progressively increased according to the patient's ability.

Although the benefits of general exercise have been described for patients with chronic SCI, no literature could be found that provides specific exercise guidelines for acute or chronic spinal cord-injured patients (Wolfe *et al.*, 2012).

Rehabilitation of the patient during the sub-acute and chronic phases of SCI is beyond the scope of this text, and the reader is referred to Section 8.11 and Appendix III for further reading on this topic.

8.9.2.5. *Paediatric considerations*

Pain affects about 6% of children with SCI and may be radicular, musculoskeletal or dysesthetic. Management is directed at the cause of the pain using medical, surgical or therapeutic interventions. Therapeutic interventions include physiotherapy and occupational therapy, conditioning, hydrotherapy, psychotherapy and TENS in older children (Zidek and Srinivasan, 2003).

Spasticity can severely impact on function in children with SCI. The evaluation and management of spasticity, which is often more severe in children with incomplete lesions, should address the impact on developmentally appropriate function, comfort or ease of caregiving (Zidek and Srinivasan, 2003). Spasticity can be addressed indirectly by appropriate positioning, splinting, weight bearing, and active or facilitated movement. This is in addition to medical management, summarised previously.

8.9.3. *Patient response to treatment*

Outcomes measures and markers to assess the response of a patient with SCI to treatment interventions are summarised in Chapter 4 (Section 4.3). The choice of test will be determined by the patient's type and level of lesion and the particular stage of recovery that the patient is in at the time of assessment.

8.10. Clinical Case Scenarios

8.10.1. *Case scenario of an adult patient*

A 30-year-old man was involved in a motorcycle accident and sustained a complete SCI at level T5. He has no significant past medical history and took part in sporting activities such as cycling and swimming prior to the accident. After spinal stabilisation he was admitted to the ICU and has been in the unit for two weeks. A tracheostomy was performed and he is currently receiving pressure-controlled synchronised intermittent mandatory ventilation. The ventilator circuit is humidified by an attached heat moisture exchanger. He is receiving six breaths per minute from the ventilator and, in addition, he is doing 10 breaths per minute spontaneously. Chest x-ray shows lung volume loss in both left and right lung fields, with consolidation over the right middle lobe. The nursing staff reports that creamy-yellow thick sputum plugs are being removed from his airways during suction and that he has a weak cough. His vital signs are stable. He has a tracheostomy, is awake and able to follow commands.

- What treatment goals would you aim to achieve for this patient during the remainder of his stay in the ICU?
- What precautions or contraindications would you consider during physiotherapy intervention for this patient?

8.10.1.1. *Discussion*

8.10.1.1.1. Treatment goals

The complete SCI at level T5 has left this patient with intact diaphragm function, innervation of the upper internal and external intercostal muscles and full upper limb function. The abdominal muscles, however, will not be innervated with this type of lesion and therefore he will struggle with forced expiration and coughing, as reported by the nursing staff. An important aim of physiotherapy intervention would be to assess the patient's ability to cough spontaneously and to educate him and the nursing staff on cough augmentation techniques, such as assisted cough manoeuvres using bilateral lower chest wall compression or abdominal compression during coughing.

Another important aim of treatment would be to assist with the mobilisation and clearance of infected retained secretions, especially from the right middle lobe. Adjustment of the patient's humidification from a heat moisture exchanger to a heated water humidification system will limit the thickness of the secretions. Mycolitic therapy can also be considered to assist with thinning retained secretions. Modified postural drainage positions that target the middle lobe, as well as other lung segments in which secretions are identified during assessment, can be used in combination with manual chest clearance techniques such as chest percussion, chest wall shaking and vibrations, as well as MHI, to facilitate the mobilisation of secretions. Secretion removal can be achieved through the use of suction and assisted cough manoeuvres, as mentioned above, to enhance the patient's cough efficacy.

Optimisation of lung volumes and lung capacities and improving lung compliance are important goals for this patient's treatment. This can be achieved through the use of body position changes together with increases in pressure support delivered through the ventilator during physiotherapy treatment sessions. Manual or ventilator hyperinflation can be used to restore lung volume and compliance. The patient can be encouraged to increase his own tidal volume through deep breathing by using ventilator graphics as biofeedback while proprioception is given by the physiotherapist's hands, placed over the upper lung segments that have muscle innervation. When spinal shock subsides, standing the patient in a tilt table (using an abdominal binder if indicated) with gradual increases in the inclination of the table may further assist with increasing lung volumes if pressure support is increased to facilitate the distribution of pressure to more lung segments.

The patient has been in the ICU for two weeks and is awake and responsive and able to do a fair amount of spontaneous breathing, so it is important that respiratory muscle training is introduced into his rehabilitation in order to assist with weaning from MV. The trigger sensitivity delivered through the ventilator can be reduced during physiotherapy treatment to supply resistance to the patient's spontaneous breathing efforts. An inspiratory muscle trainer device can be attached to the patient's tracheostomy tube when the patient is able to breathe without support from the ventilator for short time periods.

During the phase of spinal shock it is important to establish the patient's baseline ASIA and muscle strength using a muscle chart. Muscle strength should be regularly reassessed thereafter. It is important to progressively strengthen his upper limb muscles, as he will be dependent on them for performing all ADLs and transfers.

The maintenance of passive joint ROM of all joints in the lower limbs is important, as well as the prevention of contracture formation of the hamstrings, hip flexors and tendon Achilles by performing sustained stretches of these two-joint muscles daily. Splinting may also be required. Activities that are task-orientated are important to initiate as soon as spinal shock subsides. Activities such as rolling in bed, sitting up in bed and practising static and dynamic sitting balance should form part of rehabilitation in the acute care setting. If the patient has an extended stay, another goal of rehabilitation would be to start practising slide board transfers from the patient's bed to a chair or onto a custom-made wheelchair. Reconditioning the patient with a view to increasing exercise endurance should form part of his management, and this may be achieved through the progression of the duration of each treatment session, increasing the frequency of treatment sessions each day, as well as the progression of the intensity and frequency of muscle strength training.

Communication with and handover to the physiotherapist in the spinal ward is vital to ensure the effective continuation of rehabilitation for this patient after discharge from the ICU.

8.10.1.1.2. Precautions or contraindications to treatment interventions in the ICU

- The physiotherapist should adhere to the infection control policy of their local ICU.
- The nasogastric feed should be temporarily switched off during treatment to prevent aspiration of food into the lungs during position changes in bed.
- It is important to monitor the patient's vital signs closely during the treatment session so that the physiotherapist is immediately alerted to adverse responses from the patient to treatment received, in particular bradycardia as a result of vasovagal response to suction or hypertension and cardiac arrhythmia due to autonomic dysreflexia.
- The patient should be log rolled during body position changes until the surgeon is satisfied that spinal stabilisation was successful.
- Precautions related to the suction procedure include the pre-oxygenation of the patient prior to suctioning and the use of a sterile

suction technique. Pre-oxygenation is especially important to avoid bradycardia following the stimulation of the vagal nerve during suction.

- The physiotherapist should aim to keep the area around the tracheostomy tube clean and not to pull on the tracheostomy tube with the ventilator circuit during position changes in the treatment session.
- Care should be taken with the tracheostomy tube and the ventilator circuit during task-oriented activities, to avoid the dislodgement of the tube or disconnection from the ventilator circuit.

8.10.2. *Case scenario of a paediatric patient*

An eight-year-old boy with achondroplasia and associated ligamentous laxity was admitted after a minor fall, during which he sustained a C1–C2 subluxation with partial SCI. Initially he was in complete spinal shock with no active movement and no spontaneous ventilation. He therefore underwent a tracheostomy and was completely dependent on mechanical positive pressure ventilation. He underwent spinal stabilisation two days after admission and, after six weeks of log rolling, was cleared by the neurosurgeons for graded mobilisation.

Developmentally he was normal for an eight-year-old, despite being hypermobile. He was independently ambulant and enjoyed swimming and playing with his peers. He was cognitively normal and enjoyed school at a mainstream facility.

- Consider treatment options during the following stages of recovery.
  - During the first six weeks in paediatric ICU, he developed nosocomial pneumonia, with left lung collapse and increased ventilator requirements. His spine was still considered unstable despite the operative intervention.
  - After six weeks he started regaining active movement in his extremities (initially his thumb) and this gradually progressed to all limbs, trunk and respiratory muscles.
- What precautions should you take at each stage?

8.10.2.1. *Discussion*

8.10.2.1.1. Treatment during the acute stage after injury (ventilator dependent)

General precautions to consider in the paediatric ICU include infection control principles, especially hand washing. Spinal cord precautions for a potentially unstable spine must be taken, including log rolling, ensuring that a second person supports the head in a full head hold whilst doing manually assisted coughing (using chest compression only) and ensuring that the head and neck are well aligned in side-lying positions. Prevent hypoxia through pre-oxygenation with suctioning. Careful monitoring of vital signs throughout treatment is essential, as well as ensuring the integrity of invasive devices and lines.

Treatment should involve preventing deformities by maintaining ROM of all joints with passive movements, stretches and splinting. It is important to liaise with the nursing staff to ensure regular changes in position and to check skin integrity.

Treat lung collapse and retained secretions with bilateral manual chest vibrations in a supine position and assisted cough manoeuvres (precautions itemised above). Suction via tracheostomy using standard precautions. Interdisciplinary holistic care is essential and therefore the extended interdisciplinary team (including teacher, occupational therapist, social worker or psychologist) should be included in goal setting. Referral of the child to a speech therapist is important early on, in order to devise an effective alternative communication technique (e.g. using eye glance). Central to the interdisciplinary team is the patient and his family and they should also be involved in clinical decision making and goal setting.

8.10.2.1.2. Treatment options after six weeks

At this stage the child is likely to present with the return of some active movement. Precautions to consider include infection control and lines attached to the patient, as well as other precautions mentioned above. Be aware of neck muscle flaccidity when mobilising to upright positions, as this constitutes a risk for re-injury. A neck collar (type of collar discussed with the surgeon) should be placed prior to mobilisation. Postural hypotension is likely when moving to the upright posture and should therefore be done gradually using a tilt table test.

Treatment should include a graded strengthening programme of skeletal and respiratory muscles. Attempts should be made to wean ventilator settings to encourage spontaneous breathing. Ventilator dependence should be reduced gradually, as tolerated, and only as and when respiratory muscle function returns. The physiotherapist should focus treatment on facilitating ADL and play activities. Weight-bearing through the legs (supported standing) and arms (supported sitting) should be encouraged. Continue maintenance therapy as before, but introduce active breathing exercises such as ACBT. Other methods to facilitate inspiratory muscle training may also be used.

Progress the child's rehabilitation to independent ADL, including wheelchair transfers into the custom-made wheelchair and tracheostomy care. Improve his exercise tolerance and muscle strength by increasing duration and intensity of exercises as indicated. An important part of pre-discharge management is advice and education to the child and caregivers to prepare them for home care.

8.11. Suggested Reading Material for Further Study

Structure of the spinal cord (Gondim, 2013; Kahle and Frotscher, 2003); paediatric cervical spine injuries (Mortavazi *et al.*, 2011; Krey *et al.*, 2012); secondary mechanisms of injury following spinal cord trauma (Kwon *et al.*, 2004); autonomic dysreflexia (Consortium for Spinal Cord Medicine, 1997); respiratory care protocol for the management of patients with acute SCI (Consortium for Spinal Cord Medicine, 2008); rehabilitation of a patient with SCI after discharge from the acute care setting (Spinal Cord Injury Rehabilitation Evidence, 2012; Zidek and Srinivasan, 2003).

8.12. Conclusion

Patients with acute SCI suffer from respiratory compromise due to the detrimental effects of cervical or high-thoracic lesions on the innervation of the muscles of respiration. Hypoxia is one of the main causes for secondary damage to the spinal cord. It is the duty of the physiotherapist, as a member of the interdisciplinary team in the ICU, to prevent or manage respiratory complications that arise, quickly and effectively, in order to reduce the effects of hypoxia on the injured spinal cord. The information provided in this chapter should enable the physiotherapist to have a better understanding of the acute presentation and management of a patient with traumatic SCI and to provide the treatment required by each individual patient in an effective and safe manner.

Bibliography

Ackery, A., Tator, C., and Krassioukov, A. (2004). A global perspective on spinal cord injury epidemiology, *J. Neurotrauma,* **21**, 1355–1370.

American Spinal Cord Injury Association. (2003). *Reference Manual of the International Standards for Neurological Classification of Spinal Cord Injury*, Chicago, IL.

Baydur, A., Adkins, R.H., and Milic-Emili, J. (2001). Lung mechanics in individuals with spinal cord injury: effects of injury level and posture, *J. Appl. Physiol.,* **90**, 405–411.

Berlly, M.B., and Shem, K. (2007). Respiratory management during the first five days after spinal cord injury, *J. Spinal Cord Med.,* **30**, 309–318.

Berney, S., Bragge, P., Granger, C., *et al.* (2011). The acute respiratory management of cervical spinal cord injury in the first six weeks after injury: a systematic review, *Spinal Cord,* **49**, 17–29.

Binder, D.K., Sonne, D.C., and Lawton, M.T. (2004). Spinal epidural hematoma, *Neurosurg. Q.,* **14**, 51–59.

Boaventura, C.M., Gastaldi, A.C., Silveira, J.M., *et al.* (2003). Effect of an abdominal binder on the efficacy of respiratory muscles in seated and supine tetraplegic patients, *Physiotherapy,* **89**, 290–295.

Boitano, L.J. (2009). Equipment options for cough augmentation, ventilation and noninvasive interfaces in neuromuscular respiratory management, *Pediatrics,* **123** [Suppl], S226–S230.

Brown, R., DiMarco, A.F., Hoit, J.D., *et al.* (2006). Respiratory dysfunction and management in spinal cord injury, *Respir. Care,* **51**, 853–870.

Call, M.S., Kutcher, M.E., Izenberg, R.A., *et al.* (2011). Spinal cord injury: outcomes of ventilator weaning and extubation, *J. Trauma,* **71**, 1673–1679.

Casha, S., and Christie, S. (2011). A systematic review of intensive cardiopulmonary management after spinal cord injury, *J. Neurotrauma,* **28**, 1479–1495.

Celik, E.C., Erhan, B., Gunduz, B., *et al.* (2013). The effect of low-frequency TENS in the treatment of neuropathic pain in patients with spinal cord injury. *Spinal Cord,* **51**, 334–337.

Cha, J.R., Park, K.B., and Ko, S.H. (2011). Post-traumatic lumbar epidural haematoma with neurology: report of 1 case, *Asian Spine J.,* **5**, 130–132.

Chin, L.S. (2014). *Spinal Cord Injuries*. Medscape. [Online] Available at: http://emedicine.medscape.com/article/793582-overview [Accessed 29 July 2014].

Choi, H.J., Paeng, S.H., Kim, S.T., *et al.* (2013). The effectiveness of early tracheostomy (within at least 10 days) in cervical spinal cord injury patients, *J. Korean Neurosurg. Soc.,* **54**, 220–224.

Clarke, E.C. (2012). 'Contrasting adult and paediatric traumatic spinal cord injuries', in Martin, A.A., and Jones, E.J. (eds), *Spinal Cord Injuries: Causes, Risk Factors and Management*, Nova Science Publishers, New York, NY, pp 251–262.

Connolly, S.J., Mehta, S., Foulon, B.L., *et al.* (2014). 'Upper limb rehabilitation following spinal cord injury', in Eng, J.J., Teasell, R.W., Miller, W.C., *et al.* (eds), *Spinal Cord Injury Rehabilitation Evidence*, Version 5.0, Vancouver, pp. 1–19. [Online] Available at: http://www.scireproject.com/rehabilitation-evidence/upper-limb [Accessed August 2013].

Consortium for Spinal Cord Medicine. (1997). *Consumer Guides: Autonomic Dysreflexia: What you should know*. Consortium for Spinal Cord Medicine. [Online] Available at: http://www.scicpg.org/cpg_cons.htm#AD [Accessed April 2014].

Consortium for Spinal Cord Medicine. (2008). Respiratory management following SCI: clinical practice guideline, *J. Spinal Cord Med.,* **31**, 403–479.

Cotton, B.A., Pryor, J.P., Chinwalla, I., *et al.* (2005). Respiratory complications and mortality risk associated with thoracic spine injury, *J. Trauma,* **59**, 1400–1409.

Cripps, R.A., Lee, B.B., Wing, P., *et al.* (2011). A global map for traumatic spinal cord injury epidemiology: towards a living data repository for injury prevention, *Spinal Cord,* **49**, 493–501.

Denton, M., and McKinlay, J. (2009). Cervical cord injury and critical care, *Contin. Educ. Anesth. Crit. Care Pain,* **9**, 82–86.

DiMarco, A.F. (2005). Restoration of respiratory muscle function following spinal cord injury. Review of electrical and magnetic stimulation techniques, *Respir. Physiol. Neurobiol.,* **147**, 273–287.

DiMarco, A.F., Kowalski, K.E., Geertman, R.T., *et al.* (2009). Lower thoracic spinal cord stimulation to restore cough in patients with spinal cord injury: results of a national institutes of health-sponsored clinical trial. Part I: clinical outcomes, *Arch. Phys. Med. Rehabil.*, **90**, 717–725.

DiMarco, A.F., Onders, R.P., Ignagni, A., *et al.* (2006). Inspiratory muscle pacing in spinal cord injury: case report and clinical commentary, *J. Spinal Cord Med.,* 29, 95–108.

Ditunno, J.F., Little, J.W., Tessler, A., *et al.* (2004). Spinal shock revisited: a four-phase model, *Spinal Cord,* **42**, 383–395.

Ditunno, F., Young, W., Donovan, W.H., *et al.* (1994). The international standards booklet for neurological and functional classification of spinal cord injury, *Paraplegia,* **32**, 70–80.

Domingo, A., Lam, T., Wolfe, D.L., *et al.* (2014). 'Lower limb rehabilitation following spinal cord injury', in Eng, J.J., Teasell, R.W., Miller, W.C., *et al.* (eds), *Spinal Cord Injury Rehabilitation Evidence*, Version 5.0, Vancouver, pp. 1–55. [Online] Available at: http://www.scireproject.com/rehabilitation-evidence/lower-limb [Accessed August 2013].

Duhem, R., Tonnelle, V., Vinchon, M., *et al.* (2008). Unstable upper pediatric cervical spine injuries: report of 28 cases and review of the literature, *Child. Nerv. Syst.,* **24**, 343–348.

Dumont, R.J., Okonkwo, D.O., Verma, S., *et al.* (2001). Acute spinal cord injury part I: pathophysiologic mechanisms, *Clin. Neuropharmacol.,* **24**, 254–264.

Eng, J., and Chan, C. (2013). *American Spinal Injury Association impairment scale (AIS): International Standards for Neurological Classification of Spinal Cord Injury*. SCIRE. [Online] Available at: http://www.scireproject.com/outcome-measures-new/american-spinal-injury-association-impairment-scale-ais-international-standards [Accessed 23 June 2014].

Farcy, J.P.C., and Schwab, F.J. (2009). *Index of Surgical Procedures*. Orthospine. [Online] Available at: http://www.orthospine.com/index.php/component/content/article/57 [Accessed 20 June 2014].

Finder, J.D. (2010). Airway clearance modalities in neuromuscular disease, *Paediatr. Respir. Rev.,* **11**, 31–34.

Furlan, J.C. (2013). Autonomic dysreflexia: a clinical emergency, *J. Trauma Acute Care Surg.,* **75**, 496–500.

Gollee, H., Hunt, K.J., Allan, D.B., *et al.* (2008). Automatic electrical stimulation of abdominal wall muscles increases tidal volume and cough peak flow in tetraplegia, *Technol. Health Care,* **16**, 273–281.

Gondim, F.d.A.A. 2013. *Topographic and functional anatomy of the spinal cord*. [Online] Available at: http://emedicine.medscape.com/article/1148570-overview [Accessed 15 November 2014].

Harrop, J.S., Sharan, A., and Ratliff, J. (2006). Central cord injury: pathophysiology, management and outcomes, *Spine J.,* **6** [Suppl] , S198–S206.

Harvey, L. (2008). *Management of Spinal Cord Injury: A Guide for Physiotherapists*, Butterworth Heinemann Elsevier, Edinburgh.

Kahle, W., and Frotscher, M. (2003). *Color Atlas and Textbook of Human Anatomy: Nervous System and Sensory Organs*, 5th edn., Thieme Publishers, Stuttgart.

Kang, S.W., Shin, J.C., Park, C.I., *et al.* (2006). Relationship between inspiratory muscle strength and cough capacity in cervical spinal cord injured patients, *Spinal Cord,* **44**, 242–248.

Kawu, A.A., Alimi, F.M., Gbadegesin, A.A.S., *et al.* (2011). Complications and causes of death in spinal cord injury patients in Nigeria, *West Afr. J. Med.,* **30**, 301–304.

Kirshblum, S., Gonzalez, P., Cuccurullo, S., *et al.* (2004). 'Classification of SCI', in Cuccurullo, S. (ed), *Physical Medicine and Rehabilitation Board Review*, Demos Medical Publishing, New York, NY. pp. 498–552.

Krey, C., Johnston, T., Shakhazizian, K., *et al.* (2012). 'Spinal cord injury', in Campbell, S., Palisano, R., and Orlin, M. (eds), *Physical Therapy for Children*, 4th edn., Elsevier Saunders, St. Louis, MO, pp. 644–678.

Kwon, B.K., Tetzlaff, W., Grauer, J.N., *et al.* (2004). Pathophysiology and pharmacological treatment of acute spinal cord injury, *Spine J.,* **4**, 451–464.

Lauweryns, P. (2010). Role of conservative management of cervical spine injuries, *Eur. Spine J.,* **19** [Suppl], S23–S26.

Lavy, C., James, A., Wilson-MacDonald, J., *et al.* (2009). Cauda equina syndrome, *Br. Med. J.,* **338**, b936. [Online] Available at: http://www.bmj.com/content/338/bmj.b936.long [Accessed 15 November 2014].

Lee, B.B., Boswell-Ruys, C., Butler, J.E., *et al.* (2008). Surface functional electrical stimulation of the abdominal muscles to enhance cough and assist tracheostomy decannulation after high-level spinal cord injury, *J. Spinal Cord Med.,* **31**, 78–82.

Longo, U.G., Denaro, L., Campi, S., *et al.* (2010). Upper cervical spine injuries: indications and limits of the conservative management in halo vest. A systematic review of efficacy and safety, *Injury,* **41**, 1127–1135.

Magerl, F., Aebi, M., Gertzbein, S.D., *et al.* (1994). A comprehensive classification of thoracic and lumbar injuries, *Eur. Spine J.,* **3**, 184–201.

Marieb, E.N. (1992). *Human Anatomy and Physiology*, 2nd edn., Benjamin Cummings, San Francisco, CA.

Markandaya, M., Stein, D.M., and Menaker, J. (2012). Acute treatment options for spinal cord injury, *Curr. Treat. Options Neurol.,***14**, 175–187.

Marré, B., Ballesteros, V., Martinez, C., *et al.* (2011). Thoracic spine fractures: injury profile and outcomes of a surgically treated cohort, *Eur. Spine J.,* **20**, 1427–1433.

McKinley, W. (2014). *Cardiovascular Concerns in Spinal Cord Injury*. Medscape. [Online] Available at: http://emedicine.medscape.com/article/321771-overview#aw2aab6c14 [Accessed 20 June 2014].

McKinley, W., Santos, K., Meade, M., *et al.* (2007). Incidence and outcomes of spinal cord injury clinical syndromes, *J. Spinal Cord Med.,* **30**, 215–224.

McKinney, D. (2013). *Prevention of Thromboembolism in Spinal Cord Injury*. Medscape. [Online] Available at: http://emedicine.medscape.com/article/322897-overview#aw2aab6b7 [Accessed 19 June 2014].

Mehta, S., Teasell, R.W., Loh, E., *et al.* (2014). 'Pain following spinal cord injury', in Eng. J.J., Teasell, R.W., Miller, W.C., *et al.* (eds), *Spinal Cord Injury Rehabilitation Evidence*, Version 5.0. SCIRE project, Vancouver, pp. 1–79. [Online[Available at: http://www.scireproject.com/rehabilitation-evidence/pain-management [Accessed 15 July 2014].

Middleditch, A., and Oliver, J. (2005). *Functional Anatomy of the Spine*, 2nd edn., Elsevier Butterworth Heinemann, London.

Mietto, C., Pinciroli, R., Patel, N., *et al.* (2013). Ventilator-associated pneumonia: evolving definitions and preventive strategies, *Respir. Care,* **58**, 990–1003.

Miranda, A.R., and Hassouna, H.I. (2000). Mechanisms of thrombosis in spinal cord injury, *Hematol. Oncol. Clin. North Am.,* **14**, 401–416.

Morrow, B., Zampoli, M., Van Aswegen, H., *et al.* (2013). Mechanical insufflation-exsufflation for people with neuromuscular disorders, *Cochrane Database of Systematic Reviews,* **12**, CD010044.

Mortavazi, M., Gore, P.A., Chang, S., *et al.* (2011). Pediatric cervical spine injuries: a comprehensive review, *Child. Nerv. Syst.,* **27**, 705–717.

Newton, B.W. (2008). 'Anatomy of the spinal cord and brain', in Conn, M. (ed), *Neuroscience in Medicine*, 3rd edn., Humana Press, Totowa, NJ, pp. 25–51.

O'Dowd, J.K. (2010). Basic principles of management of cervical spine trauma, *Eur. Spine J.,* **19** [Suppl], S19–S22.

Oh, S.H., Han, I.B., Koo, Y.H., *et al.* (2009). Acute spinal subdural hematoma presenting with spontaneously resolving hemiplegia, *J. Korean Neurosurg. Soc.,* **45**, 390–393.

Oskouian, R.J. (2012). *Spinal Hematoma*. Medscape. [Online] Available at: http://emedicine.medscape.com/article/247957-overview [Accessed 30 June 2014].

Oyinbo, C.A. (2011). Secondary injury mechanisms in traumatic spinal cord injury: a nugget of this multiply cascade, *Acta Neurobiol. Exp.,* **71**, 281–299.

Pang, D., and Wilberger, J.E. (1982). Spinal cord injury without radiographic abnormalities in children, *J. Neurosurg.,* **57**, 114–129.

Pape, K.E. (2012). Developmental and maladaptive plasticity in neonatal SCI, *Clin. Neurol. Neurosurg.,* **114**, 475–482.

Paralyzed Veterans of America. (2005). *Respiratory Management following Spinal Cord Injury: A Clinical Practice Guideline for Health Care Professionals.* Paralyzed Veterans of America. [Online] Available at: http://www.pva.org/site/c.ajIRK9NJLcJ2E/b.6357755/apps/s/content.asp?ct=8824707 [Accessed 19 June 2014].

Parent, S., Mac-Thiong, J-M., Roy-Beaudry, M., *et al.* (2011). Spinal cord injury in the pediatric population: a systematic review of the literature, *J. Neurotrauma,* **28**, 1515–1524.

Patel, J.C., Tepas, J.J., Mollitt, D.L., *et al.* (2001). Pediatric cervical spine injuries: defining the disease, *J. Pediatr. Surg.,* **36**, 373–376.

Pickett, G.E., Campos-Benitez, M., Keller, J.L., *et al.* (2006). Epidemiology of traumatic spinal cord injury in Canada, *Spine,* **31**, 799–805.

Pullarkat, V.A., Kalapura, T., Pincus, M., *et al.* (2000). Intraspinal hemorrhage complicating oral anticoagulant therapy: an unusual case of cervical hematomyelia and a review of the literature, *Arch. Intern. Med.,* **160**, 237–240.

Rahimi-Movaghar, V., Sayyah, M.K., Akbari, H., *et al.* (2013). Epidemiology of traumatic spinal cord injury in developing countries: a systematic review, *Neuroepidemiol.,* **41**, 65–85.

Reid, W.D., Brown, J.A., Konnyu, K.J., *et al.* (2010). Physiotherapy secretion removal techniques in people with spinal cord injury: a systematic review, *J. Spinal Cord Med.,* **33**, 353–370.

Rodesch, G., Hurth, M., Alvarez, H., *et al.* (2004). Angio-architecture of spinal cord arteriovenous shunts at presentation. Clinical correlations in adults and children. The Bicêtre experience on 155 consecutive patients seen between 1981–1999, *Acta Neurochir. Wien,* **146**, 217–227.

Romero, J., Vari, A., Gambarrutta, C., *et al.* (2009). Tracheostomy timing in traumatic spinal cord injury, *Eur. Spine J.,* **18**, 1452–1457.

Roth, E.J., Stenson, K.W., Powley, S., *et al.* (2010). Expiratory muscle training in spinal cord injury: a randomized controlled trial, *Arch. Phys. Med. Rehabil.,* **91**, 857–861.

Schilero, G.J., Spungen, A.M., Bauman, W.A., *et al.* (2009). Pulmonary function and spinal cord injury. *Respir. Physiol. Neurobiol.,* **166**, 129–141.

Schmidt, O.I., Gahr, R.H., Gosse, A., *et al.* (2009). ATLS and damage control in spine trauma. *World J. Emerg. Surg.,* **4**, 9. [Online] Available at: http://www.wjes.org/content/4/1/9 [Accessed 15 November 2014].

Scivoletto, G., and Di Donna, V. (2009). Prediction of walking recovery after spinal cord injury, *Brain Res. Bull.,* **78**, 43–51.

Sekhon, L.H.S., and Fehlings, M.G. (2001). Epidemilogy, demographics and pathophysiology of acute spinal cord injury, *Spine,* **26** [Suppl], S2–S12.

Sharma, H., Alilain, W.J., Sadhu, A., *et al.* (2012). Treatments to restore respiratory function after spinal cord injury and their implications for regeneration, plasticity and adaptation, *Exp. Neurol.,* **235**, 18–25.

Shavelle, R.M., DeVivo, M.J., Strauss, D.J., *et al.* (2006). Long-term survival of persons ventilator dependent after spinal cord injury, *J. Spinal Cord Med.,* **29**, 511–519.

Shears, E., and Armitstead, C.P. (2010). Surgical versus conservative management for odontoid fractures, *Cochrane Database Syst. Rev.,* **4**, CD005078.

Sheel, A.W., Reid, W.D., Townson, A.F., *et al.* (2008). Effects of exercise training and inspiratory muscle training in spinal cord injury: a systematic review, *J. Spinal Cord Med.,* **31**, 500–508.

Spinal Cord Injury Rehabilitation Evidence. (2012). *Rehabilitation Evidence: Physical Activity*. SPIRE. [Online] Available at: http://www.scireproject.com/rehabilitation-evidence/physical-activity [Accessed April 2014].

Staheli, L. (2001). *Practice of Pediatric Orthopedics*, Lippincott Williams and Wilkins, Seattle, WA.

Stephenson, R.O. (2013). *Autonomic Dysreflexia in Spinal Cord Injury*. Medscape. [Online] Available at: http://emedicine.medscape.com/article/322809-overview [Accessed 17 June 2014].

Stepp, E.L., Brown, R., Tun, C.G., *et al.* (2008). Determinants of lung volume in chronic spinal cord injury, *Arch. Phys. Med. Rehabil.,* **89**, 1499–1506.

Tedde, M.L., Filho, P.V., Hajjar, L.A., *et al.* (2012). Diaphragmatic pacing stimulation in spinal cord injury: anesthetic and perioperative management, *Clinics,* **67**, 1265–1269.

Terson de Paleville, D.G.L., McKay, W.B., Folz, R.J., *et al.* (2011). Respiratory motor control disrupted by spinal cord injury: mechanisms, evaluation and restoration, *Transl. Stroke Res.,* **2**, 463–473.

Thibault-Halman, G., Casha, S., Singer, S., *et al.* (2011). Acute management of nutritional demands after spinal cord injury, *J. Neurotrauma,* **28**, 1497–1507.

Thim, T., Krarup, N.H.V., Grove, E.L., *et al.* (2012). Initial assessment and treatment with the airway, breathing, circulation, disability, exposure (ABCDE) approach, *Int. J. Gen. Med.,* **5**, 117–121.

Uustal, H., and Baerga, E. (2004). 'Spinal orthoses', in Cuccorullo, S. (ed), *Physical Medicine and Rehabilitation Board Review*, Demos Medical Publishing, New York, NY. pp. 409–488.

Van Houtte, S., Vanlandewijck, Y., and Gosselink, R. (2006). Respiratory muscle training in persons with spinal cord injury: a systematic review, *Respir Med.,* 100, 1886–1895.

Vásquez, R.G., Sedes, P.R., Farina, M.M., *et al.* (2013). Review article: respiratory management in the patient with spinal cord injury, *BioMed Res. Int.,* Article ID 168757. [Online] Available at: http://dx.doi.org/10.1155/2013/168757 [Accessed 19 June 2014].

Wolfe, D.L., McIntyre, A., Ravenek, K., *et al.* (2012). 'Physical activity and SCI', in Eng, J.J., Teasell, R.W., Miller, W.C., *et al.* (eds), *Spinal Cord Injury Rehabilitation Evidence*, Version 4.0. SCIRE Project, Vancouver, pp. 409–488. [Online] Available at: http://www.scireproject.com/rehabilitation-evidence/physical-activity [Accessed 29 July 2014].

Wong, S.L., Shem, K., and Crew, J. (2012). Specialized respiratory management for acute cervical spinal cord injury: a retrospective analysis, *Top. Spinal Cord Inj. Rehabil.,* **18**, 283–290.

Wuermser, L.A., Ho, C.H., Chiodo, A.E., *et al.* (2007). Spinal cord injury medicine. 2. Acute care management of traumatic and non-traumatic injury, *Arch. Phys. Med. Rehabil.,* **88** [Suppl], S55–S61.

Wyndaele, M., and Wyndaele, J.J. (2006). Incidence, prevalence and epidemiology of spinal cord injury: what learns a worldwide literature survey, *Spinal Cord,* **44**, 523–528.

Zidek, K., and Srinivasan, R. (2003). Rehabilitation of a child with a spinal cord injury, *Semin. Pediatr. Neurol.,* **10**, 140–150.

Zimmer, M.B., Nantwi, K., and Goshgarian, H.G. (2007). Effect of spinal cord injury on the respiratory system: basic research and current clinical treatment options, *J. Spinal Cord Med.,* **30**, 319–330.

Chapter 9

Traumatic Brain Injury

Written by R. Roos, B.M. Morrow and H. van Aswegen

Traumatic brain injury (TBI) is a problem worldwide, due in part to the high prevalence of road traffic accidents and the presence of violence such as civil unrest and wars. Prior to the twentieth century, severe head injury was most often fatal, but now, due to improved medical management, patients are surviving and the need for rehabilitation services has increased (Cifu *et al.*, 2010). Traumatic brain injury can result in significant impairments, physical limitations and participation restrictions that require rehabilitation. The rehabilitation services available are often limited depending on the country in which the injury occurs. Medical and therapeutic strategies to enhance brain protection in the early phase following TBI is therefore of extreme importance to try and lessen mortality and improve functional outcome.

The information covered in this chapter is focused on the acute care management of a patient with TBI and includes:

- The causes and mechanisms of injury.
- The types of TBI.
- Primary and secondary damage associated with TBI.
- The severity of injury.

(Continued)

(Continued)

- Medical and surgical management of a patient who sustained TBI.
- The physiotherapy aims for the management of a patient who sustained TBI in the intensive care unit and neurosurgical ward.
- The contraindications and precautions related to the physiotherapy management of a patient with TBI.
- Physiotherapy interventions for patients who suffered TBI.
- Adult and paediatric clinical case scenarios.

There is a wealth of information related to the rehabilitation of individuals with TBI in the later stages of rehabilitation. Information for further reading on chronic rehabilitation of a patient with TBI is provided in Section 9.10.

9.1. Causes and Mechanisms of Injury

9.1.1. *Injury in adults*

Traumatic brain injury is defined as an alteration in brain function or other evidence of brain pathology caused by an external force (CDC, 2011). Events that can lead to TBI include falls, motor vehicle accidents (MVA) and assault (CDC, 2011). Other causes of TBI include blast-related injuries and gun shots. Sixty percent of blast-related injuries will result in TBI due to the primary blast wave alteration in atmospheric pressure, flying shrapnel and the propulsion of an individual against a hard object (Cifu *et al.*, 2010). Motor vehicle accidents are the most common cause of TBI in teenagers and young adults, whereas falls occur more in children or older adults. Individuals more at risk of TBI are males, the elderly and children younger than four years (Marik *et al.*, 2002; CDC, 2011).

9.1.2. *Injury in paediatrics*

Children are more predisposed to TBI than adults because they have a larger head in relation to body size and lax spinal ligaments. These factors predispose young children to *coup* and *contre-coup* brain lesions. It is rare for a child with multiple injuries to present without an associated head injury (Dykes, 1999). The immature brain is more prone to injury and the protective cranial bones are thinner than in adults. Children may lose large volumes of blood with scalp lacerations, which may predispose them to hypovolaemic shock. Scalp lacerations may be accompanied by deeper and more serious head injuries because of the relative lack of protection of the child's brain through anatomical structures (Weiner and Weinberg, 2000).

Abusive head trauma remains an important cause of trauma death in children under three years old in developed and developing countries, and is an important cause of morbidity in infants and young children (Duhaime *et al.*, 1998; John *et al.*, 2013). Compared to children and adults with accidental head injury, victims of non-accidental head injury are likely to present with more severe symptoms (such as cardiorespiratory compromise, seizures, altered mental status), which lead to severe brain injuries, worse neurologic outcomes and higher mortality (Herman *et al.*, 2011).

Falls are the most common cause of TBI in children between two and four years of age, as they explore higher surfaces such as furniture or jungle gyms. In younger children devices like highchairs and walkers, designed to protect them, have been associated with significant head injuries when the child falls from them. In older children, vehicle-related accidents become a more frequent cause of head injury (bicycles, passengers in cars and victims of pedestrian MVA) (Weiner and Weinberg, 2000).

Crush injuries often occur at home when heavy objects pulled by small children land on their heads (Weiner and Weinberg, 2000). Violent penetrating injuries in children are still relatively uncommon in most geographical areas, but in turbulent communities it is not uncommon for a child to be caught in cross-fire and sustain a gunshot wound. In cases of domestic violence a child may even be used as a human shield. Accidental penetrating injuries may occur as a result of a fall onto a sharp object (Weiner and Weinberg, 2000).

Traumatic brain injury involving adults or children can be classified according to a number of factors, such as the mechanics of injury, location (e.g. configuration of the skull, specific brain pathology), extent (e.g. diffuse or focal injury, primary or secondary damage) and severity of injury (patient level of consciousness).

9.1.3. *Forces related to traumatic brain injury*

Primary injury refers to the initial traumatic force applied to the head that results in neuronal damage (refer to Section 9.3). Mechanisms related to primary TBI include forces of high or low velocity that result in compression, traction or shearing of brain tissue (Paz and West, 2009). These forces are categorised as deceleration forces (e.g. being struck by a blunt object), acceleration forces (e.g. fall from a height), coup and contre-coup forces (e.g. collision of the head with the steering wheel of a motor vehicle, in which the impact moves the head into extension resulting in posterior contact with the seat) and, lastly, rotational forces (e.g. rolling of a motor vehicle causing torsion of vascular structures). The latter three incidences could result in significant orthopaedic (e.g. multiple rib fractures with pulmonary contusions) and additional neurologic (e.g. spinal cord) injury that may complicate the acute care management of a patient. The physiotherapist working in a trauma ICU should therefore have the necessary translational physiotherapy skills to manage cardiopulmonary as well as orthopaedic or specific neurological complications in a trauma victim who presents with multi-system involvement.

9.2. Types of Traumatic Brain Injury

9.2.1. *Open or closed injury*

A patient with TBI may present with damage to the skull and brain tissue or structures of the brain only. An open injury results in a brain injury in the presence of a skull fracture. Penetrating injuries such as gunshot or stab injuries result in open head injury. The presence of skull fractures implies that a large force was applied to the patient's head, and the likelihood of an intracerebral haematoma is increased in such a situation (Fig. 9.1). In a closed injury there is damage to the brain but the skull remains intact, such as in an MVA, assault to the head or sports-related injury (Marik *et al.*, 2002; Paz and West, 2009).

Skull fractures are common during infancy because the cranium is relatively thin. Most simple, undisplaced skull fractures are not associated with underlying brain injury; however, if this has occurred, separation of

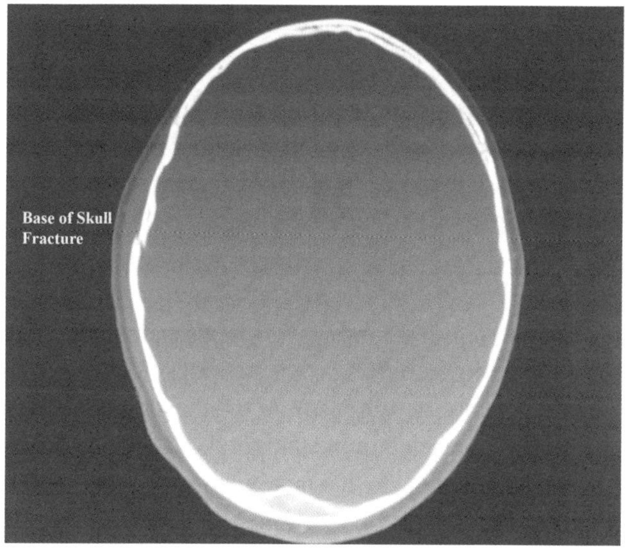

Fig. 9.1: Computed tomography scan of a patient with a base-of-skull fracture.

the edges of the fractured skull may indicate brain swelling or raised intracranial pressure (ICP) (Weiner and Weinberg, 2000).

Diastatic fractures occur uniquely in children when there is traumatic separation of the cranial sutures (most often lamboidal). Growing fractures are sometimes seen, particularly in the toddler age group, in which a diastatic fracture grows as the brain herniates through the torn dura into the fracture site. This type of fracture often presents some time after the acute injury and there is persistent welling or a pulsatile mass of herniated tissue palpable. Urgent repair of the dura is required in such cases (Weiner and Weinberg, 2000).

In adults and children, every case of TBI should be screened for the presence of cervical spine injury, both clinically and radiologically.

9.2.2. *Focal or diffuse injury*

In addition to being described as an open or closed injury, TBI can also be described as diffuse or focal. These terms are used to describe whether the injury is gross or specific in nature.

9.2.2.1. *Focal injury*

A focal injury is an injury to a specific part of the brain. The types of focal injuries can be specified as epidural, subdural, subarachnoid and intracerebral haematomas (Marik *et al.*, 2002; Morton *et al.*, 2005). A description of each type is provided below.

9.2.2.1.1. Epidural haematoma

An epidural haematoma develops when blood accumulates between the skull and dura mater. Road traffic accidents, falls, assault or laceration of the middle meningeal artery will result in the development of such a haematoma. It is most often found in the temporal or temporo-parietal region. Quick surgical evacuation of the haematoma usually results in favourable outcomes (Bullock *et al.*, 2006).

9.2.2.1.2. Subdural haematoma

A subdural haematoma develops with bleeding between the dura mater and arachnoid meninges. It occurs more often in a trauma victim than epidural haematoma. Haematoma formation occurs due to damage inflicted on the bridging veins between the cerebral cortex and venous sinus. A subdural haematoma appears as a crescent-shaped collection between the brain and dura on computerised tomography (CT) scan.

Subdural haematomas are the most common forms of intracranial bleeds that occur in infants. In this age group they most commonly occur in the fronto-parietal area by a tearing of the bridging meningeal veins. Subdural haematomas are frequently associated with significant underlying parenchymal damage. Clinically, infants with subdural haematomas often present with initial loss of consciousness and a depressed mental state or they may be comatose. Following CT confirmation of the diagnosis, urgent surgical review and prompt surgical intervention when required is essential. All young children presenting with subdural haematomas should be investigated for possible non-accidental injury (e.g. shaken-baby syndrome), particularly when associated with retinal haemorrhage (Levin, 2010).

9.2.2.1.3. Subarachnoid haematoma

Subarachnoid haematoma refers to bleeding in the subarachnoid space due to the tearing and shearing of micro-vessels. Subarachnoid haematomas often accompany other severe brain injuries, adding to poorer outcomes (Bullock *et al.*, 2006) (Fig. 9.2). Subarachnoid haemorrhage also has non-traumatic causes such as ruptured aneurysm; reports from most clinical settings indicate that a large number of patients with this type of haemorrhage are seen.

9.2.2.1.4. Intracerebral haematoma

Intracerebral haematomas are commonly seen with moderate to severe TBI (Fig. 9.3). The majority of lesions occur in the frontal and temporal lobes. Intracerebral haemorrhage may also be related to a ruptured aneurysm, as mentioned above.

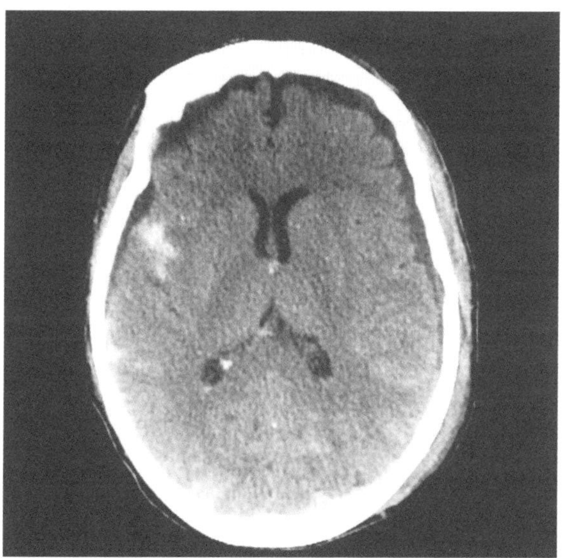

Fig. 9.2: CT scan of a patient with subarachnoid haemorrhage (bright white spots in brain tissue).

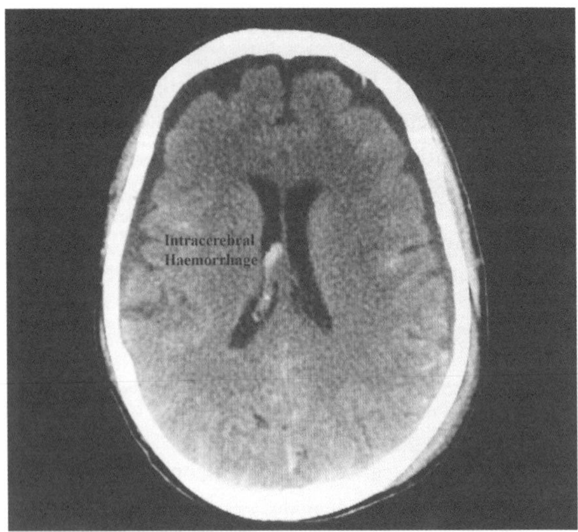

Fig. 9.3: CT scan of a patient with intracerebral haemorrhage.

9.2.2.2. *Diffuse injury*

A diffuse injury such as diffuse axonal injury (DAI) may occur when the head is struck with an object. The rapid acceleration and deceleration forces cause the brain to move forwards and backwards in the skull and different areas of the brain are compressed and stretched. These shearing forces affect axons that transverse a large area of the brain stem. It results in dysfunction of the reticular activating system. This type of injury is often not visible on initial CT scan. It may cause immediate and prolonged unconsciousness and patients may also have a high mortality rate. If they survive, their morbidity is high (Marik *et al.*, 2002; Morton *et al.*, 2005).

9.3. Primary and Secondary Injury Associated with Traumatic Brain Injury

The extent of TBI should be evaluated according to the pathophysiology related to primary and secondary damage. As mentioned previously, the initial traumatic force applied to the head (e.g. fall, assault, penetrating injury) is the primary injury that results in neuronal damage due to contusion, damaged blood vessels and axonal injury. This is the direct mechanical damage caused by the injury and cannot be influenced by therapy received after injury (Werner and Engelhard, 2007).

Secondary injury is the delayed non-mechanical damage that develops over hours and days after the primary injury. The degree of secondary brain injury that the patient develops is related to the extent and duration of cerebral ischaemia and intracranial hypertension (Bullock and Povlishock, 2007; Werner and Engelbrand, 2007; Shirley, 2009). Factors that lead to cerebral ischaemia include hypoxaemia (e.g. pulmonary infection, atelectasis and blood volume loss), systemic hypotension (e.g. blood volume loss due to trauma), cerebral hypoperfusion (e.g. cerebral vasospasm), inflammatory processes (e.g. release of proinflammatory cytokines and free oxygen radicals) and intracranial hypertension. Intracranial hypertension is caused by cerebral hyperperfusion, often as a result of hypercarbia, and cerebral oedema (Werner and Engelbrand, 2007). Figure 9.4 gives an outline of the factors that influence secondary brain injury.

Two groups of patients are more at risk of developing secondary brain damage. These are women, as they are more prone to develop cerebral oedema leading to increased ICP, and also patients with TBI who received anticoagulation therapy on admission (Protheroe and Gwinnutt, 2011).

Intensive care unit (ICU) management of a patient with TBI therefore focuses on limiting secondary damage by managing ICP and cerebral perfusion pressure (CPP) and promoting optimal oxygenation in order to limit cellular injury (Meyer *et al.*, 2010).

9.3.1. *Intracranial pressure*

Intracranial pressure is the pressure within the cranium and is influenced by the volume occupied by the brain tissue, cerebrospinal fluid (CSF) and cerebral blood flow. The interdependence between ICP and the contents of the rigid skull can be explained using the Monro-Kellie hypothesis. This hypothesis describes the volume-pressure relationship between the brain tissue, CSF and cerebral blood flow. If there is an increase in the volume or amount of either one of these components (brain tissue, CSF or cerebral blood flow), there will be a decrease in one or both of the other components in an attempt to maintain normal ICP. Of the components that

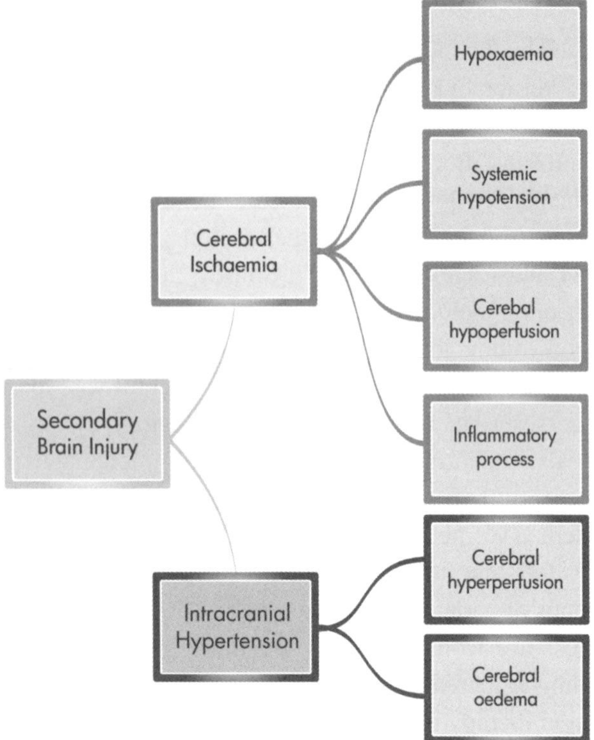

Fig. 9.4: Factors that influence secondary brain injury.

take up volume in the skull, CSF can be displaced most rapidly into the spinal epidural space. Alternatively, the absorption rate of CSF can be rapidly increased in an attempt to maintain ICP within normal limits (Mokri, 2001; Dunn, 2002). A rise in ICP will be initiated when this compensatory mechanism becomes exhausted, as is the case with TBI. After TBI the volume of brain tissue increases due to oedema formation and haemorrhage and blood supply to the brain is disturbed. Increased pressure in the skull will lead to a lack of blood supply to the brain cells and eventual hypoxia. Hypoxia in itself is a stimulus for the blood vessels to dilate and for blood pressure (BP) to be raised to allow greater blood flow to the brain, which in turn will contribute to a further rise in ICP (Dunn, 2002). It is known today that aggressive ICP monitoring and treatment in patients with severe TBI lessens mortality and leads to favourable outcomes following critical illness (Stein *et al.*, 2010).

Patients with TBI that present the signs and symptoms in Table 9.1 should undergo ICP monitoring.

Various methods can be used to monitor ICP, including: a) epidural sensor; b) subdural bolt; c) subarachnoid bolt; d) parenchymal catheter; and e) intraventricular catheter (Morton *et al.*, 2005) (Fig. 9.5). The ventricular catheter is the most accurate of the abovementioned devices (Bullock and Povlishock, 2007).

Table 9.1: Indications for ICP monitoring*.

Indications
• Glasgow coma scale score less than 9 out of 15
• Prolonged non-neurosurgical surgery
• Abnormal findings on CT scan
• Age over 40 years with uni- or bilateral motor posturing
• Age over 40 years with systolic blood pressure less than 90 mmHg

*(Fakhry *et al.*, 2004; Bullock and Povlishock, 2007; Mejaddam and Velmahos, 2012).

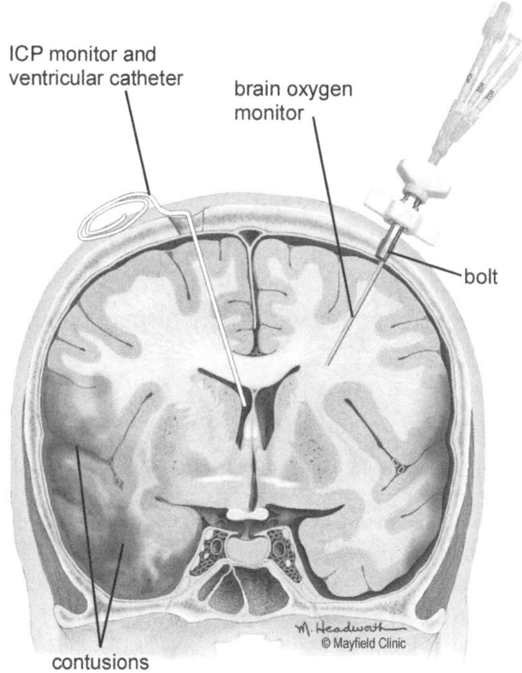

Fig. 9.5: Intracranial pressure monitoring devices. Printed with permission from The Mayfield Clinic.

Early signs of raised ICP in a self-ventilating patient with TBI include restlessness, agitation, headaches, vomiting, photophobia and neck stiffness (Paz and West, 2009). The normal value for ICP in adults and children is less than 15 millimetres of mercury (mmHg). The physiological and treatment threshold value for ICP is 20–25 mmHg. Secondary brain injury has a significantly negative impact on the patient's outcome, with sustained levels of ICP above 25 mmHg (Weiner and Weinberg, 2000; Bullock and Povlishock, 2007).

Certain pathophysiological changes occur with a raise in ICP and are outlined in Table 9.2 (Morton *et al.*, 2005).

It is important to note that with handling, be it nursing procedures or physiotherapy, ICP will most likely fluctuate.

Key Message

Physiotherapy treatment should not proceed in cases in which ICP is sustained above 25 mmHg despite the administration of additional sedative or paralysing drugs. However, if sputum accumulation in the lungs is the cause for the high ICP, physiotherapy treatment to effectively clear the patient's airways should be commenced without delay.

Late signs of increased ICP include changes in the level of consciousness, pupil size and reactivity, motor response and vital signs. Examples of late signs of increased ICP are listed in Table 9.3.

Children with open cranial sutures may display bulging of the fontanelles in response to raised ICP.

Table 9.2: Pathophysiological changes associated with increased ICP.

- The microcirculation in the brain parenchyma becomes compromised when ICP increases to 15–20 mmHg
- Venous return is impeded and oedema starts to develop in the non-injured brain tissue when ICP increases to 30–35 mmHg
- As ICP increases above 40 mmHg, cerebral perfusion can no longer be maintained and brain death is inevitable if these levels of increased pressure are sustained

Table 9.3: Late signs of increased ICP*.

Sign	Patient presentation
Level of consciousness	Coma
Pupil size and reactivity	Papilledema or ipsilateral fixed and dilated pupil or bilateral fixed and dilated pupils in the presence of brain herniation
Motor response	Abnormal posturing or flaccidity if brain herniation has occurred
Vital signs	Cushing's response, which includes hypertension, bradycardia, altered respiratory pattern and increased temperature

*(Paz and West, 2009).

9.3.2. *Cerebral perfusion pressure*

Cerebral perfusion pressure refers to the BP gradient across the brain. It is calculated with the equation CPP = mean arterial pressure (MAP) — ICP. If MAP is not recorded on the patient's chart or displayed on the heart rate monitor, it can be calculated using the equation MAP = diastolic blood pressure (DBP) + [(systolic blood pressure (SBP) — DBP)/3]. In a healthy state, cerebral blood flow is maintained at a constant level over a range of CPP through the process of autoregulation. When autoregulation is disrupted, such as with TBI, changes in BP or ICP will directly impact cerebral blood flow. If autoregulation remains intact after TBI, changes in ICP or BP may influence blood volume (e.g. dilatation or constriction of blood vessels) and influence ICP. Increases in ICP without a concomitant increase in MAP may lead to a decrease in CPP (Dunn, 2002; Toledo *et al.*, 2008).

A normal adult CPP value is more than 70 mmHg. The threshold value for CPP in adults is 50 mmHg, as the effect of secondary brain injury has a marked influence on patient outcome with sustained CPP levels below 50 mmHg. If CPP is maintained at threshold value, blood flow to the brain becomes inadequate and neural hypoxia and brain death can occur (Morton *et al.*, 2005). It is suggested that a CPP of 60–70 mmHg in a patient with TBI is sufficient to maintain cerebral oxygenation (Shirley, 2009). Other authors have noted that if CPP is kept at 70–80 mmHg, mortality in patients with severe TBI is less than 35% (Guha, 2004). The aim of medical management of an adult patient with TBI is therefore to maintain CPP above 70 mmHg. It is essential that ICP and MAP be maintained within normal limits in order to prevent cerebral ischaemia.

Secondary brain injury is a frequent occurrence in severe paediatric head trauma, leading to raised ICP. All head-injured children with Glasgow coma scale (GCS) less than eight, evidence of intracranial mass lesions or brain contusion, shearing or DAI require ICP monitoring (Weiner and Weinberg, 2000; Kochanek *et al.*, 2012). In children, CPP should generally be maintained above 40 mmHg (Alterman and Geibel, 2011; Kochanek *et al.*, 2012). Age-related critical threshold levels for CPP have been reported by Chambers *et al.* (2006), who suggest that CPP be maintained above 48 mmHg (ages 2–6), 54 mmHg (ages 7–10) and 58 mmHg (ages 11–15).

9.4. Severity of Injury

Severity of injury is evaluated using GCS. The GCS evaluates consciousness by reviewing eye, verbal and motor responses to stimuli. The eye response gives an understanding of arousal or wakefulness; the verbal response information on alertness and awareness; and motor response reveals the extent of motor activity (Palmer and Knight, 2006; Matis and Birbilis, 2008) (Table 9.4). The maximum GCS score is 15/15 and indicates full consciousness; the minimum score is 3/15, which indicates no response to stimuli. If a person is mechanically ventilated, GCS grading is out of a total of 10, as the verbal response is excluded from scoring due to the presence of an artificial airway.

A severe head injury is graded as a GCS score less than 8/15, moderate injury a score between 9/15 and 12/15 and mild injury between 13/15 and 14/15. A mild injury is commonly diagnosed as a concussion and could be further assessed by evaluating the severity of amnesia. The extended GCS (GCS-E) serves as an additional tool to evaluate and monitor mild injuries (Nell *et al.*, 2000; Matis and Birbilis, 2008). In children less than three years of age, the paediatric GCS should be used to evaluate consciousness due to communication skills not being fully developed in very young children (Table 9.5).

Table 9.4: Glasgow coma scale for adult patients*.

Eye response

4 — spontaneous opening of eyes
3 — opens eyes on response to speech
2 — opens eyes on pain stimulus
1 — no response elicited

Verbal response

5 — orientated and converses normally
4 — confused and disorientated
3 — utters inappropriate words
2 — makes inappropriate sounds
1 — makes no sound

Motor response

6 — obeys commands
5 — localises to painful stimulus
4 — flexes or withdraws to painful stimulus
3 — abnormal flexing to painful stimulus (decorticate response)
2 — extension to painful stimulus (decerebrate response)
1 — no motor response present

*Adapted from Palmer and Knight (2006).

Abnormal flexion and extension on the GCS indicates abnormal posturing. Abnormal flexion is noted when a patient exhibits the following movement pattern: adduction of the upper limbs, flexion of the arm, wrist and fingers with extension and internal rotation of the lower limbs and plantar flexion of the feet. This is called decorticate posturing. Abnormal extension is demonstrated as adduction and hyperpronation of the upper limbs with extension of the lower extremities and plantar flexion. The head and neck may also be arched backwards. This is decerebrate posturing (Matis and Birbilis, 2008). Both these abnormal postures indicate loss of higher motor control function and poor outcomes (Palmer and Knight, 2006).

9.5. Medical and Surgical Management

Effective management of the patient with TBI is dependent on interdisciplinary team work. The interdisciplinary team in the acute care setting

Table 9.5: Paediatric Glasgow coma scale.

Eye opening response		
≤2 years	*Score*	*>2 years*
Spontaneous	4	Spontaneous
To speech	3	To voice
To pain	2	To pain
None	1	None
Verbal response		
≤2 years	*Score*	*>2 years*
Coos and babbles	5	Oriented
Irritable and cries	4	Confused
Cries to pain	3	Inappropriate
Moans to pain	2	Incomprehensible
None	1	None
Motor Response		
≤2 years	*Score*	*>2 years*
Normal, spontaneous	6	Obeys commands
Withdraws to touch	5	Localises pain
Withdraws to pain	4	Withdraws to pain
Abnormal flexion	3	Flexion to pain
Abnormal extension	2	Extension to pain
None	1	None

includes paramedics, medical doctors (trauma surgeon, neurosurgeon, ICU consultant or orthopaedic surgeon), nursing staff and physiotherapists. Additional therapeutic specialists, such as occupational therapists and speech and language therapists, and counsellors are included in the team as the patient's condition improves and they move into the sub-acute and chronic phases of recovery. Family members and caregivers form part of the team and should be educated regarding their role throughout the patient's recovery, even if it only includes sensory stimulation of the patient by touch and speech during the acute phase. Lastly, the patient is central to this team once consciousness is regained, and active participation in physical activity can be encouraged in the acute care setting.

9.5.1. *Primary survey and resuscitation of vital functions*

The airways, breathing, circulation, disability, exposure (ABCDE) approach to assessment and care provided during the primary survey for patients with suspected TBI consists of a similar approach to that described in the previous chapters of this book (Chapter 5, Section 5.3.1). The establishment of a patent airway as well as assessment for disability using the alert, voice responsive, pain responsive or unresponsive (AVPU) (Chapter 5, Section 5.3.1) approach and GCS are of particular importance during the primary survey of a patient with TBI.

9.5.2. *Secondary survey as adjunct to primary survey*

The secondary survey of a patient with TBI consists of similar assessment and management approaches as that described in the previous chapters of this book (Chapter 5, Section 5.3.2). Computed tomography scanning or three-dimensional CT (if available) is performed for all patients with TBI to assess the extent of the injury and to identify those in need of immediate surgical intervention (Coles, 2007). Assessment for other injuries is also performed, especially in relation to the spinal cord (Thim *et al.*, 2012).

9.5.3. *Definitive care*

9.5.3.1. *Care provided in the ICU*

Monitoring of a patient with TBI forms an integral part of the care provided in the ICU. Monitoring includes routine physiological parameters and also more specific neurological parameters such as ICP, CPP, pupil size and reactivity and assessment for the presence of neurogenic pulmonary oedema. These neurological parameters are concepts that physiotherapists, working with patients with TBI, should know and understand well, as they influence the management of such patients. Critical care management of the patient with TBI also includes prevention of secondary brain insults related to hyponatraemia, hypotension, hypoxaemia, hypercarbia and raised ICP, as well as early diagnosis and treatment of newly developed medical and surgical problems (Mauritz *et al.*, 2007; Timmons, 2012).

The following strategies are implemented to limit secondary brain insults during ICU stay.

- The patient is nursed in a 30° upright (angle of the head on an ICU bed) position with the head in midline. This position facilitates ventilation, reduces ICP by encouraging venous drainage, improves CPP and limits the onset of ventilator-associated pneumonia, as the risk for aspiration is reduced in this position (Meyer *et al.*, 2010; Haddad and Arabi, 2012).
- Compression of the jugular veins with tight tape fixation of the endotracheal tube (ETT) is avoided as this might impede cerebral venous drainage and lead to an increase in ICP (Haddad and Arabi, 2012).
- Sedatives such as morphine and fentanyl are first-line drugs in the management of a patient with TBI in the ICU. Propofol is also used in some trauma centres to reduce ICP. These drugs are particularly important to reduce the effect of manual handling on ICP and CPP during nursing procedures and physiotherapy treatment (Haddad and Arabi, 2012; Mejaddam and Velmahos, 2012).
- Neuromuscular blocking agents (paralysing drugs) may be prescribed as a means to inhibit the cough reflex and induce muscle relaxation in an attempt to control ICP (Guha, 2004).
- The prescription of barbiturates assists in lowering ICP by suppressing cerebral metabolism. This is achieved by lowering cerebral metabolic demands and cerebral blood volume. An adverse result of barbiturates is the subsequent reduction in BP that can cause a fall in CPP. Close monitoring of cardiovascular status of the adult and paediatric patient with TBI is therefore required during administration of barbiturates (Bullock and Povlishock, 2007; Roberts and Sydenham, 2009; Kochanek *et al.*, 2012).
- The use of corticosteroids to reduce ICP is associated with high mortality in both adult and paediatric patients with TBI and is not recommended (Bullock and Povlishock, 2007; Kochaneck *et al.*, 2012; Rosenfeld *et al.*, 2012).

- Hyperosmolar therapy such as mannitol or hypertonic saline is transfused to assist with managing cerebral oedema and lowering ICP in the adult patient (Bullock and Povlishock, 2007; Wakai *et al.*, 2007). Hypertonic saline is frequently used in paediatric patients with severe TBI to control ICP (Kochanek *et al.*, 2012).
- Anti-seizure prophylaxis is given, using phenytoin in both adult and paediatric patients to reduce the number of early posttraumatic seizure episodes. It is recommended that phenytoin be used only during the first seven days after TBI in order to prevent the onset of its side-effects (Bullock and Povlishock, 2007; Kochaneck *et al.*, 2012; Mejaddam and Velmahos, 2012).
- An external ventricular drain (EVD) may be positioned to drain excess CSF (Meyer *et al.*, 2010) (Figs 9.6A and B).
- The patient is mechanically ventilated to ensure adequate oxygenation and reduce metabolic demand. Hyperventilation (partial pressure of

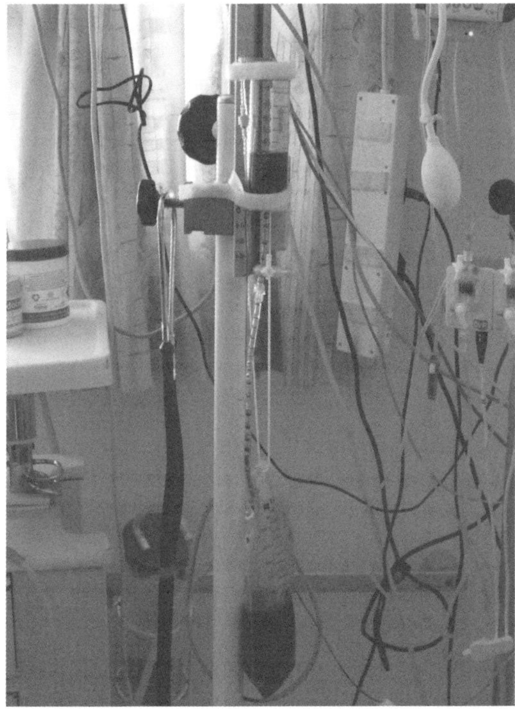

Fig. 9.6A: External ventricular drain.

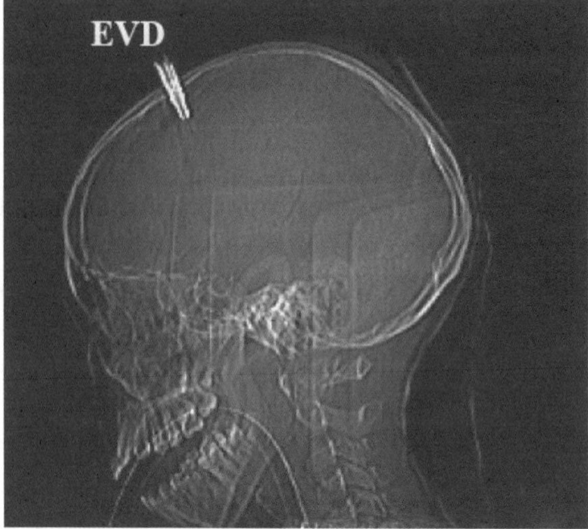

Fig. 9.6B: Fixed CT scan image of a nine-year-old girl with severe head injury and EVD after a motor vehicle accident.

carbon dioxide in arterial blood ($PaCO_2$) 30–35 mmHg (3.9–4.6 kPa)) is employed for only brief periods to manage episodes of acute neurological deterioration in order to reduce ICP by creating cerebral vasoconstriction and reduce cerebral blood flow. The use of hyperventilation in the first 24 hours after admission is, however, not advocated due to the reduction in cerebral blood flow in brain tissue that might already be close to ischaemic threshold (Bullock and Povlishock, 2007; Robert and Schierhout, 2009). Adequate ventilation should ensure arterial blood gas values as follows: $PaCO_2$ of 35–40 mmHg (4.7–5 kPa), partial pressure of oxygen in arterial blood (PaO_2) greater than 80 mmHg (10 kPa) and oxygen saturation equal to or greater than 95% (Arabi *et al.*, 2010). As with the adult, prolonged hyperventilation should be avoided in the head-injured child to prevent secondary ischaemic brain injury. Hyperoxia should be avoided, as this has been associated with poor outcome in adult and paediatric studies (Kochanek *et al.*, 2012).

- Early tracheostomy is advocated for adult patients with TBI in order to reduce the number of mechanical ventilation (MV) days (Bullock and Povlishock, 2007).

- Traumatic brain injury is associated with an increase in blood glucose concentration and correlates with the severity of injury and outcome. It is suggested that an elevated blood glucose level promotes anaerobic metabolism in the brain, resulting in an increased level of lactic acid, which promotes secondary brain damage. Tight glycaemic control in the adult patient with severe TBI is therefore important (Protheroe and Gwinnutt, 2011). The effect of tight glycaemic control in the paediatric patient with TBI is unknown (Kochanek *et al.*, 2012).
- Body temperature is controlled to a mild to moderate hypothermic state for up to 48 hours to lessen secondary brain damage (Peterson *et al.*, 2008; Meyer *et al.*, 2010). This appears to be especially efficacious with young adults (younger than 45 years), but results from paediatric trials showed no benefits (De Deyne, 2010; Alterman and Geibel, 2011).
- Prophylaxis for deep venous thrombosis in adult patients with TBI is achieved with the use of graduated compression stockings and low molecular weight heparin (Bullock and Povlishock, 2007).
- Patients who present with neurological deterioration more than 24 hours after admission undergo repeat CT scanning in order to identify the cause for the deterioration (Brown *et al.*, 2007; Kochanek *et al.*, 2012).

In addition to the strategies outlined above, special attention is given to the monitoring of pupil size and reactivity and the development of neurogenic pulmonary oedema.

9.5.3.1.1. Pupil size and reactivity

Evaluation of pupil size and reactivity provides information regarding the integrity of the third cranial nerve and thus brain stem function. The size of the pupils is observed as well as their reaction to light. Pupil size is measured in millimetres and reactivity in terms of ‘brisk’, ‘sluggish’ or ‘fixed’ by observing response to light (Morton *et al.*, 2005). If assessment indicates a normal response, the following acronyms are often used in ICU documentation: PEARL (pupils equal and reactive to light) or PERL (pupils equal reactive to light). Poor prognosis is reflected by fixed and dilated pupils. Examples of and explanations for abnormal pupil presentations in patients with TBI are summarised in Table 9.6.

Table 9.6: Abnormal pupil presentation in a patient with TBI*.

Pupillary presentation	Possible explanations
Pinpoint pupils	• Medication such as opiates • Eye drops for glaucoma • Small reactive pupils indicative of metabolic abnormalities • Small reactive pupils indicating bilateral dysfunction of the diencephalon • Damage to the pons if pupils non-reactive
Dilated pupils	• Seizures • Sedative drugs such as thiopentone • Recreational drugs such as cocaine • Fear and panic • Unilateral non-reactive dilated pupil ('blown pupil') indicative of third cranial nerve damage following herniation of the uncal portion of the temporal lobe • Bilateral fixed dilated non-reactive pupils due to brain herniation

*(Morton *et al.*, 2005; Paz and West, 2009).

9.5.3.1.2. Neurogenic pulmonary oedema

Neurogenic pulmonary oedema is a clinical syndrome that develops following a significant central nervous system insult, such as TBI, and presents as acute pulmonary oedema. Patients with TBI are therefore at risk of developing neurogenic pulmonary oedema. Individuals in whom the neurological insult occurred in an abrupt and rapid manner, resulting in a sudden increase in ICP, appear to be at the greatest risk of developing neurogenic pulmonary oedema. Autonomic response to the rapid rise in ICP results in a release of catecholamines, leading to blood volume shift from the systemic circulation to the pulmonary circulation. Increased pressure in the pulmonary circulation results in pulmonary oedema. It is also suggested that, during the above process, barotrauma occurs at the alveolar-capillary membrane, which results in persistent vascular leaks (Davison *et al.*, 2012). The early form of neurogenic pulmonary oedema develops within minutes to hours after injury; the delayed form develops within 12 to 24 hours following injury.

Clinical signs and symptoms of neurogenic pulmonary oedema are similar to other causes of pulmonary oedema and include dyspnoea, tachypnoea, hypoxia, cough productive of pink frothy liquid (not sputum) and gravity-dependent bilateral crackles on auscultation. Chest x-ray features include bilateral hyperdense infiltrates widespread over both lung fields, similar to that seen in acute respiratory distress syndrome. Signs and symptoms often resolve spontaneously, but in patients with severe TBI and elevated ICP, neurogenic pulmonary oedema may persist (Davison *et al.*, 2012).

9.5.3.2. *Surgical interventions*

Surgical intervention is considered in cases in which conservative management alone is not effective in controlling ICP (e.g. ICP sustained at values greater than 25 mmHg). It may also be indicated when neurological deterioration is detected in spite of optimal conservative management of the patient. Craniotomy or decompression craniectomy may be performed for adult or paediatric patients under these conditions in order to prevent further secondary brain injury.

9.5.3.2.1. Craniotomy

Craniotomy is a cut that opens the skull. A bone flap (section of the skull) is removed to allow the neurosurgeon access to the dura and the brain underneath. Craniotomy can be small-sized (coin-sized) or large. Small-sized craniotomy is called burr hole or keyhole surgery and is performed for the insertion of an ICP monitor or ventricular drain. Large-sized craniotomy is called skull base surgery and is usually performed after penetrating trauma (gunshot or stab injury) to the head that resulted in a skull fracture and brain injury. After the procedure the bone flap is replaced and secured to the skull with small plates and screws (Warnick, 2013).

9.5.3.2.2. Decompression craniectomy

Decompression craniectomy involves the removal of a segment of the skull bone to allow the swelling brain to expand without compression. It is a last resort therapy to prevent herniation of the brain. The skull bone is only replaced several days later, when brain swelling has subsided. It is recommended that decompression craniectomy is performed in the early stages of the patient's management in order for the patient to derive optimal benefits from this procedure (Kochanek *et al.*, 2012). Decompression craniectomy may lead to better control of ICP, but results from studies investigating the long-term outcomes in patients who underwent this procedure are discouraging: neurologic function is reported to be more affected in these patients at six months after discharge than in those who didn't undergo decompression craniectomy (Mejaddam and Velmahos, 2012; Rosenfeld *et al.*, 2012). The randomised evaluation of surgery with craniectomy for uncontrollable elevation in intracranial pressure (RESCUEicp) trial is a multicentre trial currently investigating whether decompression craniectomy is effective in the management of uncontrollable ICP. Results from this trial are awaited (Hutchinson *et al.*, 2011).

After either of the abovementioned surgical procedures, the patient will be returned to the ICU for monitoring and care.

9.5.3.3. *Brain stem death*

Brain stem death is a clinical syndrome, whereby reflexes that have pathways through the brain stem cease to function. Death of the patient is therefore certified when brain stem death is confirmed, as the patient would have permanently lost consciousness as well as the ability to breathe spontaneously (Wijdicks *et al.*, 2010). A multi-centre study in Canada found that brain herniation was the most common cause for withdrawal of life-saving treatment for patients involved in MVAs with severe TBI (Cote *et al.*, 2013).

The determination of brain stem death is done in some countries by a neurologist or neurosurgeon and in other countries by two doctors who are registered with the Health Professions Council of that specific country but who may not necessarily specialise in neurology. There are certain prerequisites that need to be in place before brain stem testing can be conducted, and these are summarised in Table 9.7.

The neurologic assessment for brain stem death consists of four steps (Wijdicks *et al.*, 2010):

- assessment for coma (patient must lack all evidence of responsiveness; thus no eye or motor responses to painful stimuli);
- assessment for absence of brain stem reflexes (Table 9.8);

Table 9.7: Prerequisites for brain stem testing*.

- Determination of the cause of coma
  - CT scan diagnosis
  - Exclusion of the presence of central nervous system depressant drugs and neuromuscular blocking agents in the patient's circulation
  - No electrolyte, endocrine and acid-base levels abnormalities
- Patient's core body temperature must be within normal limits
- Patient's SBP must be within normal limits

*(Wijdicks *et al.*, 2010).

- apnoea test (Table 9.8); and
- confirmation of the irreversibility of these findings by repeated measure.

Once brain stem death is confirmed and the family consents to organ donation, the medical team may request continuation of physiotherapy treatment to optimise secretion clearance and promote optimal oxygenation in preparation for organ procurement (Bugge, 2009). Treatment modalities such as manual chest clearance techniques (e.g. percussions, vibrations, shaking), manual hyperinflation (MHI) and body position changes with suctioning would be indicated to assist with optimising respiratory function of the potential organ donor.

9.6. Physiotherapy Aims of Management

The role of the physiotherapist as a member of the interdisciplinary team in the adult and paediatric ICU includes accurate assessment of physiological and functional parameters to identify deficiencies in the critically ill patient. Formulation and implementation of an appropriate therapeutic treatment plan based on the needs of each individual patient, monitoring patient response to treatment interventions and modification of intervention as required is integral to physiotherapy management. Provision of effective communication, education and support to the patient and family members are important skills required of the physiotherapist in the ICU setting. Education with the family members and caregivers should include information on the role of the physiotherapist in the management of the patient with TBI in the acute, sub-acute and chronic stages of care. It should also

Table 9.8: Tests performed to assess for cranial nerve function and respiratory effort in a patient with severe TBI*.

Name of test	Cranial nerve(s) tested	Test description
Pupil reaction	Cranial nerve (CN) II (optic) and CN III (occulomotor)	A bright light is shone into each eye. In brain stem death both pupils are mid-dilated or dilated and non-reactive to light.
Doll's eye movement		Two reflexes are tested, namely the occulocephalic and occulovestibular reflexes.
	• CN VI (abducens)	• The occulocephalic reflex is tested by moving the patient's head up and down and from side to side rapidly. In brain stem death no eye movement will be seen during head movements.
	• CN IV (trochlear) and CN VIII (vestibulocochlear)	• The occulovestibular reflex is tested by irrigating the patient's ear with ice cold water in a 30º head elevated position. No eye movement will be detected if the patient has brain stem death.
Corneal test	CN V (trigeminal)	The cornea is touched with a piece of tissue paper or a cotton swab. Corneal reflex is absent and no eyelid movement is present in brain stem death.
Pain reflex	CN VII (facial)	Deep pressure is applied over the supraorbital ridge or the condyles of the temperomandibular joint. No grimacing or facial movement will be observed with brain stem death.
Pharyngeal and tracheal test	CN IX (glossopharyngeal) and CN X (vagal)	• The gag (pharyngeal) reflex is assessed by touching the back of the throat with a suction catheter or tongue blade. In brain stem death no gag reflex will be observed. • The cough (tracheal) reflex is assessed by suctioning the trachea down to the level of the carina or by up and down movement of the ETT in the airway. No cough reflex indicates brain stem death.

(*Continued*)

Table 9.8. *(Continued)*

Name of test	Cranial nerve(s) tested	Test description
Apnoea test (absence of respiratory drive)		A carbon dioxide challenge test is performed. • Prior to the test the patient's $PaCO_2$ must be 35–45 mmHg (4.6–6 kPa). • The patient is preoxygenated for a minimum of 10 minutes on 100% oxygen until PaO_2 is greater than 200 mmHg (26.7 kPa). Ventilator frequency is then reduced to 10 breaths/minute and positive end expiratory pressure (PEEP) is reduced to five cmH_2O. If pulse oximetry remains higher than 95% an arterial blood gas (ABG) is performed. • The patient is then disconnected from the ventilator and oxygen therapy is administered to them through an insufflation catheter placed inside the ETT at the level of the carina. The insufflation catheter is connected to the oxygen flow meter set at six L/minute and delivers continuous oxygen to the patient. • The patient is then closely observed for eight to 10 minutes to see if any respiratory movements (e.g. gasp or abdominal or chest wall movements) take place. • The test is stopped if SBP falls below 90 mmHg or if pulse oximetry falls below 85% for more than half a minute. • If no respiratory movement is observed after 10 minutes, ABG is repeated. If $PaCO_2$ is greater than 60 mmHg (7.9 kPa) or more than 20 mmHg (2.6 kPa) above the baseline level and no respiratory movements were observed, the apnoea test is positive.

*Adapted from Wijdicks *et al*. (2010).

consist of advice regarding activities that they can perform to enhance patient recovery. The National Institute of Health and Care Excellence (NICE) clinical practice guidelines described in Chapter 5 (Section 5.4) should form the foundation for management of a critically ill patient with TBI in the acute care setting.

In addition to the above, specific aims of physiotherapy in the management of a patient with TBI in ICU are summarised in Table 9.9.

As the patient's condition stabilises and intensive monitoring of the patient is no longer required, transfer to the neurological or neurosurgical ward will be considered. Prior to discharge from the ICU, the physiotherapist should re-assess each individual patient to identify their rehabilitation needs as care is continued on the ward. The results of each patient's 'prior to ICU discharge' assessment, as well as a summary of rehabilitation provided in the ICU, should be communicated with the physiotherapist on the neurology ward. Possible aims of physiotherapy management of patients with TBI in the ward setting are summarised in Table 9.10.

Each patient is unique and responds differently to treatment and therefore the aims of physiotherapy intervention will differ between patients and within patients as their condition stabilises or deteriorates. Regular re-assessment of each patient is vitally important to ensure that effective physiotherapy rehabilitation is provided in the acute care setting.

Table 9.9: Aims of physiotherapy management for patients with TBI in the ICU.

- Liaison with the interdisciplinary team members in the ICU regarding the status of the patient, aims of general management and progress of the patient
- Adequate humidification of the airways to ensure optimal functioning of the mucociliary escalator
- Optimisation of alveolar ventilation to ensure adequate oxygenation in order to limit secondary brain injury from hypoxia
- Prevention of secondary chest complications through effective mobilisation and removal of retained secretions
- Optimisation of lung and chest wall compliance in order to prevent secondary chest complications
- Maintenance or restoration of passive range of motion (ROM) of all limbs in order to prevent or reduce joint stiffness in patients who are intubated and sedated
- In cases of increased muscle tone, aim to normalise muscle tone as able
- Initiation of early mobility programmes, dependent on the stability of the patient's condition

Table 9.10: Aims of progression of management for patients with TBI in the neurology or neurosurgical ward setting.

- Continue to normalise muscle tone for those with abnormal tone, as able
- Improve the patient's proprioception as well as static and dynamic balance
- Improve the patient's ability to perform transfers with minimal assistance
- Improve the patient's self-dependence with progression of the mobility programme initiated in the ICU
- Improve cardiorespiratory exercise endurance in order to obtain the health benefits of exercise
- Ensure adequate humidification of the airways until the patient's oxygen therapy is discontinued
- Ensure excessive retained secretions are adequately cleared from the patient's airways or from the tracheostomy tube
- Optimise lung compliance and lung volumes to prevent the onset of hospital-acquired infections

9.6.1. *Functional assessment prior to discharge*

A functional assessment should be performed for any adult or paediatric patient with TBI prior to discharge home to identify physical and non-physical limitations and their impact on the patient's ability to perform activities of daily living (ADL). Based on these findings, rehabilitation goals for post-discharge rehabilitative care should be discussed with the patient and their family and agreed on.

9.7. Precautions and Contraindications Related to Physiotherapy Management

Recommendations provided here are mostly based on expert opinion derived from clinical practice due to paucity in the literature in certain aspects of patient care in the acute care setting.

9.7.1. *General precautions related to physiotherapy in intensive care*

The reader is referred to Chapter 5 (Section 5.5.1) for a list of general precautions that should be adhered to during the treatment of any trauma patient in the ICU.

9.7.2. *Specific precautions related to physiotherapy in patients with traumatic brain injury*

9.7.2.1. *Adult patients*

When evaluating the need for treatment of a patient with TBI, the benefit of treatment should always outway the risks posed to the patient by treatment. A strong consideration of the following should be made before the initiation of physiotherapy intervention.

- Cardiovascular instability such as MAP greater than 120 mmHg or MAP less than 60 mmHg; any new electrocardiograph abnormalities requiring medical intervention; excessive inotropic support, e.g. noradrenaline or adrenaline administered at 30 mg per hour or more (Patman *et al.*, 2009; Gosselink *et al.*, 2011). If cardiovascular instability is primarily caused by the retention of excessive amounts of sputum, physiotherapy intervention is indicated.
- Neurological instability characterised by sustained levels of ICP greater than 25 mmHg and sustained levels of CPP less than 70 mmHg (Patman *et al.*, 2009). If neurological instability is primarily caused by the retention of excessive amounts of sputum, physiotherapy intervention is indicated.
- Non-reactive fixed dilated pupils. In the case of organ donation physiotherapy chest treatment is still indicated.
- Temperature greater than 40°C due to high metabolic rate and increased oxygen requirements at tissue level (Gosselink *et al.*, 2011).
- Haematological instability indicated by platelet count less than 30,000 cells/mm^3 (Hanekom *et al.*, 2011).
- Nasal suction should not be performed when the patient has a base-of-skull fracture, as the physiotherapist might be clearing CSF instead of secretions.
- Manual chest clearance techniques are contraindicated when a patient presents with neurogenic pulmonary oedema, as the physiotherapist will be clearing pulmonary oedema fluid (pink frothy fluid) and not pulmonary secretions. This may contribute to hypoxemia as the airways collapse due to the removal of surfactant in the oedema fluid.

In addition, suctioning may exacerbate pulmonary oedema through the removal of positive pressure that serves to counteract increases in pulmonary vascular pressures. Other physiotherapy techniques such as positioning and passive movements could be continued if the patient is cardiovascularly and neurologically stable.

During physiotherapy treatment of an adult patient with TBI the following precautions should be followed.

- Ensure adequate analgesia is provided, as painful stimuli and stress increase metabolic demands, BP and ICP.
- If a patient's ICP level is above the normal value, ask for an extra bolus of sedation or paralysing agent to be given to the patient prior to physiotherapy intervention and suction to minimise the increase in ICP.
- Endotracheal suction should be kept brief (up to two suction catheter passes) when ICP is raised (Moore, 2003; Haddad and Arabi, 2012).
- During the first 72 hours following admission to the ICU, maintain the 30° head-up position (bed tilted to a 30° angle) with the head in a neutral spine position. No side flexion or rotation of the head is advised, as these movements will influence venous drainage and alter ICP (Haddad and Arabi, 2012). When turning the patient into side lying, maintain the neutral head position with a towel or pillow, positioned prior to turning, so that the patient's head is adequately supported.
- If a decompression craniectomy was performed, ensure the patient's head is not positioned directly on this area, as the protective mechanism of the brain is removed.
- During movement of the patient be aware of ICP monitor leads to prevent dislodging of the equipment while handling the patient.
- If the patient has an EVD, discuss the precautions regarding this drain during physiotherapy treatment with the neurosurgeon, as precautions may differ between units and surgeons.
- As discussed previously, patients with TBI most likely will have additional traumatic injuries to the spinal cord, trunk or limbs, and the treating physiotherapist should implement those additional precautions. Refer to the other chapters in this book for a revision of suggested precautions.

- Patients recovering from TBI may be agitated and irritable, thus management strategies for such situations should be in place to improve the effectiveness of physiotherapy intervention.
- If you are unsure whether physiotherapy intervention is indicated for the patient, discuss this with the patient's neurosurgeon or the consultant in the ICU as well as the senior physiotherapist in the unit.

9.7.2.2. *Paediatric patients*

The scenarios listed below are contraindications to physiotherapy treatment of children with TBI.

- Cardiovascular instability characterised by BP above or below the normal age-specific range or fluctuating BP; bradycardia or tachycardia; bradycardia with hypertension is of particular concern as it may indicate a Cushing's response with potential coning or herniation of the brain through the brain stem; high levels of inotropic drug support; fluctuations of any vital signs by more than 20% within the previous 12 hours.
- Sustained CPP less than 40 mmHg and ICP greater than 25 mmHg indicating neurological instability.

All other precautions and contraindications listed above for adults can be applied to the management of the paediatric patient with TBI.

9.8. Physiotherapy Interventions

The physiotherapy treatment of a patient with TBI in the acute care setting is most often aimed at minimising impairments and physical activity limitations. The extent of the impairments may be related to a number of factors, such as age of the patient, presence of other co-morbidities (e.g. chronic obstructive pulmonary disease or HIV), severity of TBI, presence of other traumatic injuries, length of MV, development of secondary complications and, in children, whether aspiration has occurred during the injury (e.g. deciduous teeth, vomitus or food).

Physiotherapy treatment alters during the course of the management of a patient with TBI depending on the critical nature of the individual, impairments identified, the appropriateness of a mobility programme and stage of initiation of a mobility programme. Physiotherapy treatment should align with the overall ICU management goals of the patient at any specific time to reflect the interdisciplinary team approach. At the very acute stage, physiotherapy would focus on improving oxygenation to try and lessen secondary brain damage, balancing this potential gain against the risk of causing raised ICP and further injury. As the patient responds to management, the focus of treatment could shift to encouraging active breathing exercises to facilitate weaning off MV. Treatment focus should also shift to the implementation of mobility programmes to address body deconditioning. Rehabilitation is dependent on cooperation from the patient, as agitation in a patient recovering from TBI is a possibility (Lombard and Zafonte, 2005).

The first 72 hours following TBI is often seen as the period in which cerebral oedema develops and secondary brain damage escalates. Less is more at this stage, and if oxygenation is adequate and there are no focal chest problems a hands-off approach is advised for the first 72 hours. When intervention is indicated, for example with retention of secretions due to aspiration pneumonia or a history of smoking, special attention to body positioning of the patient during physiotherapy intervention should be made (refer to Section 9.7).

9.8.1. *Respiratory system*

A patient with TBI is at risk of developing impairments such as retention of secretions, reduction in lung volumes, ventilation and/or perfusion mismatch, change in work of breathing secondary to site of injury resulting in altered breathing pattern, respiratory rate or both and, lastly, respiratory muscle weakness due to prolonged ventilation. Physiotherapists should be aware of these complications, and methods to manage these complications are suggested below. These suggestions are based on research evidence, where available, as well as expert opinion in the absence of research evidence.

9.8.1.1. *Oxygenation*

Ventilation and perfusion are both optimal when a person assumes an upright and moving body position. As ventilation and perfusion improve, so does oxygenation. In previous chapters the effects of body position on ventilation and perfusion and ultimately oxygenation were discussed. A patient with severe TBI is not able to assume the upright and moving position due to the acuteness and nature of their injury and, as described previously in this chapter, should be managed in a 30º upwards bed tilt position while the head is maintained in a neutral position (nose in line with the sternum), especially during the first 72 hours after admission. Regular body position changes (with the aforementioned precautions in mind) from supine to side lying assist with ventilation of the posterior lung segments that are often unable to expand optimally in the supine position (Haddad and Arabi, 2012).

As the patient's ICP stabilises and they become haemodynamically stable, a 60º head-up sitting position in bed can be utilised to improve functional residual capacity (FRC) (Chapter 4, Section 4.2.3.1). As FRC increases, ventilation/perfusion (V/Q) matching is improved and oxygenation increases. Progression from this position would involve sitting the patient up over the edge of the bed, in a chair by the bedside and eventually standing upright. In the upright seated or standing position, the posterior and lateral lung segments can expand without restriction; ventilation therefore improves further and oxygenation becomes optimal.

9.8.1.2. *Humidification*

Nebulisation with mucolytics such as carbocystine or isotonic saline could assist with humidification of the airways and thereby assist with the clearance of excessive secretions. The reader is referred to Chapter 5 (Section 5.6.1.2), in which other methods of humidification of the airways are described. These methods are also applicable to the management of patients with TBI in the acute care setting.

9.8.1.3. *Management of pulmonary secretions*

9.8.1.3.1. Intubated patient

Modified postural drainage positions can be used to facilitate the drainage of secretions from the lung periphery to the central airways. The patient with TBI may be positioned in a modified postural drainage position for secretion mobilisation, such as 30° upwards bed tilt with alternate side-lying positions, during the first 72 hours. When ICP has stabilised, modified postural drainage positions can be adjusted by introducing a horizontal bed position (supine) during alternate side lying. Position changes to side lying from supine assist with drainage of secretions from the posterior lung segments. This type of position change also influences ventilation and perfusion in different lung segments, as previously described. Body position changes are, however, dependent on the stability of the patient who has multiple injuries.

Manual chest clearance techniques, such as percussions, chest wall shaking and chest wall vibrations, can be implemented together with modified postural drainage positions to loosen and mobilise secretions to the central airways. The reader is referred to Chapter 4 (Section 4.2.4) for information on how to perform manual chest clearance techniques effectively and safely. These techniques can influence ICP, CPP and SBP if combined in one treatment (Paratz and Burns, 1993). Percussions have been shown to decrease ICP when used in isolation (Paratz and Burns, 1993), and bilateral chest wall vibrations (in 30° upwards bed tilt position) do not increase ICP during chest physiotherapy treatment of patients with severe head injury (Toledo *et al.*, 2008). Thus, when ICP is already elevated above normal prior to treatment, it would be more advantageous to use percussion or vibrations in isolation and not combined with other manual chest clearance techniques in the same treatment session. The mechanical vibromat may also be used to mobilise and drain pulmonary secretions when the patient's ICP is raised above normal. Respiratory physiotherapy can be used safely in patients with TBI if ICP is less than 30 mmHg (Thiesen *et al.*, 2005).

Manual hyperinflation can be used to assist with sputum clearance and enhance lung volumes, as used in studies conducted by Paratz and Burns (1993) and Patman *et al.* (2009) in patients with acute head injury. The former authors did, however, note that MHI could increase ICP and SBP. It is important to note that the MHI manoeuvre used in their study was performed in a horizontal bed position; therefore it is possible that just the change of body position from 30° head up to horizontal influenced ICP before the MHI manoeuvre was started. It is suggested that performing

MHI in a 30° upwards bed tilt position (if ICP is above normal) may reduce its detrimental effects on ICP, as the effect of gravity on cerebral venous drainage is preserved. Manual hyperinflation, however, increases intrathoracic pressures due to the increase in alveolar pressures and pulmonary volumes, which, together with an inspiratory hold, can collaborate to decrease venous return. When ICP and CPP are already of concern (sustained levels close to threshold values) prior to treatment, routine MHI may not be appropriate due to its effect on ICP, but could be implemented during treatment at a later stage when the patient is more stable.

Patman *et al.* (2009) did, however, note that routine treatment with MHI combined with positioning and suction did not alter ICU length of stay, number of MV days or lessen the development of ventilator-associated pneumonia (VAP) in patients with TBI. In their study, the MHI technique was performed in the 30° head-up position, thereby lessening its effect on ICP. Manual hyperinflation remains a physiotherapy technique that assists with sputum clearance, enhances lung volumes, improves lung compliance and reduces airflow resistance, as suggested by researchers who studied its effects in other ICU populations (Choi and Jones, 2005; Gosselink *et al.*, 2008; Dennis *et al.*, 2012). It should, therefore, not be excluded as a possible means to address such problems in a patient with TBI when the patient is cardiovascularly and neurologically stable. Reports from clinicians support the use of MHI to address respiratory complications in patients with TBI, during the first 72 hours after injury, in cases in which sudden partial or complete atelectasis caused an acute increase in ICP. The temporary use of MHI under these circumstances assists with the restoration of lung volumes and a decrease of ICP to baseline levels. The reader is referred to Chapter 4 (Section 4.2.6.1) for information on the safe and effective application of MHI.

Thiesen *et al.* (2005) reported that endotracheal suction increased ICP in patients with TBI, regardless of the level of ICP prior to suction. Suction to remove secretions mobilised to the central airways can be used in the patient with TBI, provided that precautions and contraindications, as listed in Section 9.7, are adhered to. Close monitoring of changes in the patient's MAP and CPP values during and after suction is important. The reader is referred to Chapter 4 (Section 4.2.7.1) for information on suction of artificial airways.

9.8.1.3.2. Spontaneously breathing patient with a tracheostomy

Some patients with TBI may experience a prolonged period of inability to protect their own airways despite being able to breathe spontaneously. After discharge from the ICU, these patients are managed with tracheostomy tubes in the ward. All the above-mentioned physiotherapy techniques would be applicable to use in this situation to mobilise and clear excessive secretions from the airways. In addition, the physiotherapist should understand and be able to perform tracheostomy care when the need arises (Chapter 5, Section 5.3.4.1). The physiotherapist should also work closely with the speech and language therapist when swallow assessments are performed and when decisions are being made by the attending physician regarding the downsizing and removal of the tracheostomy.

9.8.1.3.3. Spontaneously breathing patient without an artificial airway

After the removal of the tracheostomy tube, the patient's ability to understand instructions and carry out these instructions effectively will determine whether the physiotherapist should continue to use manual chest clearance techniques and modified postural drainage positions for secretion removal, or if another approach can be considered. Methods such as active cycle of breathing technique (ACBT), flutter device, active exercises and active coughing may be used for secretion clearance. If the patient's own cough effort is not effective enough to clear secretions, nasotracheal or orotracheal suction should be performed. The reader is referred to Chapter 4 (Section 4.2) for information on the safe and effective application of ACBT, use of the flutter device and nasotracheal and orotracheal suction.

9.8.1.4. *Lung capacity and volumes*

9.8.1.4.1. Intubated patient

Body position changes can be used to improve lung volumes and FRC, and MHI can be used to optimise lung volumes and pulmonary compliance, as previously mentioned.

Neurophysiological facilitation techniques such as peri-oral stimulation and intercostal stretching (Figs 9.7A and B), as well as passive movements, are reported to improve minute ventilation and peripheral oxygen saturation in patients with head injuries (Chang *et al.*, 2002). These techniques can be used with patients who are able to perform spontaneous breathing, with an artificial airway or without.

Thirteen patients with a GCS less than 11, tracheostomy and haemodynamic stability took part in the study reported by Chang *et al.* (2002). In this experimental trial the order of interventions was randomised. Peri-oral stimulation was performed using the horizontal placement of the physiotherapist's finger against the patient's top lip and nose (using the pad of the finger) (Fig. 9.7A), followed by the application of moderate pressure for 10 seconds. This was followed by intercostal stretching. Intercostal stretching was performed bilaterally on the anterior chest wall on ribs two and three. Moderate pressure was applied onto these ribs during expiration with the direction of the pressure down towards the next rib and not inwards towards the patient's back (Fig. 9.7B). Intercostal stretching was applied for 20 seconds. This cycle was repeated for three minutes (Chang *et al.*, 2002). This is the only recent study that could be found on the effect of neurophysiological facilitation on lung mechanics and therefore the results should be interpreted with caution.

Once the patient's sedation is stopped and they are able to follow commands, active deep breathing exercises can be initiated if the patient

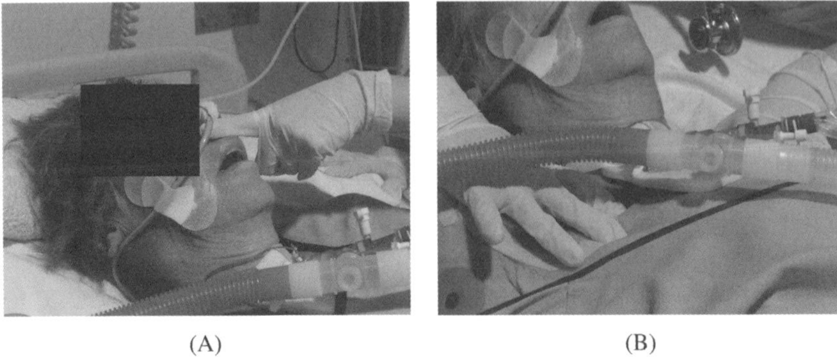

(A) (B)

Fig. 9.7: Neurophysiological facilitation techniques. A) Peri-oral stimulation; B) Intercostal stretching.

is on continuous positive airway pressure (CPAP) ventilation. The tidal volume curve display on the ventilator panel provides visual feedback to the patient during deep breathing (biofeedback) and serves as encouragement for the patient to breathe even deeper. Posterior-anterior thoracic movements can be added to the patient's deep breathing to improve basal ventilation. These movements are facilitated by the physiotherapist as they place their hands on the posterior aspects of the patient's thorax and gently lift the thorax during inspiration.

9.8.1.4.2. Spontaneously breathing patient

After extubation, active deep breathing or ACBT can be continued, and other adjuncts to physiotherapy such as incentive spirometry (Chapter 4, Section 4.2.2.1) may be used if the patient is able to understand how the device should be used. No research evidence could be found in which the effect of incentive spirometry on lung function in patients with TBI was investigated. Breath stacking (Chapter 4, Section 4.2.1.3) may be used to increase lung volumes in spontaneously breathing patients with TBI without intracranial hypertension; research evidence of the effectiveness of this technique in this patient population is, however, also lacking.

Anecdotal evidence suggests that intermittent positive pressure breathing (IPPB) (Chapter 4, Section 4.2.2.2) may contribute to a raise in ICP in patients with closed TBI. Cerebral venous return is thought to be impeded by the increase in intrathoracic volumes and pressures that are created with IPPB during the inspiratory phase of breathing; however, no research evidence could be found to support or refute this assumption. If IPPB is indicated for a patient with closed TBI, the physiotherapist should discuss its potential effect on ICP with the neurosurgeon or neurologist in charge of the patient before IPPB is used; if permission is granted to continue with IPPB, close observation of the patient for signs of raised ICP should be made during the treatment session.

Functional residual capacity increases through the use of positive expiratory pressure (PEP) such as non-invasive CPAP or oscillating PEP devices (Chapter 4, Section 4.2.2.4). No research evidence could be found to support or refute the effectiveness of oscillating PEP or non-invasive CPAP in the management of patients with TBI with normal ICP. Since oscillating PEP and non-invasive CPAP create an increase in intrathoracic pressure during expiration and inspiration, close monitoring of the patient with closed TBI should be done for signs of raised ICP during the treatment session. If the patient presents with any of these signs, treatment with PEP should immediately be terminated and the patient's neurosurgeon informed.

9.8.1.5. *Respiratory muscle training*

Weakness of the respiratory muscles may develop in a patient with TBI who requires prolonged MV, particularly those with additional injuries. Respiratory muscle weakness will affect the patient's ability to wean effectively from MV. The reader is referred to Chapter 4 (Section 4.2.1.5) for information on the various methods that may be employed to enhance respiratory muscle strength for patients who struggle to wean from MV. Similar methods may be used for patients with TBI.

9.8.1.6. *Paediatric considerations*

Caution must be taken with manual chest therapy techniques in young children, as dynamic compression of the very compliant chest wall and the airways may lead to obstruction, deoxygenation and associated increases in ICP (Hess, 2002). Percussion of the chest, as well as shaking with large amplitudes, is likely to cause translational movement of the head and neck, which may cause further brain injury in the young child (Harding *et al.*, 1998); therefore low-amplitude techniques like vibrations are preferable for this patient group. Some clinicians use head holding when applying manual chest clearance techniques in children in order to reduce the likelihood of further brain injury.

Some physiotherapists use MHI in paediatric ICU practice, therefore this is a note of caution. Owing to the differences in anatomy and physiology (Chapter 2), children have increased risk of barotrauma or volutrauma and therefore great care should be taken when applying MHI to paediatric practice. No paediatric studies of MHI in cases of TBI have been published to date. Only two studies have been published on this technique in the general paediatric ICU population. One paediatric study of MHI showed that manual chest compression-vibrations combined with MHI in sedated, fully ventilated children increased peak expiratory flow rates and hence secretion clearance (Gregson *et al.*, 2012). However, it was concerning that the highest inflation volumes and pressures recorded during physiotherapy exceeded those believed to cause lung injury and, furthermore, PEEP was not used during MHI. It is also possible that the chest compression could reduce FRC and cause alveolar derecruitment or atelectasis. There are currently no studies that adequately address the safety and efficacy of MHI in children and it therefore cannot be recommended as a standard treatment modality in ventilated children. Children following TBI are at particular risk of severe neurological sequelae, which could occur from inappropriate chest treatment. Manual hyperinflation should therefore be used with caution during the treatment of children with TBI until adequate data supporting its use are obtained. If it is necessary to use MHI, a pressure manometer must be attached to the MHI circuit to carefully monitor the pressures delivered to the child's airways.

Airway suction may be indicated to assist with clearance of retained secretions for children with TBI who have an ineffective cough effort (Fig. 9.8). Specific precautions and guidelines for paediatric endotracheal

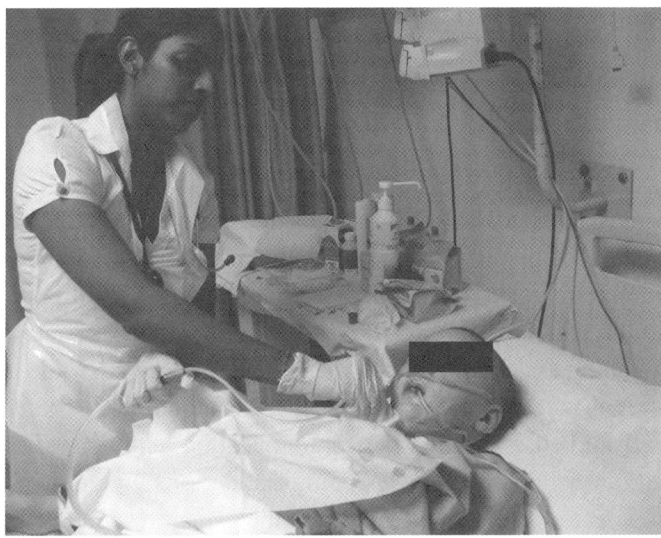

Fig. 9.8: Sterile suctioning of the tracheostomy of a 10-year-old girl with moderate severity TBI.

suctioning are provided in a review and guideline paper (Morrow and Argent, 2008).

As sedation is stopped and consciousness improves, ACBT can be done in older, cooperative children. After extubation, breathing exercises in the awake, cooperative child can be performed using blowing games (e.g. bubbles and windmills).

It is important for the physiotherapist to remember that each adult or paediatric patient responds differently to treatment. Therefore each patient should be closely monitored for signs of adverse effects to treatment interventions used for respiratory system management.

9.8.2. *Neuromusculoskeletal system*

A patient with TBI is at risk of developing various impairments, such as an alteration in the level of consciousness, an alteration in muscle tone, a reduction in static and dynamic balance, an alteration in volitional movement, reduced joint range of motion (ROM), diminished muscle length, muscle weakness and a reduction in exercise tolerance. Physiotherapists should be aware of these complications, and methods to manage these complications are suggested below. These suggestions are based on research evidence, where available, as well as expert opinion in the absence of research evidence.

9.8.2.1. *Patient orientation*

As the patient responds to medical management and sedation is lessened and ultimately stopped, orientation of the patient to their environment becomes important. The physiotherapist can contribute to this process by informing the patient daily regarding the day of the week, date and time prior to initiating treatment. It is also beneficial to speak at an adequate tone of voice to enhance communication over the loud noises in the ICU, such as alarms from bedside monitors. Communication with the patient before and during an activity aids in lessening patient anxiety, as it allows the patient to prepare for the intervention. As the patient responds to treatment and ICP is no longer being monitored, changes in body position including movement out of bed aid in addressing musculoskeletal deconditioning and enhance sensory stimulation and orientation (Jones and Dean, 2004; Gosselink *et al.*, 2008).

9.8.2.2. *Altered muscle tone*

Traumatic brain injury is one of the causes of the development of spasticity, due to anoxic injury to the cerebral cortex, cerebellum and basal ganglia. In the acute phase of TBI, muscle tone may be flaccid with hyporeflexia and may fluctuate dramatically. Spasticity gradually sets in and can be identified through the presence of clonus, hyperreflexia, Babinski sign and flexor spasms (Vanek, 2012). Spasticity increases the patient's risk for developing contractures and physiotherapy intervention is important to prevent contracture formation. Interventions such as muscle stretching and splinting can be used to inhibit muscle spasticity in the acute care setting. Ankle foot orthoses (AFO) are often used in the ICU to position the ankle in a neutral comfortable position and avoid the formation of plantar-flexion contractures. Physiotherapy should be performed together with the use of AFO, as AFO on their own are not effective enough to prevent plantar-flexion contractures (Kobayashi *et al.*, 2011). Hand splints can also be used to maintain functional grip positions.

9.8.2.3. *Joint range of motion*

9.8.2.3.1. Intubated unresponsive patient

Initiating early activity is important in a bedridden patient to lessen deconditioning and maintain joint ROM and muscle length. Physiotherapy movement modalities during early ICU admission should include passive joint ROM (to end-of-range) and muscle stretches (Irdesel *et al.*, 2007). Passive exercises are reported to reduce the likelihood of contractures in the neurosurgical patient (Vanek, 2012). Others noted that passive movements were safe to perform and did not affect ICP significantly (Brimioulle *et al.*, 1997). The recommendations by Brimioulle *et al.* (1997) concerning the notion that passive exercise can be carried out without detriment to the neurosurgical patient can be taken forward with conditions. Experienced clinicians advise that ICP should be stable prior to the initiation of passive exercise. This viewpoint is supported by other researchers, who advise that passive movements should be left until 48–72 hours after injury, as this is the acute phase in which medical management is aimed at stabilising and optimising the patient's condition (Paratz and Burns, 1993). During this time no extreme hip flexion should be performed, as this may cause neural stretch that can impact on ICP. All parameters should be monitored whilst movements are carried out.

9.8.2.3.2. Responsive and cooperative patient

Once sedation is lessened, ICP no longer monitored and the patient starts to interact, active-assisted and active ROM exercises should be encouraged.

9.8.2.4. *Muscle strength*

A patient with TBI and spasticity may have underlying muscle weakness. Muscle-strengthening exercises should therefore be incorporated into the patient's acute care management as soon as the patient is awake and responsive enough to perform such exercises (Vanek, 2012). The patient can be shown exercises whereby body weight is initially utilised for resistance training. The progression of strengthening exercises should include the use of resistance bands or ankle or wrist weights. The number of repetitions per exercise, as well as the frequency of exercise, should gradually be increased according to each patient's ability.

9.8.2.5. *Functional ability, mobilisation and exercise endurance*

Once sedation is reduced or stopped, an increased dependence with bed mobility, transfers in and out of bed or in and out of a chair and early ambulation may be found. At this stage, more movement pattern abnormalities might be identified, e.g. a patient with a subarachnoid haemorrhage may present with a hemiplegic movement pattern.

Active movement aids in the prevention of pressure sores, normalising patterns of movement, decreasing or increasing muscle tone and improving sitting and standing balance. Once sedation is lessened, active participation of the patient in bed mobility activities and transfers should be encouraged, as this may be a stimulus to increase their awareness. Functional activities such as rolling in bed, bridging, sitting up over the side of the bed, standing upright and performing stepping transfers from bed to chair should all form part of a physiotherapy rehabilitation programme. These activities can commence when the patient's condition has stabilised, even while they are still intubated and ventilated. The patient may initially require assistance from one or two physiotherapists to safely perform these activities, but as the patient's condition improves, the aim is to assist them to become more independent (Fig. 9.9).

Graded mobilisation should also be encouraged (Hellweg and Johannes, 2008). Early ICU mobility frameworks are available for guidance when early rehabilitation is implemented, such as the 'start to move' protocol (Gosselink *et al.*, 2011) and the four phases programme (Perme and Chandrashekar, 2009). Various ICU physiotherapy algorithms are available for reviewing specific safety issues that should be considered when the physiotherapist starts implementing active mobility programmes in the ICU (Stiller and Phillips, 2003; Korupolu *et al.*, 2009; Hanekom *et al.*, 2011).

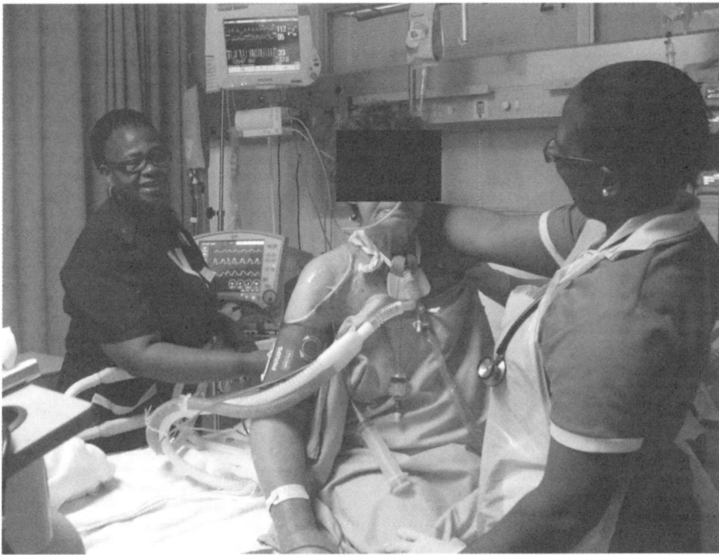

Fig. 9.9: A patient with TBI sitting up over the edge of the bed in the ICU with assistance from a physiotherapist.

These should be taken into consideration when mobilising patients with TBI. Functional activities such as sit-to-stand from the edge of the bed or from a chair can be used as a strengthening exercise in the acute care setting, and will have a beneficial effect on the patient's cardiovascular endurance. As the patient's ability to cooperate in functional activities improves, the frequency and duration of treatment sessions per day should be increased. This will assist with further improving the patient's exercise tolerance.

9.8.2.6. *Paediatric considerations*

In the acute care setting, similar rehabilitation approaches to alter muscle tone, improve muscle strength and increase participation in functional abilities and mobilisation may be used as suggested for adults (Figs 9.10 and 9.11).

Traumatic brain injury may lead to neurodevelopmental regression in young children and infants, especially if the lesion is subcortical (Bonnier *et al.*, 2007). The physiotherapist should, therefore, be able to incorporate the principles of neurodevelopmental therapy in relation to motor function into the acute care rehabilitation of such children.

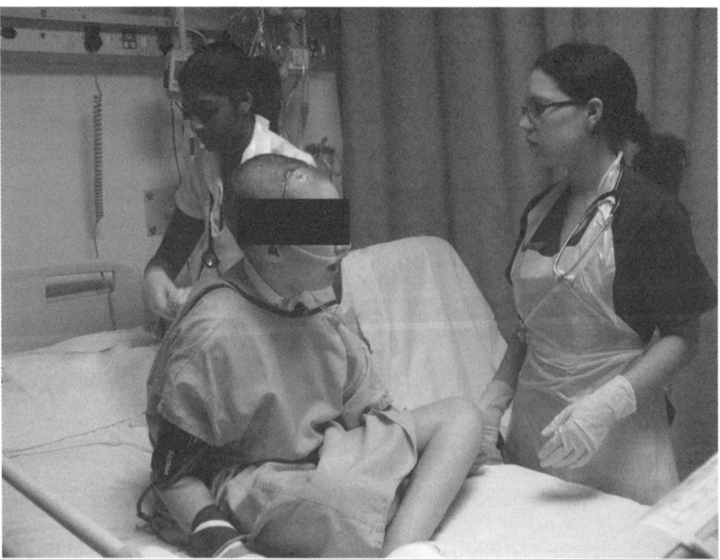

Fig. 9.10: A paediatric patient with TBI sitting up in bed prior to mobilisation out of bed.

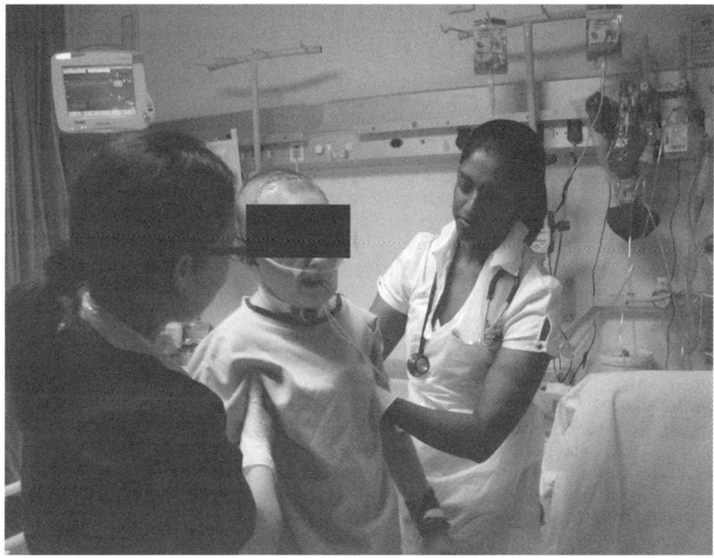

Fig. 9.11: A paediatric patient with TBI transferring out of bed to a chair for the first time with assistance from two physiotherapists.

In the critical care setting there have been clinical reports of some TBI paediatric patients who developed myositis ossificans, especially of the bicep muscle. The exact cause for its development is mostly unknown. The physiotherapist who works in the paediatric ICU should therefore be aware of this phenomenon and be gentle when performing passive ROM in children with TBI.

9.8.3. *Patient response to treatment*

During rehabilitation of adult and paediatric patients with TBI in the acute care setting, it is important for the physiotherapist to remember that patients respond differently to treatment. Therefore each patient should be closely monitored for signs of adverse effects to treatment interventions used, and the physiotherapist should be able to alter interventions as necessary. Resources related to the rehabilitation of patients with TBI in the sub-acute and chronic stages after injury are listed in Section 9.10.

Outcome measures that would be appropriate for use in a patient with TBI should include instruments that can evaluate the progress in such a patient from the very acute to the early rehabilitation phase. The reader is referred to Chapter 4 (Section 4.3) for a list of subjective and objective markers, as well as outcome measurement tools to use for the evaluation of the effectiveness of treatment interventions used during the management of patients with TBI.

9.9. Clinical Case Scenarios

9.9.1. *Adult case scenario*

A 28-year-old man was admitted to a level one trauma ICU two days ago following a MVA. He sustained the following injuries: right subarachnoid haemorrhage, right temporal skull fracture, right clavicle fracture, posterior fractures of ribs four to seven on the right chest wall and haemopneumothorax. His GCS on scene was 5/15. The medical team at the hospital suspects that aspiration pneumonia occurred at the time of injury due to features of consolidation in the right middle lobe on chest x-ray after hospital admission. Medical management included the immediate insertion of two intercostal drains (ICD) into the right chest wall to address the haemopneumothorax. In an attempt to control the ICP, the patient was intubated and placed on MV (settings: fraction of inspired oxygen (FiO_2) 0.6, PEEP five cmH_2O, pressure support 10 cmH_2O, peak inspiratory pressure (PIP) 15 cmH_2O, expiratory tidal volume 450 ml and ventilator rate 16 breaths per minute). An ICP monitoring device was inserted into the patient's skull. Sedative drugs, namely Dormicum and Morphine, were prescribed, as well as other medication, including an osmotic diuretic, anticonvulsant and paralysing agent, to administer when the patient is handled during physiotherapy or nursing care activities.

On day one after admission, you note that the patient is receiving a blood transfusion and ICP is 15 mmHg with GCS of 2/10. The latest recorded vital signs show heart rate (HR) of 110 beats per minute (sinus rhythm), BP of 110/65 mmHg (MAP of 80 mmHg), peripheral oxygen saturation (SpO_2) of 94% and body temperature of 38°C. Arterial blood gas results on FiO_2 of 0.6 are pH 7.34, PaO_2 85 mmHg (11.3 kPa), $PaCO_2$ 46 mmHg (6.1 kPa), HCO_3 24 mmol/l and base excess −1.5. On auscultation you find coarse crackles in the right middle lobe, with significantly reduced air entry in the right lower lobes. The patient is a known smoker and has been smoking approximately 20 cigarettes per day for 10 years.

- Calculate the patient's cerebral perfusion pressure.
- Identify the physiotherapy impairments (problems) that the patient is at risk of developing.
- Would you treat this patient today?
- What precautions would you implement if you decide to treat this patient?

9.9.1.1. *Discussion*

9.9.1.1.1. Cerebral perfusion pressure

The correct equation to use for this calculation is CPP = MAP — ICP. Thus, CPP is 65 mmHg and slightly less than the ideal (CPP greater than 70 mmHg). Satisfactory cerebral oxygenation can, however, still be provided with CPP of 65 mmHg.

9.9.1.1.2. Physiotherapy-related impairments

This patient presents with impairments such as retention of secretions in the right middle lobe, as supported by auscultation and chest x-ray (CXR) findings, reduced lung volumes, as supported by decreased breath sounds in the right lower lobes, and decreased oxygenation capacity. Oxygenation capacity is affected by the reduced SpO_2, PaO_2, oxygen content (dissolved oxygen + oxygen bound to Hb) and PaO_2/FiO_2 ratio (see Appendix II); all of which will directly influence this patient's overall prognosis.

9.9.1.1.3. Physiotherapy intervention

Yes, it would be appropriate to treat this patient. No contraindications to treatment are currently present, as ICP and CPP values are not critical. The clearance of the retained secretions in the right middle lobe should assist with improving lung ventilation and breath sounds in the right middle and lower lobes, thereby contributing to an improvement in oxygenation capacity. Physiotherapy treatment may therefore contribute to reducing secondary brain damage.

9.9.1.1.4. Precautions to physiotherapy intervention

- Infection control precautions must be adhered to, such as wearing a clean apron, gloves and eye protection.
- Increase the QRS complex volume on the bedside monitor to be aware of changes in the patient's cardiovascular status during treatment.
- No manual vibrations or shaking should be performed on the right side of the chest wall. These techniques compress the chest wall and the patient has multiple rib fractures on this side, which may lacerate the underlying pulmonary structures.
- Control right upper limb movements and try to maintain a 'sling position' as this patient has a right clavicle fracture.
- No head-down tilt position beyond the supine position as ICP is high.
- Maintain the patient's head in a neutral position (no side flexion or rotation) to ensure optimal cerebral venous drainage to lessen the effect on changes in ICP. Ensure the head is fully supported and kept in midline when the patient's position in bed is changed.
- Ask that the prescribed paralysing agent be administered prior to treatment if the patient has had problems with ICP during handling. An added bolus of sedation could be administered during the suction procedure to lessen the effects of coughing on changes in ICP.
- Precautions related to the ICD systems should be maintained during treatment (Chapter 5, Section 5.5.3).
- Preoxygenate the patient a few minutes prior to as well as during the suction procedure to minimise episodes of hypoxaemia.
- Monitor the patient's vital signs and ICP values during the treatment session and evaluate the patient's reaction to treatment.
- If the patient presents with seizures, physiotherapy treatment should be stopped and assistance sought from the medical and nursing personnel.
- Pay attention not to dislodge any lines or tubes connected to the patient during the treatment session.

9.9.2. *Paediatric case scenario*

A six-month-old baby girl presented to the trauma unit with an acute closed head injury two days ago. Following resuscitation she was admitted to the paediatric ICU. The initial history was of a fall from the changing table but after careful examination and social worker consultation, it emerged that the baby had been shaken by the mother in the early hours of the morning. As a result she sustained a subdural haemorrhage with retinal haemorrhages. There are no associated injuries on the CT scan. She has had a decompressive craniectomy and has an ICP monitor *in situ*. Currently ICP is 20 mmHg but the ICU nursing sister reports that this increases to over 40 mmHg when she is suctioned. She is generally hypotonic but has brisk lower limb reflexes.

She was intubated (size 3.5 ETT) and ventilated on synchronised intermittent mandatory ventilation with respiratory rate of 30 breaths per minute, FiO_2 0.6, PIP of 20 cmH_2O and PEEP of five cmH_2O. She is only making minimal spontaneous respiratory efforts herself and her GCS is 5/10. She does have a cough reflex. She is positioned in supine with the bed raised to 30° head-up tilt position. On assessment her vital signs are body temperature 38.2°C, HR 150 beats per minute, SpO_2 90% and BP 100/60 mmHg (MAP 73 mmHg). Arterial blood gas results on FiO_2 0.6 reveal PaO_2 of 57 mmHg (7.65 kPa), $PaCO_2$ 93.8 mmHg (12.5 kPa) and pH of 7.34. Today her septic markers are raised and her secretions have changed from small quantities of loose, clear secretions to moderate amounts of thick, yellowish secretions. On chest x-ray there is right upper lobe collapse and consolidation with scattered patchy opacifications throughout the rest of the lung fields. On auscultation there are reduced breath sounds over the right upper zone and scattered coarse crackles throughout the rest of the lung fields.

- Tabulate the risks and potential benefits of treatment as the baby presents now in order to determine whether treatment would be appropriate.
- If you consider treatment to be appropriate, what modalities would you use and why?

9.9.2.1. Discussion

9.9.2.1.1. Risks and benefits of treatment

9.9.2.1.2. Treatment modalities

Initially, the patient should be treated in supine with the head kept in midline and the bed raised to 30° in order to determine her response to handling.

Table 9.11: Risks and benefits of treatment.

Risks	Benefits
Risk of further raising the ICP, potentially leading to brain herniation and further secondary damage.	$PaCO_2$ is high and PaO_2 is low and could aggravate the ICP. By clearing obstructive secretions and reinflating collapsed lung segments, these values could improve, which could lead to improved ICP as well as work of breathing. Once oxygenation improves, the FiO_2 could also be turned down, which would prevent hyperoxia-associated injury.
Currently febrile, with increased metabolic requirements.	A tracheal aspirate could be sent to identify the organism responsible for the respiratory infection. Appropriate directed antibiotic therapy could then address this issue. Treatments could be short in order to avoid further increasing oxygen consumption.
SpO_2 is low, potential for exacerbating hypoxia, which could contribute to further increases in ICP.	From the first point above, appropriate treatment could improve oxygenation, which should reduce ICP. Short-term desaturation could be avoided by adequate analgesia, sedation and brief periods of preoxygenation.
Potential to cause further brain injury by shaking of the head during chest manipulations.	This is preventable by choice of therapy and head stabilisation throughout.

Decision: potential benefits outweigh risks of treatment.

Vital signs (HR, BP, SpO_2), ICP and CPP should be monitored at all times. Discussion with the nursing and medical staff is essential to determine whether the child is sufficiently sedated and if pain is well-controlled with analgesia.

Gentle vibrations would be the optimal treatment, over all lung zones, concentrating on the atelectatic region (right upper zone). After vibrating and suctioning in supine, the child should be reassessed. If the air entry has improved on the right and there are no crackles, then treatment should be discontinued at this stage and the FiO_2 turned back to pre-treatment levels.

If there is not adequate improvement, and the child has tolerated treatment up until that point, then careful turning onto the side (with the head stabilised in the midline) is warranted. First turn the child onto the left side in order to loosen obstructive secretions on the right, suction and then reassess before carefully turning her onto the right side. After allowing her to rest, repeat the same treatment. After the acute phase of the patient's injury had lapsed (first 72 hours), passive movements may be applied to all limbs. Care should be taken not to overstretch, especially at the shoulder. This could be done during a separate session from the chest treatment if ICP is labile.

9.10. Suggested Reading Material for Further Study

Discharge planning after TBI (Wagner *et al.*, 2003); rehabilitation of a patient with TBI after discharge from an acute care facility (British Society of Rehabilitation Medicine, 2002, 2009; New Zealand Guidelines Group, 2006).

9.11. Conclusion

Physiotherapists may find the management of patients with TBI in the acute care setting daunting. This is due to the patient's relative instability during the first 72 hours after the primary injury and the increased risk of them developing secondary brain injury, which would negatively impact on their outcome. The information shared in this chapter should assist the physiotherapist to make an informed decision as to whether physiotherapy intervention is warranted during the first 72 hours of a particular patient's stay in the ICU. It should also assist the physiotherapist to provide effective and safe care for patients with TBI during the early acute phase of injury until they are transferred to a rehabilitation setting for further management during the sub-acute and chronic phases of recovery.

Bibliography

Alterman, D.M., and Geibel, J. (2011). *Considerations in Pediatric Trauma.* Medscape. [Online] Available at: http://emedicine.medscape.com/article/435031-overview [Accessed May 2014].

Arabi, Y.M., Haddad, S., Tamim, H.M., *et al.* (2010). Mortality reduction after implementing a clinical practice guidelines-based management protocol for severe traumatic brain injury, *J. Crit. Care,* **25**, 190–195.

Bonnier, C., Marique, P., Van Hout, A., *et al.* (2007). Neurodevelopmental outcome after severe traumatic brain injury in very young children: role of subcortical lesions, *J. Child Neurol.,* **22**, 519–529.

Brimioulle, S., Moraine, J.J., Norrenberg, D., *et al.* (1997). Effects of positioning and exercise on intracranial pressure in a neurosurgical intensive care unit, *Phys. Ther.,* **77**, 1682–1689.

British Society of Rehabilitation Medicine. (2002). *Standards for Specialist In-Patient and Community Rehabilitation Services.* BSRM. [Online] Available at: http://www.bsrm.co.uk/publications/BSRMStandardsforRMServices2002.pdf [Accessed September 2013].

British Society of Rehabilitation Medicine. (2009). *BSRM Standards for Rehabilitation Services.* BSRM. [Online] Available at: http://www.bsrm.co.uk/publications/StandardsMapping-Final.pdf

Brown, C.V., Zada, G., Salim, A., *et al.* (2007). Indications for routine repeat head computed tomography (CT) stratified by severity of traumatic brain injury, *J. Trauma,* **62**, 1339–1344.

Bugge, J.F. (2009). Brain death and its implications for management of the potential organ donor, *Acta Anaesthesiol. Scand.,* **53**, 1239–1250.

Bullock, M.R., and Povlishock, J.T. (2007). Guidelines for the management of severe traumatic brain injury 3rd edition, *J. Neurotrauma,* **24** [Suppl], S1–S106.

Bullock, M.R., Chesnut, R., Ghajar, J., *et al.* (2006). Surgical management of TBI, *Neurosurg.,* **58**, S2-1-S2-111.

Centers for Disease Control (CDC). (2011). *Injury Prevention and Control: Traumatic Brain Injury.* CDC. [Online] Available at: www.cdc.gov/traumaticbraininjury [Accessed July 2014].

Chambers, I.R., Jones, P.A., Lo, T.Y.M., *et al.* (2006). Critical thresholds of intracranial pressure and cerebral perfusion pressure related to age in paediatric head injury, *J. Neurol. Neurosurg. Psychiatry,* **77**, 234–240.

Chang, A., Paratz, J., and Rollston, J. (2002). Ventilatory effects of neurophysiological facilitation and passive movement in patients with neurological injury, *Aust. J. Physiother.,* **48**, 305–309.

Choi, J.S.P., and Jones, A.Y.M. (2005). Effects of manual hyperinflation and suctioning on respiratory mechanics in mechanically ventilated patients with ventilator-associated pneumonia, *Aust. J. Physiother.,* **51**, 25–30.

Cifu, D.X., Cohen, S.I., Lew, H.L., *et al.* (2010). The history and evolution of traumatic brain injury rehabilitation in military service members and veterans, *Am. J. Med. Rehabil.,* **89**, 688–694.

Coles, J.P. (2007). Imaging after brain injury, *Br. J. Anaesth.,* **99**, 49–60.

Cote, N., Turgeon, A.F., Lauzier, F., *et al.* (2013). Factors associated with the withdrawal of life-sustaining therapies in patients with severe traumatic brain injury: a multicentre cohort study, *Neurocrit. Care,* **18**, 154–160.

Davison, D.L., Terek, M., and Chawla, L.S. (2012). Neurogenic pulmonary edema, *Crit. Care,* **16**, 1–7.

De Deyne, C.S. (2010). Therapeutic hypothermia and traumatic brain injury, *Curr. Opin. Anaesthesiol.,* **23**, 258–262.

Dennis, D., Jacobs, W., and Budgeon, C. (2012). Ventilator versus manual hyperinflation in clearing sputum in ventilated intensive care unit patients, *Anaesth. Intensive Care,* **40**, 142–149.

Duhaime, A.C., Christian, C.W., Rorke, L.B., *et al.* (1998). Non-accidental head injury in infants — the 'shaken-baby syndrome', *N. Engl. J. Med.,* **338**, 1822–1829.

Dunn, L.T. (2002). Raised intracranial pressure, *J. Neurol. Neurosurg. Psychiatry,* **73**, i23–i27.

Dykes, E.H. (1999). Paediatric trauma, *Br. J. Anaesth.,* **83**, 130–138.

Fakhry, S.M., Trask, A.L., Waller, A.L., *et al.* (2004). Management of brain-injured patients by an evidence-based medicine protocol improves outcomes and decreases hospital charges, *J. Trauma,* **56**, 492–500.

Gosselink, R., Bott, J., Johnson, M., *et al.* (2008). Physiotherapy for adult patients with critical illness: recommendations of the European Respiratory Society and European Society of Intensive Care Medicine Task Force on Physiotherapy for Critically Ill Patients, *Intensive Care Med.,* **34**, 1188–1199.

Gosselink, R., Clerckx, B., Robbeets, C., *et al.* (2011). Physiotherapy in the intensive care unit, *Neth. J. Crit. Care,* **5**, 66–75.

Gregson, R.K., Shannon, H., Stocks, J., *et al.* (2012). The unique contribution of manual chest compression-vibrations to airflow during physiotherapy in sedated, fully ventilated children, *Pediatr. Crit. Care Med.,* **13**, e97–e102.

Guha, A. (2004). Management of traumatic brain injury: some current evidence and applications, *Postgrad. Med. J.,* **80**, 650–653.

Haddad, S.H., and Arabi, Y.M. (2012). Critical care management of severe traumatic brain injury in adults, *Scand. J. Trauma Resus. Emerg. Med.,* **20**, 12. [Online] Available at: http://www.sjtrem.com/content/20/1/12 [Accessed July 2014].

Hanekom, S., Dean, E., Ambrosino, N., *et al.* (2011). The development of a clinical management algorithm for early physical activity and mobilization of critically ill patients: synthesis of evidence and expert opinion and its translation into practice, *Clin. Rehabil.,* **25**, 771–787.

Harding, J.E., Miles, F.K.I., Becroft, D.M.O., *et al.* (1998). Chest physiotherapy may be associated with brain damage in extremely premature infants, *J. Pediatr.,* **132**, 440–444.

Hellweg, S., and Johannes, S. (2008). Physiotherapy after traumatic brain injury: systematic review of the literature, *Brain Injury,* **22**, 365–373.

Herman, B.E., Makoroff, K.L., and Corneli, H.M. (2011). Abusive head trauma, *Pediatr. Emerg. Care,* **27**, 65–69.

Hess, D.R. (2002). Secretion clearance techniques: absence of proof or proof of absence? *Respir. Care,* **47**, 757–758.

Hutchinson, P.J., Kolias, A.G., Timofeev, I., *et al.* (2011). Update on the RESCUEicp decompressive craniectomy trial, *Crit. Care,* **15**, P312.

Irdesel, J., Aydiner, S.B., and Akgoz, S. (2007). Rehabilitation outcome after traumatic brain injury, *Neurocirugia,* **18**, 5–15.

John, S.M., Kelly, P., and Vincent, A. (2013). Patterns of structural head injury in children younger than 3 years: a ten-year review of 519 patients, *J. Trauma Acute Care Surg.,* **74**, 276–281.

Jones, A.Y.M., and Dean, E. (2004). Body position change and its effect on hemodynamic and metabolic status, *Heart Lung,* **33**, 281–901.

Kobayashi, T., Leung, A.K.L., and Hutchins, S.W. (2011). Design and effect of ankle-foot orthoses proposed to influence muscle tone: a review, *J. Prosthet. Orthot.,* **23**, 52–57.

Kochanek, P.M., Carney, N., Adelson, P.D., *et al.* (2012). Guidelines for the acute medical management of severe traumatic brain injury in infants, children and adolescents — 2nd edition, *Paediatr. Crit. Care Med.,* **13** [Suppl], S1–S82.

Korupolu, R., Gifford, J.M., and Needham, D.M. (2009). Early mobilization of critically ill patients: reducing neuromuscular complications after intensive care, *Contemp. Crit. Care,* **6**, 1–12.

Levin, A.V. (2010). Retinal hemorrhage in abusive head trauma, *Pediatrics,* **126**, 961–970.

Lombard, L.A., and Zafonte, R. (2005). Agitation after traumatic brain injury, *Am. J. Phys. Med. Rehabil.,* **84**, 797–812.

Marik, P.E., Varon, J., and Trask, T. (2002). Management of head trauma, *Chest,* **122**, 699–711.

Matis, G., and Birbilis, T. (2008). The Glasgow coma scale: a brief review past, present and future, *Acta Neurol. Belg.,* **108**, 75–89.

Mauritz, W., Janciak, I., Wilbacher, I., *et al.* (2007). Severe traumatic brain injury in Austria IV: intensive care management, *Wien. Klin. Wochenschr.,* **119**, 46–55.

Mejaddam, A.Y., and Velmahos, G.C. (2012). Randomised controlled trials affecting polytrauma care, *Eur. J. Trauma Emerg. Surg.,* **38**, 211–221.

Meyer, M.J., Megyesi, J., Meythaler, J., *et al.* (2010). Acute management of acquired brain injury part 1: and evidence-based review of non-pharmacological interventions, *Brain Injury,* **24**, 694–705.

Mokri, B. (2001). The Monro-Kellie hypothesis: applications in CSF volume depletion, *Neurology,* **56**, 1746–1748.

Moore, T. (2003). Suctioning techniques for the removal of respiratory secretions, *Nurs. Stand.,* **18**, 47–53.

Morrow, B., and Argent, A. (2008). A comprehensive review of pediatric endotracheal suctioning: effects, indications and clinical practice, *Pediatr. Crit. Care Med.,* **9**, 465–477.

Morton, P.G., Fontaine, D.K., Hudak, C.M., *et al.* (2005). *Critical Care Nursing: A Holistic Approach*, 8th edn., Lippincott, Williams and Wilkins, Philadelphia, PA.

Nell, V., Yates, D.W., and Kruger, J. (2000). An extended Glasgow coma scale (GCS-E) with enhanced sensitivity to mild brain injury, *Arch. Phys. Med. Rehabil.,* **81**, 614–617.

New Zealand Guidelines Group. (2006). *Traumatic Brain Injury: Diagnosis, Acute Management and Rehabilitation. Evidence-based Best Practice Guideline*. Ministry of Health. [Online] Available at: http://www.health.govt.nz/publication/traumatic-brain-injury-diagnosis-acute-management-and-rehabilitation [Accessed September 2013].

Palmer, R., and Knight, J. (2006). Assessment of altered conscious level in clinical practice, *Br. J. Nurs.,* **15**, 1255–1259.

Paratz, J., and Burns, Y. (1993). The effect of respiratory physiotherapy on intracranial pressure, mean arterial pressure, cerebral perfusion pressure and end tidal carbon dioxide in ventilated neurosurgical patients, *Physiother. Theory Pract.,* **9**, 3–11.

Patman, S., Jenkins, S., and Stiller, K. (2009). Physiotherapy does not prevent, or hasten recovery from ventilator-associated pneumonia in patients with acquired brain injury, *Intensive Care Med.,* **35**, 258–265.

Paz, J.C., and West, M.P. (2009). *Acute Care Handbook for Physical Therapists*, 3rd edn., Saunders Elsevier, St. Louis, MO.

Perme, C., and Chandrasekar, R. (2009). Early mobility and walking program for patients in intensive care units: creating a standard of care, *Am. J. Crit. Care,* **18**, 212–221.

Peterson, K., Carson, S., and Carney, N. (2008). Hypothermia treatment for traumatic brain injury: a systematic review and meta-analysis, *J. Neurotrauma,* **25**, 62–71.

Protheroe, R.T., and Gwinnutt, C.L. (2011). Early hospital care of severe traumatic brain injury, *Anaesthesia,* **66**, 1035–1047.

Roberts I, and Sydenham, E. (2009). Barbiturates for acute traumatic brain injury, *Cochrane Database of Systematic Reviews,* **3**, CD000033.

Rosenfeld, J.V., Maas, A.I., Bragge, P., *et al.* (2012). Early management of severe traumatic brain injury, *Lancet,* **380**, 1088–1098.

Shirley, P. (2009). Operational critical care: intensive care and trauma, *J. Army Med. Corps,* **155**, 122–174.

Stiller, K., and Phillips, A. (2003). Safety aspects of mobilizing acutely ill patients, *Physiother. Theory Pract.,* **19**, 239–257.

Stein, S.C., Georgoff, P., Meghan, S., *et al.* (2010). Relationship of aggressive monitoring and treatment to improved outcomes in severe traumatic brain injury, *J. Neurosurg.,* **112**, 1105–1112.

Thiesen, R.A., Dragosavac, D., Roquejani, A.C., *et al.* (2005). Influence of respiratory physiotherapy on intracranial pressure in severe head trauma patients, *Arq. Neuropsiquiatr.,* **63**, 110–113.

Thim, T., Krarup, N.H.V., Grove, E.L., *et al.* (2012). Initial assessment and treatment with the airway, breathing, circulation, disability, exposure (ABCDE) approach, *Int. J. Gen. Med.,* **5**, 117–121.

Timmons, S.D. (2012). An update on traumatic brain injuries, *J. Neurosurg. Sci.,* **56**, 191–202.

Toledo, C., Garrico, C., Troncoso, E., *et al.* (2008). Effects of respiratory physiotherapy on intracranial pressure and cerebral perfusion pressure in severe traumatic brain injury patients, *Rev. Bras. Ter. Intensiva,* **20**, 339–343.

Vanek, Z.F. (2012). *Spasticity*. Medscape. [Online] Available at: http://emedicine.medscape.com/article/2207448-overview [Accessed July 2014].

Wagner, A.K., Fabio, T., Roos, D., *et al.* (2003). Physical medicine and rehabilitation consultation: relationships with acute functional outcome, length of stay, and discharge planning after traumatic brain injury, *Am. J. Phys. Med. Rehabil.,* **82**, 526–536.

Wakai, A., Roberts, I.G., and Schierhout, G. (2007). Mannitol for acute traumatic brain injury, *Cochrane Database Syst. Rev.,* **1**, CD001049.

Warnick, R. (2013). *Craniotomy*. Mayfield Clinic. [Online] Available at: http://www.mayfieldclinic.com/PE-Craniotomy.htm [Accessed July 2013].

Weiner, H.L., and Weinberg, J.S. (2000). 'Head injury in the pediatric age group', in Cooper, P.R., and Golfinos, J.G. (eds), *Head Injury*, 4th edn., McGraw-Hill, New York, NY, pp. 419–456.

Werner, C., and Engelhard, K. (2007). Pathophysiology of traumatic brain injury, *Br. J. Anaesth.,* **99**, 4–9.

Wijdicks, E.F.M., Varelas, P.N., Gronseth, G.S., *et al.* (2010). Evidence-based guideline update: determining brain death in adults, *Neurology,* **74**, 1911–1918.

Chapter 10

Quality of Life of Survivors of Trauma

Written by H. van Aswegen

Over the last two decades many more people have survived an episode of critical illness and injury than before, due to the major advances made in the quality of care provided to them in the intensive care unit (ICU). Traditionally the success of ICU management was measured in relation to the patient's survival from critical illness, but the quality of their lives after discharge from the ICU and from hospital was largely overlooked. A number of years ago, the 2002 Brussels Roundtable discussions among intensive care practitioners concluded that survivors of critical illness suffered from poor functional capability, decreased quality of life (QOL) and few returned to work. Subsequently, they placed an increased burden and considerable stress on families and informal caregivers, resulting in increased economic costs for the patient, their families and society (Angus and Carlet, 2003). Therefore, the importance of health-related QOL after an episode of critical illness has become the focus of many investigations over the past few years.

In this chapter information is shared on:

- The definition of quality of life.
- The assessment of quality of life.
- The quality of life of survivors of critical illness.
- The quality of life of survivors of trauma and critical illness.
- Rehabilitation for survivors of critical illness.
- The suggestions for exercise rehabilitation for survivors of trauma and critical illness.
- The potential challenges to exercise rehabilitation of survivors of trauma.

10.1. Definition of Quality of Life

There is no universally accepted definition of QOL. Socrates stated in an Athenian court that he feared some things more than death, and that it was not merely life itself but the QOL that counted most (Eales *et al.*, 2004). The World Health Organisation (WHO) described QOL as 'an individual's perception of their position in life in the context of the culture and value systems in which they live and in relation to their goals, expectations, standards and concerns' (WHO QOL Group, 1995). The WHO went further and described health-related QOL to be 'a state of complete physical, mental and social well-being and not merely the absence of disease or infirmity' (WHO QOL Group, 1997).

10.2. Assessment of Quality of Life

Research conducted into the health-related QOL of ICU survivors provides information on these survivors' recovery from illness and often highlights the need for the development of rehabilitation services to enhance recovery (Van Aswegen *et al.*, 2011). The effect of major trauma on QOL in both adults and children has only recently become the focus of research globally; however, the effect of major trauma on children without traumatic brain injury (TBI) is particularly sparse (Janssens *et al.*, 2008). Various measurement tools in the form of questionnaires have been developed and are being used to assess QOL in the critical care population (Tables 10.1 and 10.2).

Table 10.1: Subjective QOL questionnaires used for adults.

- Satisfaction with life scale
- Life satisfaction questionnaire
- World Health Organisation QOL-BREF scale
- Perceived QOL questionnaire
- Global QOL questionnaire

Table 10.2: Objective QOL questionnaires used for adults.

- Medical outcomes study short form 36 (SF-36)
- Medical outcomes study short form 12 (SF-12)
- EuroQol-5D (EQ-5D)
- Quality of well-being
- Sickness impact profile
- Nottingham health profile
- Community integration questionnaire
- World Health Organisation QOL-BREF

Subjective QOL measures allow people to express their own individual point of view regarding their QOL status. These types of outcome measures evaluate feelings of life satisfaction or happiness (Shackman *et al.*, 2005). Examples of subjective QOL measurement tools are listed in Table 10.1.

In contrast, objective QOL measurement tools assess peoples' QOL status based on specific questions about their economic or living circumstances, with less emphasis on the individual's feelings (Table 10.2).

The QOL assessment tools summarised in Tables 10.1 and 10.2 are often referred to as 'generic', as they can be applied to any patient population, regardless of their underlying disease or condition. Only the medical outcomes study short form 36 (SF-36) and the sickness impact profile questionnaires have been extensively validated for use in the general critical care population (Dowdy *et al.*, 2005). The SF-36 has also been validated for use in the trauma population (Sluys *et al.*, 2005; Ardolino *et al.*, 2012).

Examples of disease-specific QOL questionnaires that can be used for patients who have suffered traumatic injury are listed in Table 10.3.

Table 10.3: Disease-specific QOL outcome measures used in adults who suffered trauma.

- Polytrauma outcome (POLO) chart
- QOL index spinal cord injury
- Spinal cord injury-quality of life (SCI-QOL)
- Craig hospital handicap assessment and reporting technique

Table 10.4: QOL outcome measures used in paediatric patients.

- EQ-5DY
- Pediatric QOL inventory (Peds-QL)
- KIDSCREEN-27
- Child health assessment questionnaire
- Child health questionnaire
- Health utilities index — mark 3

Adults and children interpret QOL in a different manner, and therefore paediatric QOL outcome measures were developed a number of years ago. Generic QOL outcome measures recommended in the paediatric population are listed in Table 10.4 (Janssens *et al.*, 2008; Gabbe *et al.*, 2011).

The variety of outcome measures available may seem overwhelming for the physiotherapist; however, the choice of QOL measure used should be determined by the individual patient's condition as well as objectives related to the purpose of use (Wilson *et al.*, 2011).

Researchers who investigate health-related QOL in survivors of trauma often use the SF-36 and EuroQoL-5 dimensions (EQ-5D) questionnaires (Ardolino *et al.*, 2012) in adults and the paediatric QOL inventory (PedsQL) in children, and therefore these questionnaires will briefly be discussed below.

10.2.1. *SF-36 questionnaire*

The SF-36 is suitable for self-administration or administration by a trained interviewer, in person or by telephone, to persons aged 14 years or older. It can be administered in five to 10 minutes, with a high degree of acceptability and data quality (Ware, 1996). The SF-36 uses 36 items to measure eight QOL domains. These domains are physical functioning (PF), role physical (RP) (limitations due to physical problems), bodily pain, general health (GH) perception, vitality (VT), social functioning (SF), role emotional (RE) (limitations due to emotional problems) and mental health (MH). There is a further single item that assesses changes in the respondent's health over the past year. Summary scores for physical and mental health can be calculated from the above domains. Domain and summary scores range from zero to 100. Higher scores reflect a better QOL (Dowdy *et al.*, 2005; Ringdal *et al.*, 2009). An example of the SF-36 questionnaire can be accessed at: www.sf-36.org/demos/SF-36v2.html

A shortened version of the SF-36, namely the SF-12, was developed a few years ago, but has not been used to the same extent as the SF-36 in the critical care or trauma populations.

10.2.2. *EQ-5D questionnaire*

Even though the EQ-5D has not been validated for use in the critical care population, an increasing number of researchers use it for the assessment of health-related QOL of critically ill trauma survivors, due to its simplicity and ease of administration (Granja *et al.*, 2004; Cuthbertson *et al.*, 2010; Orwelius *et al.*, 2010; Pavoni *et al.*, 2010; Ardolino *et al.*, 2012). The EQ-5D comprises five items (mobility, self-care, usual activities, pain or discomfort and anxiety or depression) as well as a visual analogue scale (VAS) for self-rated health status. Each of these items has three alternatives (1 = no problems, 2 = moderate problems, 3 = severe problems) that the subject chooses from when answering each question. The subject's answers are written down to represent a five-digit code which determines the subject's health state (Badia *et al.*, 2001). The VAS is a 20 cm vertical line and is graded from zero (worst possible health state) to 100 (best possible health state). The subject is asked to indicate their own health state on the VAS line (Orwelius *et al.*, 2010; Öster *et al.*, 2011). An example of the EQ-5D can be viewed at: www.biomedcentral.com/content/supplementary/1757-1146-5-17-S1.pdf

10.2.3. *PedsQL questionnaire*

The PedsQL is a widely used valid and reliable tool to determine the QOL of paediatric patients after traumatic injury (Varni *et al.*, 2007; Weedon and Potterton, 2011). The questionnaire is developmentally appropraite as it consists of a child self-report questionnaire as well as a parent-report questionnaire for parents of children who are too young or unable to self-report on QOL. The PedsQL consists of 23 items that collect information on physical and emotional functioning as well as social and school functioning. The emotional functioning, school functioning and social functioning scales contribute towards the psychosocial health summary score, and the physical functioning scale makes up the physical health summary score. Information about the PedsQL can be accessed at: www.pedsql.org/about_pedsql.html

It is important to remember that, whereas a disease often has a finite time of onset and duration, QOL is a lifelong continuous variable, and QOL measurements may be limited by cultural differences, ethnic groups and between groups of different socio-economic status (Schipper *et al.*, 1996).

10.3. Quality of Life of Survivors of Critical Illness

10.3.1. *Physical function-related components of quality of life*

People worldwide who have survived an episode of critical illness, sepsis or multiple organ dysfunction syndrome or even acute respiratory distress syndrome (ARDS) have reported limitations in physical components of health-related QOL in the early months (three to six months) following discharge from hospital (Herridge *et al.*, 2003; Wehler *et al.*, 2003; Granja *et al.*, 2004; Cuthbertson *et al.*, 2005; Hofhuis *et al.*, 2008). A slow improvement in the physical aspects of health-related QOL has been reported during the course of the 12 months following discharge (Herridge *et al.*, 2003; Cuthbertson *et al.*, 2005); however, these limitations may persist for a period of two to five years after hospital discharge (Heyland *et al.*, 2000; Jagodic *et al.*, 2006; Cuthbertson *et al.*, 2010; Herridge *et al.*, 2011).

Physical function-related limitations in health-related QOL do not seem to be the result of long-term pulmonary abnormalities developed from episodes of ARDS or sepsis but are attributed to extrapulmonary complications associated with prolonged immobility and muscle catabolism due to critical illness (Herridge *et al.*, 2011; Hough and Herridge, 2012). Combes *et al.* (2003) reported decreased energy levels and physical mobility and increased frequency in sleep disorders three years after hospital discharge in people who endured prolonged (more than 14 days) mechanical ventilation (MV) in the ICU. When comparing the recovery of physical function-related QOL after critical illness between previously healthy people and those with chronic illness, a difference in outcome is reported. Survivors of multiple organ dysfunction syndrome who had chronic health problems prior to admission into the ICU reported that their QOL related to physical function had returned to pre-admission levels at six months following discharge. Conversely, those survivors who were in good health prior to ICU admission reported a decrease in their health-related QOL at six months (Wehler *et al.*, 2003). This suggests that those with chronic illness already experience a lower level of physical function prior to critical illness and thus have a lower expectation of improvement in physical function-related QOL after critical illness than those who were previously healthy.

Compared with individuals who never suffered critical illness, the physical function-related aspects of QOL for critical care survivors remain below the norms reported in various countries at all time points at which health-related QOL was assessed (Heyland *et al.*, 2000; Dowdy *et al.*, 2005; Hofhuis *et al.*, 2008; Cuthbertson *et al.*, 2010). Critical illness leads to a sharp decline in all aspects of health-related QOL when measured on admission to the ICU; however, there is an improvement in reported health-related QOL that already starts at discharge from the ICU and continues after discharge from the hospital (Hofhuis *et al.*, 2008). Hofhuis *et al.* (2008) emphasised that rehabilitation should start early in the ICU and be continued even after hospital discharge. The long-term negative impact that critical illness has on physical function, as mentioned previously, should be managed along the same lines as other chronic medical conditions; in other words, with rehabilitation that continues long after discharge from the hospital setting.

10.3.2. *Mental health-related components of quality of life*

Limitations in the mental health aspects of health-related QOL after critical illness occur in the first few months after discharge from the ICU but tend to recover to levels comparable with that reported for healthy populations by six months after discharge (Herridge *et al.*, 2003; Cuthbertson *et al.*, 2005, 2010; Hofhuis *et al.*, 2008). Some speculate that the unexpectedly good levels of mental health reported by ICU survivors might be attributed to a mental 'high' as subjects feel that they managed to 'cheat' death (Cuthbertson *et al.*, 2005; Livingston *et al.*, 2009). Other authors, however, have reported that mental health aspects of health-related QOL for their patients had remained low when compared to general population norms even up to 16 months after discharge (Heyland *et al.*, 2000; Dowdy *et al.*, 2005). Factors such as an inability to work after critical illness, posttraumatic stress disorder (PTSD), cognitive dysfunction and depression can contribute to a decreased level of mental health-related QOL (Wunsch and Angus, 2010).

10.3.3. *Posttraumatic stress disorder in survivors of critical illness*

Traumatic events or injury may give rise to the development of emotional illnesses such as PTSD. People who suffer from this disorder re-experience the traumatic event or injury, tend to avoid people or things that remind them of the event and are very sensitive to normal life experiences. These people suffer from avoidance and hyperarousal behavioural patterns. The prevalence of PTSD in the general ICU population has always been thought to be low, but recently new evidence has come to light that PTSD prevalence could be as high as 19–22% and that symptoms persist over time (Davydow *et al.*, 2008). Risk factors for the development of PTSD after critical illness include pre-ICU psychopathology, high dosages of benzodiazepine sedative medication and post-ICU memories of in-ICU frightening or psychotic experiences (Davydow *et al.*, 2008; Hough and Herridge, 2012). Other general risk factors for the development of PTSD in survivors of critical illness include female gender and younger age (Davydow *et al.*, 2008; Hough and Herridge, 2012).

People with a history of depression or anxiety may be prone to in-ICU delirium and psychotic experiences and may be at risk of developing PTSD post-ICU. There seems to be no association between the severity of illness on admission to the ICU and the development of PTSD post-ICU. Survivors of critical illness who develop PTSD may experience substantial limitations to their health-related QOL (Davydow *et al.*, 2008). Physiotherapists are often engaged in longer contact time with patients than the medical personnel due to the nature of their profession; therefore, if a physiotherapist suspects that a patient might be suffering from PTSD, after critical illness and discharge from the ICU, the therapist should discuss this matter with the other interdisciplinary team members and decide the appropriateness of referral of the patient for psychological evaluation and treatment.

10.4. Quality of Life of Survivors of Trauma and Critical Illness

10.4.1. *Physical function-related components of quality of life*

As discussed in Chapter 1, trauma is the leading cause of death or disability in people under the age of 45 years (Holbrook *et al.*, 2001; Sluys *et al.*, 2005). It has been reported that people with trauma, due to their relatively young age, have longer survival after discharge from the ICU than people with other types of admission diagnoses (Fu *et al.*, 2011). The limitations in health-related QOL reported by trauma survivors are not dissimilar to that reported by survivors of critical illness, as discussed in Section 10.3. The decrease in physical aspects of health-related QOL in the trauma population is similarly ascribed to musculoskeletal problems such as those experienced by the non-injured critically ill patient, and also to pain secondary to the traumatic injury. Some researchers report that health-related QOL related to physical function recovers to levels similar to those of the general population by two years following discharge from hospital (Orwelius *et al.*, 2010, 2012), whereas others report that it remains low in comparison with population norms even at five years after discharge (Sluys *et al.*, 2005; Öster *et al.*, 2011).

Limitations that various groups of trauma survivors experience in the short and long term after discharge from the acute care setting in relation to physical function-related QOL are discussed below.

10.4.1.1. *Survivors of blunt or penetrating trauma*

Recurrent trauma related to firearm injuries is often attributed to pre-injury problems such as alcohol abuse and violent behaviour, as mentioned in Chapter 5. Penetrating trunk trauma as a result of stab or gunshot wounds, especially to the chest or trunk, frequently necessitates admission of the patient into the ICU for monitoring following surgery for the repair of damage to the internal organs. Those who survive these types of injuries and spend less than five days on MV in ICU report that their health-related QOL after discharge returns to pre-morbid levels by six months. These subjects also have a health-related QOL comparable to that of a healthy age- and sex-matched group by six months after discharge (Van Aswegen *et al.*, 2011). Those who received MV for longer than five days in the ICU, however, presented with reduced health-related QOL related to physical function at six months following discharge compared to their pre-morbid status, the healthy group and those who had a short period of MV (Van Aswegen *et al.*, 2011). The reduction in physical aspects of health-related QOL experienced by this group of survivors might be explained by persistent muscle weakness after discharge due to prolonged immobilisation in the ICU and prolonged exposure to pro-inflammatory cytokine imbalance as a result of sepsis, which likely resulted in muscle catabolism (refer to the discussion on inflammatory cytokines in Chapter 1). Survivors of penetrating trunk trauma who received prolonged MV were reported to suffer from muscle weakness and limitations in exercise capacity up to six months after discharge from the hospital (Van Aswegen *et al.*, 2010).

Two years following discharge from the ICU due to blunt trauma (including head injury), subjects in China reported health-related QOL lower than that reported for the general population (Fu *et al.*, 2011). Subjects who were older than 45 years had a lower level of physical function-related QOL than those younger than 45 years at the two-year assessment. Prolonged ICU length of stay, as well as higher severity of injury, contributed to the lower reported health-related QOL with regards to physical function (Fu *et al.*, 2011).

Survivors of blunt or penetrating trauma in Sweden had lower health-related QOL in all domains of physical function compared to an age- and sex-matched group from the general Swedish population even at five years after the traumatic event (Sluys *et al.*, 2005). Older age, number of in-hospital complications, number of surgical procedures performed and prolonged ICU and hospital stay were associated with the observed decrease in health-related QOL. Those subjects who were in full employment or had part-time work five years after the event had a higher level of health-related QOL than those who were still on sick leave or who received a disability grant. A sense of abandonment after discharge from the hospital, as reported by some subjects, was found to have a negative impact on their health-related QOL. Inadequate pain management in the ICU or surgical ward was also associated with a reduction in health-related QOL at five years after discharge. Interestingly, the authors reported that blunt trauma led to a lower health-related QOL related to physical function and that penetrating trauma led to a lower health-related QOL related to mental health (Sluys *et al.*, 2005).

10.4.1.1.1. Physical function-related QOL in paediatric patients who suffered blunt or penetrating trauma

The reader is referred to the discussion in the multiple orthopaedic trauma section.

10.4.1.2. *Survivors of burn injury*

If the nature of burn injuries is taken into account, it is reasonable to assume that people who survive this type of trauma might suffer from some form of reduction in health-related QOL, not least due to the changes in physical appearance that such persons have as a result of the injury. It has been reported that burn injuries may decrease health-related QOL and muscle strength for up to 36 months after the injury (Jarrett *et al.*, 2008). The person's level of emotional distress and the amount of pain endured during and after the injury may also decrease reported health-related QOL. The size of the burn injury may also affect functional outcomes and health-related QOL. Return to work is affected by length of hospital stay as well as the number of surgical procedures that the person undergoes (Jarrett *et al.*, 2008). Subjects under 40 years of age, who sustained fairly small total body surface area burns (less than 12%), report health-related QOL near to pre-injury levels by six months after discharge (Jarrett *et al.*, 2008).

Anzarut *et al.* (2005) assessed QOL in survivors of severe burn injuries (more than 50% total body surface area) in Canada. They found that the strongest independent predictors of physical components of QOL were the total amount of full-thickness burn injury and hand function. Hand burn injury that was severe enough to necessitate grafting lead to significant reductions in reported physical component summary (PCS) scores on the SF-36.

The physiological changes to the lung which occur as a result of inhalation burns do not result in long-term pulmonary dysfunction in the majority of burn survivors; however, cases of compromised lung function, decreased aerobic capacity and reduced participation in leisure-related physical activity have been documented up to five years after inhalation injury (Willis *et al.*, 2011).

These poor long-term outcomes of burn survivors should be an impetus for the development of more integrated rehabilitation approaches (Esselman *et al.*, 2006). Early data suggests that targeted exercise prescription can improve outcomes in the burn-injured population (Al-Mousawi *et al.*, 2010; Grisbrook *et al.*, 2012; Tan *et al.*, 2012). An individualised rehabilitation programme which focuses on strength and endurance training should be available for all burn survivors (Celis *et al.*, 2003). Such a programme should start in hospital but should also be offered after hospital discharge.

10.4.1.2.1. Physical function-related QOL in paediatric patients with burn injury

Most researchers that investigate health-related QOL of paediatric survivors of major trauma exclude patients with burn injuries from their study samples due to the impact of burns on appearance and function. For this reason, QOL studies for paediatric burn survivors are scarce. One study investigated body image, mood and QOL in burn survivors aged 11–19 years who suffered burn injury as children (Pope *et al.*, 2007). The authors compared burn survivors' data with that of an age-matched control group who had not suffered burn injury. They found that the burn survivors reported higher levels of health-related QOL than the healthy control group (Pope *et al.*, 2007). These results are based on a small group of subjects and should therefore be interpreted with caution.

Another study by Weedon and Potterton (2011) set out to establish QOL in children aged two to 12 years with burn injury one week and three months after discharge from a hospital in South Africa using the PedsQL. They reported that overall QOL was 10% short of 'optimal', as reported from developed countries, at three months. The largest improvements were seen in physical aspects of health-related QOL as the children became more active as their wounds healed. They postulated that the speedy improvement in QOL observed could be attributed to the fact that young children have a faster rate of recovery from injury than adults. They also acknowledged that if QOL is assessed over a longer time period after discharge, a reduction in scores might be observed, as burn survivors are at an increased risk of developing long-term complications (Weedon and Potterton, 2011).

10.4.1.3. *Survivors of multiple orthopaedic injuries*

Multiple orthopaedic trauma as a result of motor vehicle accidents (MVA), motor cycle crashes and falls is not just isolated to the limbs but often involves the thoracic cage structures. Multiple blood transfusions and bilateral pulmonary contusions predispose to the development of ARDS, as discussed in Chapter 5. At six months after discharge from the hospital, patients who sustained bilateral pulmonary contusions at the time of injury were reported to have more restrictions in exercise capacity than those who suffered multiple trauma but didn't have pulmonary contusion (Leone *et al.*, 2008). Pulmonary function impairments in this patient population at six months following discharge was associated with the diagnosis of ARDS during ICU stay. An obstructive lung disease pattern was identified in 44% of subjects and a restrictive disease pattern in 7% of subjects (Leone *et al.*, 2008). The authors reported that smoking history prior to injury, number of fractured ribs and ICU length of stay did not have an influence on pulmonary function test results at six months after discharge. Health-related QOL for this group of patients remained decreased at one year after discharge (Leone *et al.*, 2008).

Patients who suffered multiple fractures or fractures sustained due to high-energy transfer present with prolonged disability, which has a negative impact on return to work after discharge (Livingston *et al.*, 2009). Reasons put forward for these findings include a longer ICU stay with the risk of numerous complications due to the severity of injury, which would contribute to significant loss of muscle mass and subsequently result in poor QOL related to physical function (Livingston *et al.*, 2009). Lower extremity fractures are reported to negatively impact physical function-related QOL in the first six months after hospital discharge; more so than injury to other body regions (except the spine) (Aitken *et al.*, 2012).

Patients who sustained pelvis or isolated acetabular fractures as a result of trauma suffer from pain years after the event. Gerbershagen *et al.* (2010) showed that 64% of patients reported high-intensity posttraumatic pelvic pain when surveyed four years after the incident. Those who sustained type B or C pelvic fractures or isolated acetabular fractures reported higher pain intensity than those who sustained type A pelvic fractures. As a result, physical function-related QOL was very low in those with high pain intensity (Gerbershagen *et al.*, 2010).

10.4.1.3.1. Physical function-related QOL in paediatric patients after multiple orthopaedic injuries

The most frequent cause of orthopaedic injury in children younger than 18 years is MVAs, pedestrian accidents or falls (Winthrop *et al.*, 2005). Children do have the ability to rapidly improve over the first six months after injury; however, those older than five years who have suffered major trauma that resulted in lower extremity injuries (excluding traumatic brain injury and spinal cord injury) report limitations in physical function even at six months after discharge from a trauma centre (Winthrop *et al.*, 2005). The method of fracture management might impact physical functioning, especially in relation to femur fractures. Those managed with internal fixation report higher levels of physical function-related QOL than those children managed with a spica cast or traction (Winthrop, 2010). Children with fractures of the tibia and fibula report low levels of physical function-related QOL even at one year after hospital discharge (Winthrop, 2010).

Adolescents who suffered major trauma were assessed for QOL at various time points over the first two years after discharge. They showed progressive improvement in QOL but, compared to normative population-based data, their QOL scores remained well below the norm at all time points of assessment (Holbrook *et al.*, 2007). Older adolescents reported lower QOL compared to younger adolescents up to two years after suffering major traumatic injury. A possible explanation offered by the authors is that older children's responses to injury mature into adult responses to injury, hence the lower reported QOL (Holbrook *et al.*, 2007). Injury to multiple body regions is associated with deficits in health-related QOL for adolescents up to two years after the incident (Holbrook *et al.*, 2007).

10.4.1.4. *Survivors of spinal cord injury*

Spinal cord injury (SCI) leads to severe physical disability and people with SCI and neurological deficit may develop secondary complications (e.g. bladder and bowel dysfunction, chronic pain or depression) that significantly impact their already lowered sense of life satisfaction and well-being (Van Koppenhagen *et al.*, 2008; Wijesuriya *et al.*, 2012). Quality of life research shows that people with SCI and neurological deficit have significantly lower levels of QOL compared to healthy controls or normative population data (Middleton *et al.*, 2007; Boakye *et al.*, 2012; Schouten *et al.*, 2013). Domains of QOL, as measured with the SF-36, that seem to be more severely affected by SCI are those related to PF, RP and bodily pain (Middleton *et al.*, 2007; Boakye *et al.*, 2012). As can be expected, people with tetraplegia seem to have reduced QOL related to PF and bodily pain compared to those with paraplegia (Middleton *et al.*, 2007; Boakye *et al.*, 2012).

Many people living with SCI and neurological deficit complain of chronic fatigue, which negatively impacts their physical function (Wijesuriya *et al.*, 2012). The time since the onset of SCI seems to be the most important factor related to fatigue. Less fatigue is reported by those people with a longer time since the onset of SCI (more than nine years); higher levels of fatigue are reported by those who recently experienced SCI (Wijesuriya *et al*., 2012). A possible explanation for this finding is that those who suffered SCI a long time ago had learnt to adapt to their injury and its impairments and may exhibit better physical fitness and improved coping and participation skills (Wijesuriya *et al*., 2012).

Those with SCI without neurological deficit report a QOL that is similar to that of normative population data and have a high rate of return to work (Schouten *et al*., 2013).

10.4.1.4.1. Physical function-related QOL in paediatric patients with spinal cord injury

There is a dearth of information on the effect of SCI on physical function-related QOL in the paediatric population. The only report found showed that youth with paraplegia participated in more activities more frequently than youth with tetraplegia (Riordan *et al*., 2013).

10.4.1.5. *Survivors of traumatic brain injury*

As can be expected, health-related QOL of patients who suffered moderate to severe TBI is reported to be significantly affected when compared to that reported by a healthy population (Hawthorne *et al*., 2009; Arango-Lasprilla *et al*., 2012; Hu *et al*., 2012). Various domains of physical function-related QOL (RP, bodily pain and GH) seem to be affected by TBI (Hawthorne *et al*., 2009; Arango-Lasprilla *et al*., 2012). Elevated levels of fatigue and decreased vitality are complaints often reported by people with TBI (Wijesuriya *et al*., 2012). Two years after the traumatic event, patients diagnosed with severe TBI still exhibited significantly lower scores for PCS as measured with the SF-36 than those diagnosed with moderate TBI (Hu *et al*., 2012).

This difference in physical function-related QOL measures in patients with moderate and severe TBI seems to disappear at 10 years after the injury. Andelic *et al*. (2009) reported no significant differences in PCS scores between patients with moderate and severe TBI. They also reported higher scores for PF and RP in those patients with TBI that were employed 10 years after TBI.

10.4.1.5.1. Physical function-related QOL in paediatric patients with traumatic brain injury

Functional ability of children aged between six and 14 years who suffered TBI is negatively influenced by the severity of injury (Anderson *et al.*, 2012). These authors also found that the child's pre-injury functional level was a greater predictor of post-injury functional ability than the severity of TBI.

10.4.2. *Mental health-related components of quality of life*

Intensive care unit delirium has been reported in a small percentage of trauma survivors (up to 75% of general ICU survivors have reported delusional memories) who were assessed six to 18 months after discharge from the ICU (Ringdal *et al.*, 2009). Delirium is characterised by cerebral dysfunction that can develop due to electrolyte abnormalities, sepsis, fever, shock, certain medications (benzodiazepines, opiates or anticholenergics), infection, hypertension or anemia (Cavallazzi *et al.*, 2012). Symptoms of delirium that subjects might exhibit include hallucinations, dreams, nightmares experienced in the ICU or the incorrect perception that ICU staff are trying to hurt them. It seems to be more common in younger patients who have a prolonged ICU stay, and hence longer periods of MV, higher injury severity and greater morbidity, than other trauma sufferers. These patients reported poor health-related QOL and higher levels of anxiety and signs of depression than trauma patients who had no delusional memories (Ringdal *et al.*, 2009).

Continuous decreased levels of mental health-related QOL up to two years following trauma have been reported to be the result of pre-existing disease (Orwelius *et al.*, 2010, 2012). Pre-injury factors such as age, pre-existing mental disease, gender and socio-economic status may impact on mental health-related QOL after injury. Also, factors related to the actual injury, such as type, severity of injury and perceived threat to life, may influence mental health-related QOL after injury. Post-injury factors including health care interventions and physical and psychological consequences of the injury could impact on health-related QOL (Sluys *et al.*, 2005).

Limitations in mental health-related QOL that various groups of trauma survivors experience in the short and long term after discharge from the acute care setting are discussed below.

10.4.2.1. *Survivors of blunt or penetrating trauma*

Mental health-related QOL of survivors of penetrating trunk trauma who received prolonged MV was similar to that of a healthy group and the group who received a short period of MV at six months after discharge (Van Aswegen *et al.*, 2011). The majority of these subjects were male and reported that they were grateful to be alive, which might have contributed to the higher than expected scores. Fu *et al.* (2011) reported that female survivors of blunt trauma reported lower levels of mental health-related QOL than male survivors and that subjects with head injuries had lower levels of mental health than other blunt trauma survivors.

10.4.2.2. *Survivors of burn injury*

Anzarut *et al.* (2005) reported that age at the time of injury and the level of social support that survivors had at home after discharge from the burn centre were the strongest independent predictors of mental health component summary (MCS) scores on the SF-36. The younger the survivor, the higher their reported MH score on the SF-36 questionnaire. Interestingly, these authors found no association between facial burns requiring grafting and QOL; however, the majority of their study population was male and their results might have been different if more females participated in the study (Anzarut *et al.*, 2005).

10.4.2.3. *Survivors of multiple orthopaedic injuries*

In a cohort of patients who suffered traumatic injury, age, gender and the subject's perceived ability to control their own environment impacted most on MH status. Mental health status improved as age increased, and men had a significantly higher MH status than women. Lower perceived ability to control one's own environment was associated with lower levels of MH (Aitken *et al.*, 2012).

10.4.2.4. *Survivors of spinal cord injury*

Not all patients who suffer SCI present with limitations in QOL due to MH or RE problems. There does seem to be a smaller group of SCI sufferers who are at increased risk of developing psychological disease following the injury. These people may suffer from lowered QOL due to MH, RE and SF limitations (Middleton *et al.*, 2007; Wijesuriya *et al.*, 2012). Women seem to experience lower levels of QOL after traumatic SCI than men (Middleton *et al.*, 2007). A possible explanation for this finding is that men are more frequently involved in trauma and thus the unbalanced gender sample sizes of QOL research studies could contribute to this unusual finding (Middleton *et al.*, 2007). A person with SCI who has a strong sense of self-efficacy (belief that they can do a particular task successfully in the future) is likely to have a better level of QOL compared to someone with a low sense of self-efficacy (Middleton *et al.*, 2007).

10.4.2.4.1. Mental health-related QOL in paediatric patients with spinal cord injury

Children with SCI are at a higher risk for developing depression or anxiety disorders than those without SCI. Those who develop depression or anxiety disorders have lower levels of QOL in the long term following SCI (Garma *et al.*, 2011). Children with SCI under the age of 18 years old report significantly lower levels of QOL one year after the injury, compared with QOL reported by a healthy group without SCI (Garma *et al.*, 2011). One year after SCI the reported mental health-related QOL of children with tetraplegia and those with paraplegia is not significantly different. This suggests that the level of SCI does not directly influence QOL in children in the long term (Oladeji *et al.*, 2007).

10.4.2.5. *Survivors of traumatic brain injury*

Psychiatric disorders tend to develop in up to a third of patients after severe TBI and affects these patients' QOL (Diaz *et al.*, 2012). These authors observed the development of psychiatric disorders in patients after severe TBI over an 18-month period. Major depressive disorder, anxiety disorder and personality changes were reported to develop in a third of the study population. Patients with severe TBI and personality changes had a significant decline in general health, as well as impairments in PF and SF domains, compared to those with TBI without personality changes (Diaz *et al.*, 2012). Subjects with severe TBI and depression had significantly lower health-related QOL in all domains of the SF-36 over the 18-month period compared to those with TBI without depression (Diaz *et al.*, 2012).

The severity of TBI continues to be a major contributor to poor mental health two years after injury, as patients with severe injury exhibit significantly lower scores in MCS as measured with the SF-36 than those diagnosed with moderate TBI (Hu *et al.*, 2012). This difference in mental health-related QOL measures in patients with moderate and severe TBI seems to disappear at 10 years after the injury (Andelic *et al.*, 2009).

10.4.2.5.1. Mental health-related QOL in paediatric patients with traumatic brain injury

The severity of brain injury has a greater impact on QOL outcomes in children than age at the time of injury, premorbid functioning, family or social factors (Winthrop, 2010). Those with severe TBI often present with cognitive dysfunction in the first 12 months after injury. A substantial reduction in mental health-related QOL in the first two years after injury have been reported for children younger than 18 years who have suffered moderate or severe TBI or mild TBI with intracranial haemorrhage (Rivara *et al.*, 2011). These children presented with an impaired ability to participate in life situations and life events and an impaired ability to participate in communication and social activites in school (Rivara *et al.*, 2011). Children with TBI suffer from low levels of QOL even at three years after injury. Hispanic children seem to have even lower levels of QOL at three years after TBI than non-Hispanic white children with TBI

(Jimenez *et al.*, 2013). This suggests that there may be cultural influences on mental health-related QOL.

Children with orthopaedic injuries and severe TBI have more limitations in neuropsychological, behavioural and adaptive functioning than those with orthopaedic injuries without TBI (Winthrop, 2010). Finally, the impact of caregivers' strain on the health-related QOL of survivors of TBI should not be dismissed (Winthrop, 2010).

10.4.3. *Posttraumatic stress disorder in survivors of trauma*

10.4.3.1. *Adult population*

Symptoms of PTSD (Table 10.5) have been reported in the trauma population after discharge from the ICU. A multicentre survey on a civilian population (824 participants) in the USA who sustained trauma as a result of assault, natural disasters or MVA reported a PTSD rate of 32% (Holbrook *et al.*, 2001). Perception of threat to life was associated with the onset of PTSD. The disorder was also more commonly found in younger low-income (less than $20,000) adults, and a rate of 40% was reported among females, at six months following the event. Intentional injury such as assault and the expectation that the injury might occur again was associated with late onset PTSD. A strong association was found between PTSD and penetrating trauma. The authors concluded that PTSD resulted in a decrease in health-related QOL for this civilian population (Holbrook *et al.*, 2001).

Table 10.5: Common symptoms of PTSD*.

- Intrusive memories, including recurrent distressing memories of the event or reliving the event (flashbacks)
- Avoidance, including not talking or thinking about the event and avoiding people and places associated with the event
- Negative changes in thinking and mood, which includes feeling hopeless about the future and difficulty maintaining close relationships
- Changes in emotional reactions, such as outbursts of anger, overwhelming shame or being easily frightened

*(Mayo Clinic, 2014).

A study conducted in Sweden by Öster *et al.* (2011) reported on the health-related QOL of people who suffered burn injuries. They showed that, two to seven years after discharge, these subjects had a lower health-related QOL than the general Swedish population. A diagnosis of PTSD, substance abuse disorder, pain and a none-working status had a negative impact on health-related QOL. The majority of their subjects still reported problems with pain or discomfort at the time of assessment. In subjects who sustained severe burn injuries, longer hospital length of stay was associated with more problems related to mobility and pain and indicated a slower physical recovery (Öster *et al.*, 2011).

Symptoms of PTSD diagnosed in survivors of burn injury at one month after hospital discharge has a significantly negative impact on physical functioning at two years follow up. Furthermore, PTSD at six, 12 and 24 months after discharge is reported to interfere greatly with psychosocial aspects of QOL in burn survivors (Corry *et al.*, 2010).

Subjects who suffered mild TBI are at increased risk for developing PTSD compared to others. Posttraumatic stress disorder can develop years after the TBI event. In those that do develop PTSD, impairments related to physical and cognitive function and control of emotions are reported (Vanderploeg *et al.*, 2009).

10.4.3.2. *Paediatric population*

Acute stress disorder (ASD) and the consequent development of PTSD are also reported in adolescents and children who have suffered major traumatic injury. Perceived threat to life, intentional injury and pre-trauma psychopathology are the most significant predictors of the development of ASD and PTSD in children and adolescents following trauma (Holbrook *et al.*, 2005; Winthrop, 2010). Female adolescents who suffered major traumatic injury seem to have a higher risk for developing ASD than male adolescents, but the reasons for this finding are still unclear (Holbrook *et al.*, 2005). Low health-related QOL at one year after trauma is associated with the presence of posttraumatic stress symptoms as early as one month after the injury.

Children who suffered burn injury are at a particularly high risk for the development of PTSD (Winthrop, 2010). A prevalence rate of 10%

PTSD was found in children aged one to six years at six months following the injury. Risk factors for the development of PTSD in this group were the presence of parent posttraumatic stress symptoms, size of the burn injury and pre-injury emotional and behavioural difficulties (De Young *et al.*, 2014).

Mild to severe TBI in children aged between six and 15 years is associated with an increased risk for PTSD (Brown *et al.*, 2014). The authors reported that the presence of pain was higher in those diagnosed with PTSD even at 18 months following the injury compared to those with TBI but no PTSD.

10.5. Rehabilitation of Survivors of Critical Illness

Despite the fact that the health benefits derived from regular exercise is well known, there is a dearth of literature on the effect of exercise therapy on health-related QOL in survivors of critical illness following discharge from the hospital.

Jones *et al.* (2003) tested the effectiveness of a rehabilitation programme on the recovery of survivors of critical illness using a randomised controlled study design in the UK. They compiled a 93-page rehabilitation package that consisted of a self-directed exercise programme, diagrams and illustrations. The manual also contained advice on a wide range of psychological, psychosocial and physical problems that the ICU survivor could expect to encounter after they had recovered from critical illness. Subjects were contacted by telephone three times per week after discharge to monitor progress; subjects in the experimental group were also encouraged to use the self-help rehabilitation manual. All subjects were tested at follow-up clinics at eight weeks and six months after discharge. The authors found that the SF-36 PF score for subjects in the experimental group was closer to normal and significantly different from those in the control group (Jones *et al.*, 2003). Some critique on this study includes the fact that the authors did not objectively measure muscle strength or exercise capacity in their subjects and therefore it is difficult to draw conclusions regarding the effect of the rehabilitation manual on their musculoskeletal system recovery after critical illness.

More recently, Elliot *et al.* (2011) tested the effectiveness of an eight-week home-based rehabilitation programme on the health-related QOL and physical function recovery of survivors of critical illness using a multi-centre randomised controlled trial design in Australia. The home-based physical rehabilitation programme consisted of strength training exercises and walking. The control group received no interventions except for the three study assessment visits; the exercise group received an illustrated exercise manual to use at home for eight weeks. They also received personal visits from a health care professional experienced in exercise training on three of the eight weeks to ensure graded, individualised endurance and strength training. Telephone calls from the health care professional to the participant were performed on the remaining four non-visit weeks to ensure compliance with the exercise programme. Patient outcomes (SF-36 and six-minute walk test (6MWT)) were assessed at one, eight and 26 weeks following discharge. The authors reported that the home-based rehabilitation programme had no significant effect on physical recovery and functional status of the participants in their trial. They listed some limitations to their study, including not meeting the estimated sample size despite screening over 6000 patients; unrealistic expectations of treatment effect according to the PF domain of the SF-36; and being unable to objectively assess training compliance of subjects in the exercise group (Elliot *et al.*, 2011). They did not assess muscle strength objectively in this study and therefore it is not clear whether the intensity of strength training prescribed for the experimental group was adequate during the eight weeks of training. Inter-rater reliability of the assessors in the performance of the 6MWT and administration of the SF-36 questionnaire to study participants was not mentioned in this multi-centre trial and could have influenced the results obtained.

A unique approach to exercise rehabilitation for survivors of critical illness was reported by Denehy *et al.* (2013). They tested the effectiveness of an exercise rehabilitation programme, which was initiated in the ICU and carried through to the outpatient setting, on physical function assessed at 12 months after hospital discharge. This was a single-centre randomised controlled trial. Medical or surgical adult patients with moderate severity of illness were randomised to a usual care or intervention group. The usual care group received chest physiotherapy treatment and were mobilised out of bed and encouraged to march on the spot by the bedside in the ICU. After transfer to the acute ward, patients' physiotherapy management focus shifted to functional recovery and discharge planning. Outpatient exercise classes did not form part of usual care. The intervention group received usual care as well as strength training of the extremities and functional exercises in the ICU based on individualised patient assessment outcomes. Patients were encouraged to march by the bedside and do repeated sit-to-stand movements. These exercises were commenced on day five of ICU stay. Initially exercises were performed once daily for 15 minutes and, as the patient's condition improved, frequency of exercise was increased to twice daily for 15 minutes. On the ward, exercise duration was increased to 30 minutes twice daily with the aim of reaching 60 minutes of exercise daily. The programme consisted of cardiovascular and functional exercises and progressive resistance strength training exercises. In the outpatient setting, exercise frequency was progressed to 60 minutes of exercise twice weekly for eight weeks. Individual patient's programmes were progressed according to their re-assessment findings. No maintenance exercises were prescribed to patients in the period after completion of the outpatient programme. At 12-month follow-up, the authors found no significant differences between the intervention group and usual care group subjects in relation to physical function (measured with 6MWT) or health-related QOL (measured with SF-36). The authors put forward several limitations to their study, which included failure to reach enrolment targets for the trial, the heterogenous patient population in relation to age, comorbidities and presence of sepsis and, lastly, the low attendance at the outpatient programme (Denehy *et al.*, 2013).

Despite the slightly discouraging reports on the effects of exercise rehabilitation in survivors of critical illness, the importance of rehabilitation that starts in the ICU and is carried through to post-ICU care into the community setting is still emphasised in the literature (Hough and Herridge, 2012).

10.6. Suggestions for Exercise Rehabilitation for Survivors of Trauma and Critical Illness

Physiotherapists use exercise prescription and exercise programmes in their management of a wide range of patient populations to optimise their physical activity and minimise the health risks associated with physical inactivity (World Confederation for Physical Therapy, 2011). All the clinical chapters in this book emphasised the role of physiotherapists in providing early rehabilitation in the ICU and ward settings on a daily basis for patients who had suffered traumatic injury. A large portion of the entry-level training programmes for physiotherapists worldwide focus on education and clinical reasoning in human anatomy, physiology, pathology and exercise science. Physiotherapists are therefore also well qualified to be involved in the care of these patients in the community setting, after discharge from the hospital.

Ongoing structured rehabilitation protocols and programmes for patients with burns, orthopaedic injury, SCI or TBI after discharge from the acute care setting are well known and well established in most countries. Patients who suffered blunt or penetrating trauma, especially to the chest or trunk, regularly receive rehabilitative care during their stay in the acute care setting, but rehabilitation often ceases at discharge as the need for intensive ongoing exercise therapy in the community setting is not recognised by the patient, the physiotherapist or both. A search of the available literature revealed no studies that investigated the effects of exercise rehabilitation on the recovery of survivors of blunt or penetrating trauma. In light of the significant long-term limitations to physical function-related QOL that trauma survivors suffer, especially those who had a complicated and prolonged ICU stay, exercise rehabilitation after discharge is of great importance. The suggestions made below regarding exercise rehabilitation interventions in the community setting are aimed at this specific group of trauma survivors, but can also be applied to those recovering from burn injuries or orthopaedic injuries.

The physical and mental health benefits of exercise therapy and the principles of exercise prescription were discussed in Chapter 4 (Section 4.1). Prior to exercise prescription for any survivor of trauma in the community setting, exercise testing should be performed to establish the individual's baseline exercise endurance and muscle strength. Clinical exercise testing for assessment of endurance, such as a treadmill or cycle ergometer test, may be performed if the physiotherapist has access to such equipment. Field tests such as the 6MWT, shuttle walk test or three-minute step test may also be used. Results obtained from an exercise test will guide the physiotherapist regarding aerobic exercise prescription for each individual subject in relation to frequency, intensity and duration of exercise to be performed. Muscle strength testing may also be performed using either the one repetition maximum (RM) or five RM tests in order to guide prescription for resistance training.

The dearth of literature regarding exercise rehabilition for survivors of trauma makes it difficult to set out exercise prescription guidelines for these patients. The recommendations provided in Tables 10.6 and 10.7 are based on the American College of Sports Medicine (ACSM, 2014) guidelines for exercise prescription for deconditioned individuals and the exercise format

Table 10.6: Recommendations provided by ACSM (2014) for exercise prescription for deconditioned individuals.

Duration of exercise

- Aerobic exercise
  - Start with 15–30 minutes of moderate-intensity exercise per session
  - Gradually progress to 30–60 minutes of moderate-intensity exercise per session
  - Progress to 10–20 minutes of vigorous-intensity exercise per session, when indicated
  - Gradually progress to 60 minutes of vigorous-intensity exercise, when indicated
  - Bouts of ≥ 10 minutes of exercise spread throughout the day to total the required duration of exercise may be used
- Resistance training
  - No specific duration of training was specified

Frequency of exercise

- Aerobic exercise
  - Start with moderate-intensity exercise at least three days per week; progress to moderate-intensity exercise performed five days per week
  - Further progression to vigorous-intensity exercise performed three days per week
  - Final progression to a combination of moderate- and vigorous-intensity exercise performed 3–5 days per week
- Resistance training
  - Train each muscle group 2–3 days per week with 48 hours rest between training sessions of the same muscle group
  - Start by splitting the body into selected muscle groups that are trained in different sessions; progress to training all muscle groups in one session

(Continued)

Table 10.6: (*Continued*)

Intensity of exercise

- Aerobic exercise
  - Start with light- to moderate-intensity exercise for deconditioned individuals (30–40% of maximal heart rate (HR_{max})*
  - Progress to moderate-intensity exercise (40–60% HR_{max}) if indicated
  - Final progression to vigorous-intensity exercise (60–90% HR_{max}) when indicated
- Resistance training
  - Start with 40–50% of one RM
  - Progress to 50–70% of one RM, if indicated
  - Final progression to ≥ 80% of one RM, if indicated

Type of exercise

- Aerobic exercise
  - Exercise that involves major muscle groups, e.g. walking, leisurely cycling, jogging, running, aerobics, stepping, spinning and swimming
- Resistance training
  - Multi-joint and single-joint exercises
  - Body weight, resistance bands or free weights

Volume of exercise

- Aerobic exercise
  - 1000 kilocalories per week or 150 minutes of physical activity per week or greater than 5400–7900 pedometer steps per day
- Resistance training
  - Each muscle group should be trained for 2–4 sets to improve strength and power
  - Deconditioned individuals should start with one set per muscle group
  - 8–12 repetitions per set
  - Rest period of 2–3 minutes between each set of repetitions

*$HR_{max} = 207 - (0.7 \times \text{age})$ is a more accurate estimation of exercise intensity than $HR_{max} = 220 - \text{age}$ (ACSM, 2014).

used for survivors of critical illness in the study by Berney *et al.* (2012) (refer to Chapter 4, Section 4.1). Exercise prescription for survivors of traumatic injury should therefore follow a similar pattern, adjusting the intervention to suit each individual patient's abilities and needs.

Exercise therapy for this group of trauma survivors may be performed in a supervised hospital-based outpatient environment or at the rooms of

Table 10.7: Exercise prescription format used by Berney *et al.* (2012) for outpatient-based rehabilitation of survivors of critical illness.

Duration of exercise

- Aerobic exercise
  - 30 minutes
- Resistance training
  - 20 minutes
- Functional retraining
  - 10 minutes

Frequency of sessions

- One exercise session of 60 minutes performed twice per week

Intensity of exercise

- Aerobic exercise
  - 80% of HR_{max} or rate of perceived exertion 5–6 on modified Borg scale
  - Progression to longer work interval training for endurance
- Resistance training
  - 75% of five RM

Type of exercise

- Aerobic exercise
  - Treadmill walking and stationary bicycle
- Resistance training
  - Exercises targeting the upper limb, trunk, pelvis and lower limb
  - Dumbbells, resistance bands and own body weight
- Functional retraining
  - Sit-to-stand (loaded or using body weight), rolling, supine to sitting, trunk control and trunk balance
  - Stairs

a physiotherapist who works in private practice; or it may be performed without supervision at home, using an exercise manual with illustrations. Ideally exercise in both types of environments should be encouraged, with emphasis initially on supervised exercise to ensure safety and effectiveness of training and to monitor the patient's response to exercise; however, emphasis should shift to unsupervised training away from the physiotherapist as soon as possible to empower the patient by taking responsibility for their own health and well-being.

Walking as a form of aerobic exercise is often prescribed for survivors of critical illness to perform in their community setting (Elliot *et al.*, 2011; Berney *et al.*, 2012) as it has few, if any, side-effects. Walking develops cardiovascular endurance and fitness and strengthens the muscles of the lower trunk and legs. It is a natural activity that forms part of most peoples' activities of daily living (ADL), is well tolerated by extremely deconditioned individuals and effectively reduces the risk of death from any cause (Warburton *et al.*, 2006). It would therefore be reasonable to include walking as part of a graduated home exercise programme for survivors of trauma.

Progression of resistance and flexibility exercises of the upper and lower limbs as well as trunk muscles should be done gradually to prevent muscle injury (ACSM, 2014). Time must, however, be allowed for significant wound healing to take place prior to the introduction of trunk exercises in people who are recovering from blunt or penetrating trunk trauma and subsequently underwent a single or repeated laparotomy procedures. People with abdominal skin grafts should be advised to wear an abdominal binder (Chapter 5, Fig. 5.6) and to avoid the Valsalva manoeuvre during exercise to prevent organ protrusion.

The long-term aim of exercise rehabilitation for this group of adult patients should be for them to develop a level of fitness that meets the guidelines prescribed by ACSM (2014).

10.6.1. *Exercise prescription for children and adolescents who have suffered trauma*

Rehabilitation interventions for children should take into consideration their developmental stage. No published exercise prescription guidelines for children or adolescents recovering from critical illness or trauma could be found. Guidelines for exercise prescription for healthy children and adolescents are provided by ACSM (2014), and are summarised in Table 10.8.

The ACSM exercise guidelines summarised in Table 10.7 should be tailored to adequately meet the needs of each individual child or adolescent who is recovering from trauma-related injury. The progression of exercise duration and intensity should be done gradually to prevent muscle injury. The long-term aims of exercise intervention for this paediatric group should be for them to develop a level of fitness that meets the requirements of the ACSM (2014) exercise guidelines.

Table 10.8: Exercise prescription guidelines for healthy children and adolescents.

Duration of exercise

- Aerobic exercise
  - Start with moderate-intensity exercise for the duration of time tolerated by the child and gradually progress to 60 minutes or longer per day
- Resistance training
  - No specific duration is given, but this should form part of the 60 minutes or more training per day

Frequency of exercise

- Aerobic exercise
  - Daily
- Resistance training
  - Three days per week or more

Intensity of exercise

- Aerobic exercise
  - Start with moderate-intensity exercise that produces noticable increases in HR and respiration
  - Progress to vigorous-intensity exercise, performed at least three days per week, that produces substantial increases in HR and respiration

Type of exercise

- Aerobic exercise
  - Should be enjoyable and developmentally appropriate and could include brisk walking, running, bicycling, swimming or dancing
- Resistance training
  - Unstructured muscle strengthening activities such as climbing trees, playing on playground equipment, tug-of-war
  - Structured muscle strengthening activities such as lifting weights or using resistance bands
  - Bone strengthening activities such as rope jumping, hop-scotch, running, basketball, tennis or netball

10.7. Potential Challenges Associated with Exercise Rehabilitation of Survivors of Trauma

The physiotherapist might be faced with the following challenges when introducing exercise rehabilitation to patients after hospital discharge.

- As the majority of people who suffer blunt or penetrating trauma-related injuries are from a lower socio-economic background, they might not have the financial means to attend a structured rehabilitation programme at a hospital-based or private physiotherapy room-based gymnasium over a four- or eight-week period.

- Patients who are younger and did not develop sepsis in the ICU may be reluctant to attend outpatient exercise sessions, as they may not see the need for ongoing rehabilitation (Denehy *et al.*, 2013).
- High drop-out rates among survivors of trauma during clinical trials have been reported by a number of authors (Cuthbertson *et al.*, 2005; Winthrop *et al.*, 2005; Holavanahalli *et al.*, 2006; Jarrett *et al.*, 2008; Van Aswegen *et al.*, 2010; Denehy *et al.*, 2013).

Possible solutions for these challenges are:

- A self-help rehabilitation manual that explains all the aerobic, resistance and flexibility exercises (with illustrations) could be compiled, explained and given to trauma patients to use at home;
- Regular telephone contact may improve compliance until the date of the follow-up appointment;
- Visits to the individual person's home by a community-based physiotherapist may also improve compliance and safety regarding performance of the prescribed exercises; and
- Patient selection for post-discharge exercise rehabilitation programmes should be tailored to those that had a longer duration of stay in the ICU, episodes of sepsis, poor physical function-related QOL and impaired exercise endurance.

10.8. Conclusion

The information shared in this chapter emphasises the limitations in physical function and mental health-related QOL that survivors of critical illness as a result of traumatic injury experience months and even years after the incident. Exercise rehabilitation has proven benefits to mental and physical well-being and therefore physiotherapists involved in trauma care should be seen to play a prominent role in the general reconditioning of survivors of trauma, especially those with a complicated recovery, after discharge from the acute care setting.

Bibliography

Aitken, L.M., Chaboyer, W., Kendall, E., *et al.* (2012). Health status after traumatic injury, *J. Trauma Acute Care Surg.,* **72**, 1702–1708.

Al-Mousawi, A.M., Williams, F.N., Mlcak, R.P., *et al.* (2010). Effects of exercise training on resting energy expenditure and lean mass during pediatric burn rehabilitation, *J. Burn Care Res.,* **31**, 400–408.

American College of Sports Medicine (ACSM). (2014). *ACSM's Guidelines for Exercise Testing and Prescription*, 9th edn., Wolters Kluwer Health/Lippincott Williams & Wilkins, Philadelphia, PA.

Andelic, N., Hammergren, N., Bautz-Holter, E., *et al.* (2009). Functional outcome and health-related quality of life 10 years after moderate-to-severe traumatic brain injury, *Acta Neurol. Scand.,* **120**, 16–23.

Anderson, V., Le Brocque, R., Iselin, G., *et al.* (2012). Adaptive ability, behaviour and quality of life pre and posttraumatic brain injury in childhood, *Disabil. Rehabil.,* **34**, 1639–1647.

Angus, D.C., and Carlet, J. (2003). Surviving intensive care: a report from the 2002 Brussels Roundtable, *Intensive Care Med.,* **29**, 368–377.

Anzarut, A., Chen, M., Shankowsky, H., *et al.* (2005). Quality-of-life and outcome predictors following massive burn injury, *Plast. Reconstr. Surg.,* **116**, 791–797.

Arango-Lasprilla, J.C., Krch, D., Drew, A., *et al.* (2012). Health-related quality of life of individuals with traumatic brain injury in Barranquilla, Colombia, *Brain Injury,* **26**, 825–833.

Ardolino, A., Sleat, G., and Willett, K. (2012). Outcome measures in major trauma — results of a consensus meeting, *Injury,* **43**, 1662–1666.

Badia, X., Diaz-Prieto, A., Gorriz, M.T., *et al.* (2001). Using the EuroQol-5D to measure changes in quality of life 12 months after discharge from an intensive care unit, *Intensive Care Med.,* **27**, 1901–1907.

Berney, S., Haines, K., Skinner, E.H., *et al.* (2012). Safety and feasibility of an exercise prescription approach to rehabilitation across the continuum of care for survivors of critical illness, *Phys. Ther.,* **92**, 1524–1535.

Boakye, M., Leigh, B.C., and Skelly, A.C. (2012). Quality of life in persons with spinal cord injury: comparisons with other populations, *J. Neurosurg. Spine,* **17**, 29–37.

Brown, E.A., Kenardy, J.A., and Dow, B.L. (2014). PTSD perpetuates pain in children with traumatic brain injury, *J. Pediatr. Psychol.,* **39**, 512–520.

Cavallazzi, R., Saad, M., and Marik, P.E. (2012). Delirium in the ICU: an overview, *Ann. Intensive Care,* **2**, 49. [Online] Available at: http://www.annalsofintensivecare.com/content/2/1/49 [Accessed 15 November 2014].

Celis, M.M., Suman, O.E., Huang, T.T., *et al.* (2003). Effect of a supervised exercise and physiotherapy program on surgical interventions on children with thermal injury, *J. Burn Care Rehabil.,* **24**, 57–61.

Combes, A., Costa, M.A., Trouillet, J.L., *et al.* (2003). Morbidity, mortality and quality of life outcomes of patients requiring >14 days of mechanical ventilation, *Crit. Care Med.,* **31**, 1373–1381.

Corry, N.H., Klick, B., and Fauerbach, J.A. (2010). Posttraumatic stress disorder and pain impact functioning and disability after major burn injury, *J. Burn Care Res.,* **31**, 13–25.

Cuthbertson, B.H., Roughton, S., Jenkinson, D., *et al.* (2010). Quality of life in the five years after intensive care: a cohort study, *Crit. Care,* **14,** R6. [Online] Available at: http://ccforum.com/content/14/1/R6 [Accessed 15 November 2014].

Cuthbertson, B.H., Scott, J., Strachan, M., *et al.* (2005). Quality of life before and after intensive care, *Anaesthesia,* **60**, 332–339.

Davydow, D.S., Gifford, J.M., Desai, S.V., *et al.* (2008). Posttraumatic stress disorder in general intensive care unit survivors: a systematic review, *Gen. Hosp. Psychiatry,* **30**, 421–434.

De Young, A.C., Hendrikz, J., Kenardy, J.A., *et al.* (2014). Prospective evaluation of parent stress following pediatric burns and identification of risk factors for young child and parent posttraumatic stress disorder, *J. Child Adol. Psychop.,* **24**, 9–17.

Denehy, L., Skinner, E.H., Edbrooke, L., *et al.* (2013). Exercise rehabilitation for patients with critical illness: a randomised controlled trial with 12 months of follow-up, *Crit. Care,* **17**, R156. [Online] Available at: http://ccforum.com/content/17/4/R156 [Accessed 15 November 2014].

Diaz, A.P., Schwarzbold, M.L., Thais, M.E., *et al.* (2012). Psychiatric disorders and health-related quality of life after severe traumatic brain injury: a prospective study, *J. Neurotrauma,* **29**, 1029–1037.

Dowdy, D.W., Eid, M.P., Sedrakyan, A., *et al.* (2005). Quality of life in adult survivors of critical illness: a systematic review of the literature, *Intensive Care Med.,* **31**, 611–620.

Eales, C.J., Noakes, T.D., Stewart, A.V., *et al.* (2004). Self-responsibility predicts the successful outcome of coronary artery bypass surgery, *S. Afr. J. Physiother.,* **60**, 11–20.

Elliot, D., McKinley, S., Alison, J., *et al.* (2011). Health-related quality of life and physical recovery after a critical illness: a multi-centre randomised controlled trial of a home-based physical rehabilitation programme, *Crit. Care,* **15**, R142. [Online] Available at: http://ccforum.com/content/15/3/R142 [Accessed 15 November 2014].

Esselman, P.C., Thombs, B.D., Magyar-Russell, G., *et al.* (2006). Burn rehabilitation: state of the science, *Am. J. Phys. Med. Rehabil.,* **85**, 383–413.

Fu, X.Y., Chen, M., Yu, T., *et al.* (2011). Health-related quality of life of trauma patients after intensive care: a 2-year follow-up study, *Eur. J. Trauma Emerg. Surg.,* **37**, 629–633.

Gabbe, B.J., Simpson, P.M., Sutherland, A.M., *et al.* (2011). Functional and health-related quality of life outcomes after pediatric trauma, *J. Trauma,* **70**, 1532–1538.

Garma, S.I., Kelly, E.H., Daharsh, E.Z., *et al.* (2011). Health-related quality of life after pediatric spinal cord injury, *J. Pediatr. Psychol.,* **36**, 226–236.

Gerbershagen, H.J., Dagtekin, O., Isenberg, J., *et al.* (2010). Chronic pain and disability after pelvic and acetabular fractures — assessment with the Mainz pain staging system, *J. Trauma,* **69**, 128–136.

Granja, C., Dias, C., Costa-Pereira, A., *et al.* (2004). Quality of life of survivors from severe sepsis and septic shock may be similar to that of others who survive critical illness, *Crit. Care,* **8**, R91–R98.

Grisbrook, T.L., Wallman, K.E., Elliott, C.M., *et al.* (2012). The effect of exercise training on pulmonary function and aerobic capacity in adults with burn, *Burns,* **38**, 607–613.

Hawthorne, G., Gruen, R.L., and Kaye, A.H. (2009). Traumatic brain injury and long-term quality of life: findings from an Australian study, *J. Neurotrauma,* 26, 1623–1633.

Herridge, M.S., Cheung, A.M., Tansey, C.M., *et al.* (2003). One-year outcomes in survivors of the acute respiratory distress syndrome, *N. Engl. J. Med.,* **348**, 683–693.

Herridge, M.S., Tansey, C.M., Matté, A., *et al.* (2011). Functional disability 5 years after acute respiratory distress syndrome, *N. Engl. J. Med.,* **364**, 1293–1304.

Heyland, D.K., Hopman, W., Coo, H., *et al.* (2000). Long-term health-related quality of life in survivors of sepsis. Short form 36: a valid and reliable measure of health-related quality of life, *Crit. Care Med.,* **28**, 3599–3605.

Hofhuis, J.G.M., Spronk, P.E., Van Stel, H.F., *et al.* (2008). The impact of critical illness on perceived health-related quality of life during ICU treatment, hospital stay, and after hospital discharge: a long-term follow-up study, *Chest,* **133**, 377–385.

Holavanahalli, R.K., Lezotte, D.C., Hayes, P.H., *et al.* (2006). Profile of patients lost to follow-up in the burn injury rehabilitation model system's longitudinal database, *J. Burn Care Res.,* **27**, 703–712.

Holbrook, T.L., Hoyt, D.B., Coimbra, R., *et al.* (2005). High rates of acute stress disorder impact quality-of-life outcomes in injured adolescents: mechanism and gender predict acute stress disorder risk, *J. Trauma,* **59**, 1126–1130.

Holbrook, T.L., Hoyt, D.B., Coimbra, R., *et al.* (2007). Trauma in adolescents causes long-term marked deficits in quality of life: adolescent children do not recover pre-injury quality of life or function up to two years postinjury compared to national norms, *J. Trauma,* **62**, 577–583.

Holbrook, T.L., Hoyt, D.B., Stein, M.B., *et al.* (2001). Perceived threat to life predicts posttraumatic stress disorder after major trauma: risk factors and functional outcome, *J. Trauma,* **51**, 287–293.

Hough, C.L., and Herridge, M.S. (2012). Long term outcome after acute lung injury, *Curr. Opin. Crit. Care,* **18**, 8–15.

Hu, X.B., Feng, Z., Fan, Y.C., *et al.* (2012). Health-related quality-of-life after traumatic brain injury: a 2-year follow-up study in Wuhan, China, *Brain Injury,* **26**, 183–187.

Jagodic, H.K., Jagodic, K., and Podbregar, M. (2006). Long-term outcome and quality of life of patients treated in surgical intensive care: a comparison between sepsis and trauma, *Crit. Care,* **10**, R134. [Online] Available at: http://ccforum.com/content/10/5/R134 [Accessed 15 November 2014].

Janssens, L., Gorter, J.W., Ketelaar, M., *et al.* (2008). Health-related quality-of-life measures for long-term follow-up in children after major trauma, *Qual. Life Res.,* **17**, 701–713.

Jarrett, M., McMahon, M., and Stiller, K. (2008). Physical outcomes of patients with burn injuries: a 12 month follow-up, *J. Burn Care Res.,* **29**, 975–984.

Jimenez, N., Ebel, B.E., Wang, J., *et al.* (2013). Disparities in disability after traumatic brain injury among Hispanic children and adolescents, *Pediatrics,* **131**, e1850–e1856.

Jones, C., Skirrow, P., Griffiths, R.D., *et al.* (2003). Rehabilitation after critical illness, *Crit. Care Med.,* **31**, 2456–2461.

Leone, M., Bregéon, F., Antonini, F., *et al.* (2008). Long-term outcome in chest trauma, *Anesthesiology,* **109**, 864–871.

Livingston, D.H., Tripp, T., Biggs, C., *et al.* (2009). A fate worse than death? Long-term outcome of trauma patients admitted to the surgical intensive care unit, *J. Trauma,* **67**, 341–349.

Mayo Clinic (2014). *Diseases and Conditions: Posttraumatic Stress Disorder Symptoms*. [Online] (Updated 15 Apr 2014). Available at: www.mayoclinic.org/diseases-conditions/post-traumatic-stress-disorder/basics/symptoms/con-20022540 [Accessed July 2014].

Middleton, J., Tran, Y., and Craig, A. (2007). Relationship between quality of life and self-efficacy in persons with spinal cord injury, *Arch. Phys. Med. Rehabil.,* **88**, 1643–1648.

Oladeji, O., Johnston, T.E., Smith, B.T., *et al.* (2007). Quality of life in children with spinal cord injury, *Pediatr. Phys. Ther.,* **19**, 296–300.

Orwelius, L., Bergkvist, M., Nordlund, A., *et al.* (2012). Physical effects of trauma and psychological consequences of pre-existing diseases account for a significant portion of the health-related quality of life pattern of former trauma patients, *J. Trauma Acute Care Surg.,* **72**, 504–512.

Orwelius, L., Nordlund, A., Nordlund, P., *et al.* (2010). Pre-existing disease: the most important factor for health-related quality of life long-term after critical illness: a prospective, longitudinal, multicentre trial, *Crit. Care,* **14**, R67. [Online] Available at: http://ccforum.com/content/14/2/R67 [Accessed 15 November 2014].

Öster, C., Willebrand, M., and Ekselius, L. (2011). Health-related quality of life 2 years to 7 years after burn injury, *J. Trauma,* **71**, 1435–1441.

Pavoni, V., Gianesello, L., Paparella, L., *et al.* (2010). Outcome predictors and quality of life of severe burn patients admitted to intensive care unit, *Scand. J. Trauma Resusc. Emerg. Med.,* **18**, 24–31.

Pope, S.J., Solomons, W.R., Done, D.J., *et al.* (2007). Body image, mood and quality of life in young burn survivors, *Burns,* **33**, 747–755.

Ringdal, M., Plos, K., Lundberg, D., *et al.* (2009). Outcome after injury: memories, health-related quality of life, anxiety, and symptoms of depression after intensive care, *J. Trauma,* **66**, 1226–1233.

Riordan, A., Kelly, E.H., Klaas, S.J., *et al.* (2013). Psychosocial outcomes among youth with spinal cord injury by neurological impairment, *J. Spinal Cord Med.,* Nov 8 [E-pub ahead of print].

Rivara, F.P., Koepsell, T.D., Wang, J., *et al.* (2011). Disability 3, 12 and 24 months after traumatic brain injury among children and adolescents, *Pediatrics,* **128**, e1129–e1138.

Schipper, H., Clinch, J.J., and Olweny, C.L.M. (1996). 'Quality of life studies', in Spilker, B. (ed), *Quality of Life and Pharmacoeconomics in Clinical Trials*, 2nd edn., Lippencott-Raven, Philadelphia, PA, pp. 11–21.

Schouten, R., Keynan, O., Lee, R.S., *et al.* (2013). Health-related quality-of-life outcomes after thoracic (T1-T10) fractures, *Spine J.,* **14**, 1635–1642.

Shackman, G., Liu, Y.L., and Wang, X. (2005). *Measuring Quality of Life using Free and Public Domain Data. Social Research Update. Issue 47.* University of Surrey. [Online] Available at: http://sru.soc.surrey.ac.uk/SRU47.html [Accessed 14 April 2014].

Sluys, K., Häggmark, T., and Iselius, L. (2005). Outcome and quality of life 5 years after major trauma, *J. Trauma,* **59**, 223–232.

Tan, W.H., Goldstein, R., Gerrard, P., *et al.* (2012). Outcomes and predictors in burn rehabilitation, *J. Burn Care Res.,* **33**, 110–117.

Van Aswegen, H., Eales, C., Richards, G.A., *et al.* (2010). The effect of penetrating trunk trauma and mechanical ventilation on the recovery of adult survivors after hospital discharge, *S. Afr. J. Crit. Care,* **26**, 25–32.

Van Aswegen, H., Myezwa, H., Mudzi, W., *et al.* (2011). Health-related quality of life of survivors of penetrating trunk trauma in Johannesburg, South Africa, *Eur. J. Trauma Emerg. Surg.,* **37**, 419–426.

Van Koppenhagen, C.F., Post, M.W., Van der Woude, L.H., *et al.* (2008). Changes and determinants of life satisfaction after spinal cord injury: a cohort study in the Netherlands, *Arch. Phys. Med. Rehabil.,* **89**, 1733–1740.

Vanderploeg, R.D., Belanger, H.D., and Curtiss, G. (2009). Mild traumatic brain injury and posttraumatic stress disorder and their associations with health symptoms, *Arch. Phys. Med. Rehabil.,* **90**, 1084–1093.

Varni, J., Limbers, C., and Burwinkle, T. (2007). How young children can reliably and validly self-report their health-related quality of life? An analysis of 8591 children across age subgroups with the PedsQL 4.0 generic core scales, *Health Qual. Life Outcomes,* **5**, 1. [Online] Available at: http://www.hqlo.com/content/5/1/1 [Accessed 14 November 2014].

Warburton, D.E.R., Nicol, C.W., and Bredin, S.S.D. (2006). Prescribing exercise as preventive therapy, *Can. Med. Assoc. J.,* **174**, 961–975.

Ware, J.E. (1996). 'The SF-36 health survey', in Spilker, B. (ed), *Quality of Life and Pharmacoeconomics in Clinical Trials*, 2nd edn., Lippincott-Raven, Philadelphia, PA, pp. 337–345.

Weedon, M., and Potterton, J. (2011). Socio-economic and clinical factors predictive of paediatric quality of life post burn, *Burns,* **37**, 572–579.

Wehler, M., Geise, A., Hadzionerovic, D., *et al.* (2003). Health-related quality of life of patients with multiple organ dysfunction: individual changes and comparison with normative population, *Crit. Care Med.,* **31**, 1094–1101.

Wijesuriya, N., Tran, Y., Middleton, J., *et al.* (2012). Impact of fatigue on the health-related quality of life in persons with spinal cord injury, *Arch. Phys. Med. Rehabil.,* **93**, 319–324.

Willis, C.E., Grisbrook, T.L., Elliott, C.M., *et al.* (2011). Pulmonary function, exercise capacity and physical activity participation in adults following burns, *Burns,* **37**, 1326–1333.

Wilson, J.R., Hashimoto, R.E., Detorri, J.R., *et al.* (2011). Spinal cord injury and quality of life: a systematic review of outcome measures, *Evid. Based Spine Care J.,* **2**, 37–44.

Winthrop, A.L. (2010) Health-related quality of life after pediatric trauma, *Curr. Opin. Pediatr.,* **22**, 346–351.

Winthrop, A.L., Brasel, K.J., Stahovic, L., *et al.* (2005). Quality of life and functional outcome after pediatric trauma, *J. Trauma,* **58**, 468–474.

World Confederation for Physical Therapy. (2011). *WCPT Guideline for Curricula for Physical Therapists delivering Quality Exercise Programmes across the Life Span*. World Confederation for Physical Therapy. [Online] Available at: http://www.wcpt.org/guidelines/exercise-programmes [Accessed 16 April 2014].

World Health Organisation (WHO) QOL Group. (1995). The World Health Organisation Quality of Life Assessment (WHOQOL): position paper from the World Health Organisation, *Soc. Sci. Med.,* **41**, 1403–1409.

World Health Organisation (WHO) QOL Group. (1997). *Programme on Mental Health: WHOQOL Measuring Quality of Life*. Division of Mental Health and Prevention of Substance Abuse, World Health Organisation. [Online] Available at: http://www.who.int/mental_health/media/68.pdf [Accessed 14 April 2014].

Wunsch, H., and Angus, D.C. (2010). The puzzle of long-term morbidity after critical illness, *Crit. Care,* **14**, 121–122.

Appendix I

Normal Values for Paediatrics

Table AI.1: Normal paediatric arterial blood gas values*.

	< 2 years	> 2 years
pH	7.37–7.42	7.37–7.42
$PaCO_2$ (mmHg)	30–37	35–44
PaO_2 (mmHg)	80–100	85–100
Base excess	–5–1	–2–1
Standard bicarbonate (mmol/L)	19–23	21.5–26

*Partial pressure of carbon dioxide in arterial blood, $PaCO_2$; partial pressure of oxygen in arterial blood, PaO_2; millimetres of mercury, mmHg; millimol per litre, mmol/L.

Table AI.2: Normal paediatric haemoglobin values in grams/decilitre (g/dL)

Age	Hb (g/dL)
Birth	13.5
6 weeks	9.5
3 months	10.0
6–12 months	10.5
1–1.5 years	10.5
1.5–4 years	11.0
4–7 years	11.0
7–12 years	11.5
Post puberty	
• Males	14
• Females	12

Table AI.3: Normal values for paediatric body temperature in degrees Celsius (ºC)

Axillary	36.5
Oral	37
Rectal	37.5

Appendix II

Bedside Measures to Establish the Oxygenation Status of Critically Ill Patients

Table AII.1: Oxygenation ratio and interpretation of findings.

Oxygenation can be measured using the ratio PaO_2/FiO_2.

Interpretation of results:

- Value > 350 is indicative of good oxygenation
- Value 200–350 is indicative of the development of acute lung injury in patients with septic markers or loss of lung volume
- Value < 200 indicates the development of acute respiratory distress syndrome (ARDS) (if accompanied with other characteristic signs and symptoms of ARDS) or atelectasis of a large number of lung segments

Table AII.2: Estimation of the presence of diffusion defect at alveolar-capillary membrane level.

Diffusion defect is determined using the formula $P(A\text{-}a)O_2$; thus subtracting partial pressure of oxygen in arterial blood (PaO_2) from partial pressure of oxygen in the alveoli (PAO_2).

Partial pressure of oxygen in the alveoli (PAO_2) is calculated using the formula:

$PAO_2 = FiO_2(P_{atm} - P_{H2O}) - (PaCO_2/RQ)$
FiO_2 = fraction of inspired oxygen
P_{atm} = atmospheric pressure
P_{H2O} = water vapour pressure
$PaCO_2$ = partial pressure of carbon dioxide in arterial blood
RQ = respiratory quotient

Interpretation of results:

- A patient who breaths room air has no diffusion defect at alveolar capillary level if $P(A\text{-}a)O_2$ is less than or equal to 10
- A patient who receives additional oxygen therapy has no diffusion defect at alveolar capillary level if $P(A\text{-}a)O_2$ is less than or equal to 65

Appendix III

Functional Recovery of Patients with Spinal Cord Injury

The expected recovery of patients following cervical or thoracic SCI is outlined in Table AIII.1. The expected functional abilities are based on the assumption that the patient has a complete lesion (ASIA A), since an incomplete lesion produces varying functional abilities. Most upper extremity recovery occurs in the first six months after injury (Kirshblum and O'Connor, 1998). This has implications for respiratory complications, which may or may not develop, as recovery directly influences a patient's level of activity, and level of activity, in turn, influences respiratory function.

Gait re-education for patients with thoracic SCI is an excellent training exercise in balance, endurance and strength. Table AIII.2 outlines the three different types of gait patterns that may be used in the spinal ward for gait re-education in this patient population.

Table AIII.1: Expected functional recovery of a patient with complete cervical or thoracic spinal cord lesion.

Level of injury	Available muscles and/or difficulties	Expected functional recovery
C1–C3	• Dependent on a ventilator for breathing • Limited ability to talk • C3 = limited movement of the head and neck	Functional goals for these individuals primarily focus on • Communication and wheelchair mobility • Use of a mouth stick, head control or chin control to manoeuvre a wheelchair • Assistive device for turning the pages of a book or magazine, using the telephone and operating lights and appliances at home • Assistance needed with pressure relief
C3–C4	• Usually have head and neck control • C4 = ability to shrug shoulders (trapezius = cranial nerve XI, C3 and C4) • Initially requires a ventilator • About a third of patients with complete C4 lesions may regain antigravity bicep (C5) strength	• Limited independence in feeding with accessories • All abovementioned functions
C5	• Bicep brachii intact • Head and neck control, shoulder shrug, and shoulder control (deltoid) • Minimal serratus anterior function	• Can bend his or her elbows and turn palms face up • Independence with eating, drinking, face washing, tooth brushing, face shaving, and hair care with use of assistive devices • Push a manual wheelchair for short distances over smooth surfaces • Use a power wheelchair with hand controls for daily activities • Can perform self-assisted coughs • Can perform pressure relief to prevent sacral sore formation by leaning forward or side-to-side • May drive an adapted car

(Continued)

Table AIII.1: *(Continued)*

Level of injury	Available muscles and/or difficulties	Expected functional recovery
C6	• Extensor carpi ulnaris, extensor carpi radialis longus and brevis intact • Partial innervation of latissimus dorsi • Able to shrug shoulders, bend elbows, turn palms up and down and extend the wrists	• Very functional with less dependence • Has greater ease and independence in feeding, bathing, grooming, personal hygiene and dressing • Can use a manual wheelchair for daily chores but may need a transfer board for transfers • May independently undertake bladder and bowel management • May be independent in light housekeeping duties, transfers, and pressure reliefs, turning in bed, and driving an adapted car
C7	• Triceps brachii intact • Major part of latissimus dorsi (C6, C7 and C8) intact • Greater strength for elbow extension	• Greater independence with less use of assistive devices • Greater independence with use of manual wheelchair including transfers without a transfer board • Greater ease in performing household work and transfers • Can do wheelchair push-ups for pressure reliefs
C8–T1	• C8 = flexor digitorum profundus (mainly the distal phalanx of the middle finger) intact • T1 = abductor digiti minimi (finger abductors) intact • Has better use of fingers • Latissimus dorsi intact	• Can live independently without assistive devices in feeding, bathing, grooming, oral and facial hygiene, dressing, transferring, bladder and bowel management
T2–T6	• Has good motor function in the head, neck, shoulders, arms, hands, and fingers	• Has better trunk control hence better posture • All the above functions
T7–T12	• Better abdominal control	• Can perform better coughing • Has better ability to perform unsupported seated functional activities

Table AIII.2: Gait re-education and spinal cord injury

- Swing to gait is universal because it is both the simplest and the safest. All patients with thoracic SCI above T10 are taught this gait pattern first
- Swing through gait requires skilled balance but it is the fastest and most useful
- Four-point gait is the slowest and most difficult and can only be done on crutches by accomplished walkers. Also facilitates turning and manoeuvring in confined spaces

Bibliography

Kirshblum, S.C. and O'Connor, K.C. (1998). Predicting neurological recovery in traumatic cervical spinal cord injury, *Arch. Phys. Med. Rehabil.*, **79**, 1457–1466.

Index